PRESCRIPTION FOR INEQUALITY

Also Available from Bloomsbury Academic

Medical Firsts: Innovations and Milestones That Changed the World
Tish Davidson

Wellness around the World: An International Encyclopedia of Health Indicators, Practices, and Issues [2 volumes]
Brenda S. Gardenour Walter, Editor

Exercise and Physical Activity: From Health Benefits to Fitness Crazes
R. K. Devlin, Editor

PRESCRIPTION FOR INEQUALITY

EXPLORING THE SOCIAL DETERMINANTS OF HEALTH OF AT-RISK GROUPS

Jillian M. Duquaine-Watson

BLOOMSBURY ACADEMIC
NEW YORK • LONDON • OXFORD • NEW DELHI • SYDNEY

BLOOMSBURY ACADEMIC
Bloomsbury Publishing Inc
1385 Broadway, New York, NY 10018, USA
50 Bedford Square, London, WC1B 3DP, UK
29 Earlsfort Terrace, Dublin 2, Ireland

BLOOMSBURY, BLOOMSBURY ACADEMIC and the Diana logo are trademarks of Bloomsbury Publishing Plc

First published in the United States of America 2024

Cover images (clockwise from top left): Operation 2023/Alamy Stock Photo; RichardBakerUSA/Alamy Stock Photo; Andrew Lichtenstein/Getty; Mario Tama/Getty.

Library of Congress Cataloging-in-Publication Data
Names: Duquaine-Watson, Jillian M., author.
Title: Prescription for inequality : exploring the social determinants of health of at-risk groups / Jillian M. Duquaine-Watson.
Description: New York : Bloomsbury Academic, 2024. | Includes bibliographical references and index. | Audience: Grades: 10–12
Identifiers: LCCN 2023030518 (print) | LCCN 2023030519 (ebook) | ISBN 9781440879272 (hardback) | ISBN 9781440879289 (ebook) | ISBN 9798765109977 (epub)
Subjects: LCSH: Social status–Health aspects–United States. | Equality–Health aspects–United States. | Social medicine–United States.
Classification: LCC RA418.5.S63 D87 2024 (print) | LCC RA418.5.S63 (ebook) | DDC 362.10973–dc23/eng/20231016
LC record available at https://lccn.loc.gov/2023030518
LC ebook record available at https://lccn.loc.gov/2023030519

ISBN: HB: 978-1-4408-7927-2
ePDF: 978-1-4408-7928-9
eBook: 979-8-7651-0997-7

Typeset by Integra Software Services Pvt. Ltd.
Printed and bound in Great Britain

To find out more about our authors and books visit www.bloomsbury.com and sign up for our newsletters.

To Samara, my darling gremlin child

CONTENTS

Introduction

Within the realm of contemporary Western medical research and practice, it is widely recognized that human health and well-being are influenced by a myriad of factors. Such factors are referred to as determinants of health. They are typically organized into four broad categories: biological determinants of health, environmental determinants of health, behavioral determinants of health, and social determinants of health. The first category, biological determinants of health, refers to the composition and function of the human body and body systems, hormones, genetics, and other physiological or anatomical features. The second category, environmental determinants of health, refers to the features of the natural world (e.g., climate, water access and quality, temperature, flora, and fauna) and their impact on health and well-being. The next category, behavioral determinants of health, encompasses individual actions or activities that influence one's health status, either directly or indirectly. Some behaviors (e.g., eating a nutritious diet and regularly obtaining health screenings) can help promote good health while other behaviors (e.g., smoking, engaging in high-risk sexual activities) can be detrimental to health and well-being. In contrast, social determinants of health include the legal, economic, political, and cultural aspects of human societies. This consists of social institutions such as families, communities, the economy, educational entities, the health-care system, the government, and similar features, including how such institutions are organized and function. Attention to social determinants of health promotes understanding of the ways that laws, policies, customs, dominant ideologies, distribution of wealth and services, and other aspects of culture influence human health.

It is sometimes beneficial to examine biological, environmental, behavioral, and social determinants of health separately. For example, when the SARS-CoV-2 virus first emerged in late 2019, researchers were primarily concerned with understanding the impact of the virus from the standpoint of biological determinants of health. They examined the genome sequencing of the virus and its impact on the human body, including symptoms and progression of the disease as well as transmissibility rate, incubation period, and mortality rate. Such efforts were crucial to the development of vaccines to stimulate the immune system to create antibodies, thereby helping reduce the likelihood that those exposed to the virus will develop COVID-19. Yet since the mid-twentieth century, understanding the interconnections between the four broad categories of determinants of health has prompted an increase in interdisciplinary health research and practice. Such an approach is evident in efforts aimed at reducing COVID-19 transmission and infection rates. For example, in addition to providing information about the virus and how it impacts the human body, the "We Can Do This" campaign from the US Department of Health and Human Services promotes social distancing, wearing masks, using hand sanitizer, and vaccinations. Thus, the campaign is grounded in an understanding of biological determinants of health but also seeks to promote certain actions (behavioral determinants of health) in order to minimize morbidity and mortality rates due to COVID-19. However, the campaign also provides unique educational programming for different demographic groups based on age, race, ethnicity, disability status, religious affiliation, and other identities, thereby reflecting an understanding that social determinants influence rates of infection, adherence to social-distancing practices, and vaccination rates.

Current interdisciplinary health research and practice demonstrates that while biological, environmental, and behavioral components of health are important, social determinants of health are equally and, in some cases, even more influential in determining health status and health outcomes. However, even a cursory examination of the history of medicine illustrates that attention to social determinants of health is a relatively new phenomenon. In the early decades of the American medical profession, physicians focused primarily on the biological components of health, attempting to better understand the anatomical and physiological features of the human body. They used a variety of methods such as herbal treatments, bloodletting, emetics, diuretics, and laxatives to promote healing and minimize pain. They also conducted some surgical procedures including amputations, excision of dead tissue and tumors, closure of wounds, and methods to repair the function of or remove some organs and glands. Additionally, some doctors performed surgeries to remove fetuses that had died in utero or had become stuck in the birth canal; others drilled holes into skulls to treat those who were believed to be possessed by evil spirits (but who likely suffered from what would currently be diagnosed as epilepsy, schizophrenia, or other cognitive or developmental disorders), specifically to allow such spirits to escape the body. Following the introduction of methods to sterilize wounds as well as surgical tools in the late nineteenth century, physicians expanded their knowledge of and attention to human biology. Such knowledge was instrumental in bolstering their knowledge and skills related to the prevention and treatment of infection, thereby promoting improved health outcomes for their patients.

Attention to the biological dimensions of health was also used to delineate between different populations, particularly as a means of reinforcing social hierarchies. Indeed, biology provided what many regarded as incontrovertible evidence that certain populations were inferior to others. Such arguments were predicated on the belief that biology is destiny and were central to the scientific racism that was used by those who endorsed slavery, white supremacy, anti-immigrant legislation, and measures that sought to limit the rights of and otherwise discriminate against groups based on race and ethnicity. This is evident, for example, in arguments regarding the supposed polygenesis of racial and ethnic subgroups. It is also clear in the pseudoscientific fields of craniometry as well as eugenics, both of which were used to justify the differential treatment—medically, politically, socially, economically, and legally—of immigrants, poor populations, individuals with disabilities, and those who did not conform to cisgender and heteronormative norms. Additionally, and based on biological measures related to average height and weight as well as anatomical differences, cisgender women were believed to be biologically inferior to cisgender men. It was thought that their reproductive organs and corresponding biological functions related to menstruation, pregnancy, and childbirth destined cisgender women for weakness, frailty, and otherwise poor health.

This is not to suggest, however, that health practitioners in the seventeenth, eighteenth, and nineteenth centuries lacked awareness of environmental determinants of health or behavioral determinants of health. On the contrary, they acknowledged that prolonged exposure to extreme cold or extreme heat, wounds from animal bites, and natural disasters such as flooding, hurricanes, and wildfires could diminish health and increase risk of premature death. However, they tended to regard such factors as acts of God. Thus, within an explanatory framework shaped by religious ideology, they largely failed to address the fact that certain populations—especially those who were poor and enslaved—tended to suffer the ill effects of environmental factors differently than those with more economic and social privilege. Additionally, the types of diet regimens and activity restrictions sometimes recommended for pregnant women indicate that there was an awareness that behavior could impact health. Yet such recommendations—for example, eating only soft foods to prevent the bones of the fetus from hardening, thereby promoting an easy childbirth; intensive bed rest and social isolation to diminish overstimulation of the nervous system and reduce risk of miscarriage and complications—often lacked scientific validity. Instead, they reflected gender roles and health fads common among more affluent white populations. Correspondingly, such recommendations were not provided to racial or ethnic minority populations or those from poor or working-class backgrounds.

Yet as industrialization, urbanization, and globalization expanded and the US population increased, efforts to promote good health by preventing illness and injury also increased. Thus, public efforts to address prominent health issues emerged. Beginning in the nineteenth century, some municipalities established boards of health and health departments to improve the well-being of their citizens. Others created methods of reporting and sharing data related to infectious disease outbreaks. Still others formalized data-recording methods for mortality rates among different demographic subgroups, organizing such data by sex, income level, age, race, employment status, and geographic location. These were, in essence, some of the earliest incarnations of formal public health in the United States. Initially, the primary concerns of such initiatives included issues of sanitation, industrial injuries, and outbreaks of infectious diseases such as smallpox, yellow fever, typhus, scarlet fever, tuberculosis, syphilis, malaria, influenza, and cholera. In 1912, efforts within the federal government as related to public health—including those of the Marine Hospital Service (MHS) as well as the Public Health and Marine Hospital Services (PHMHS)—were consolidated to create the US Public Health Services (PHS). As the century progressed, and due to expanding legislation as well as increased government spending on health issues, the number and scope of public health entities increased.

The expansion of public health—both in the United States and globally—continued throughout the twentieth century. Central to this expansion was increased awareness of social determinants of health. Global political discourse regarding human rights helped promote such awareness, particularly as such discourse formed in response to the atrocities of Nazi Germany. This is evident in the founding of the United Nations and creation of seminal documents such as the Universal Declaration of Human

Rights (1948); the International Covenant on Civil and Political Rights (1966); the International Covenant on Economic, Social, and Cultural Rights (1966); and special declarations regarding the rights of children, Indigenous populations, and rural populations. Such documents established the right to health and to medical care as basic human rights. Similar sentiments were expressed in the Declaration of Alma-Ata, endorsed by the World Health Organization in 1978. However, of equal importance, such documents explicitly acknowledged that persistent social inequities are responsible for the health disparities that persist throughout the world. Such sentiments were echoed by US social and political movements that strengthened in the post–World War II era, including movements for racial and ethnic equality as well as the feminist movement, environmental movement, and anti-poverty movement. Similarly, attention to systemic inequities and their impact on the health and well-being of human populations were a central component of both the Millennium Development Goals (2000) and the Sustainable Development Goals (2015). Such efforts also contributed to the development of population health, a subset of public health that is concerned with fostering improved health for specific groups (e.g., sexual and gender minorities, people with disabilities, and incarcerated populations).

Attention to health disparities is central to both public health and population health. Health disparities are the differences in health status and health outcomes of one demographic group—sometimes referred to as a population subset—when compared to another demographic group or when compared to overall trends and averages for the total population of a country, region, state, or municipality. Analysis of health disparities offers insight into the various ways that health is affected by the economic, educational, social, political, and legal dimensions of society. Thus, it is common for public health and population health researchers and practitioners to examine the ways in which housing, neighborhood conditions, education, access to and quality of food, employment, relationships between different demographic groups, the organization and operation of the US health-care system, exposure to violence and conflict, and other social factors promote health for some populations while posing health risks for others. Of equal importance, such researchers and scholars offer recommendations for how such social determinants of health can be addressed in ways that rectify health disparities and, in doing so, promote more equitable health outcomes. Thus, examination of social determinants of health within the realm of contemporary public health and population health includes attention to (1) relative access to power and resources of different demographic groups; (2) the ways in which access to and exercise of power is connected to health and well-being; and (3) options for promoting more equitable access to power and resources as a means of fostering improved health and well-being for marginalized populations.

Research demonstrates that when power and resources are allocated in an equitable manner, health disparities are diminished. However, when there is an imbalance in political, social, and economic power, the incidence and severity of health disparities are amplified. Put another way, societies with greater disparities in power and access to resources also experience greater gaps in health between different demographic groups. Thus, overall health and well-being is better for those with more power and more resources while it is measurably worse for those with reduced access. This relationship between the distribution of power/resources and health disparities has been recognized by the National Academies of Sciences, Engineering, and Medicine as well as the US Center for Disease Control and Prevention. Furthermore, the World Health Organization, the Pan American Health

Organization, and numerous American and international health-based nongovernmental organizations have acknowledged the relationship between access to various types of societal power and health outcomes, thereby attesting to the fact that existing health disparities are the result of both historical and contemporary patterns of unequal access to resources.

It is clear that health disparities in the United States—and, indeed, throughout the world—are not natural or inevitable. Instead, they are the preventable by-products of the systemic and structural inequities that persist in the twenty-first century, including inequities that are evident in social institutions (e.g., political, economic, familial, and religious entities) and that can be measured in patterns related to income and wealth, access to and quality of education, access to and quality of health care, living environment, and social context. In other words, social *inequities* constitute a prescription for inequality that virtually guarantees health *disparities*. Such disparities run counter to contemporary medical ethics, principles of public health and population health, and anti-discrimination legislation. They are also associated with diminished quality of life as well as increased risk and severity of chronic and infectious diseases, injuries, birth defects, sexually transmitted diseases, and mental health disorders. Furthermore, those who are most affected by such disparities are also at increased risk of disabilities, suicidal ideation, certain types of violence, long-term hospitalization, and premature death.

This book focuses on social determinants of health in the United States, illustrating how systemic inequities function in ways that create, sustain, and aggravate health disparities. By attending to the experiences of those groups that are marginalized based on sex, gender identity, race, sexuality, ethnicity, country of origin, age, disability status, and other socially constructed identities, it explores the contours of social determinants of health, including both causes and consequences. It also provides insight into how such determinants have changed over time. Relying on an interdisciplinary framework, this project draws on both contemporary and historical research from fields such as public health, population health, feminist theory, critical studies of race and ethnicity, poverty studies, disability studies, aging studies, cultural competence, legal studies, sociology, and medical anthropology. Furthermore, and in recognition of the reality that health disparities are the result of a complex interplay of forces and structural factors that permeate various social and economic dimensions of American culture, analysis extends beyond the realm of health care to include attention to education, work and employment, politics, living environment, and other aspects of society.

Each of the forthcoming chapters focuses on a particular demographic group, specifically those groups that encounter significant and persistent marginalization in US society. Organizing information in this manner promotes attention to health disparities as they relate to sex, gender identity and expression, sexuality, race, ethnicity, ability, age, and other socially constructed identities. Yet diverse identities and experiences exist within every demographic group. For example, although elderly populations tend to experience some common health-related needs and challenges, there are also important differences when comparing the needs and experiences of elderly populations of different racial and ethnic groups or when comparing elderly populations that are poor with those who are more affluent. Consequently, attention to the intersection of socially constructed identities is woven throughout each chapter. This not only promotes increased understanding of similarities and differences within each demographic group but also facilitates a more nuanced understanding of the complex dimensions of social determinants of health and related health disparities. To begin, each chapter provides a discussion of the most prominent health issues among the specific population that is being examined, including issues related to physical, mental, and social well-being. That discussion is followed by subsections that address economic factors, educational access and quality, health-care access and quality, and living environment and social context, with specific attention to how such considerations influence health and well-being.

Ultimately, this volume provides a comprehensive introduction to social determinants of health and related health disparities in the United States. In doing so, it promotes an increased understanding of how access to societal power and resources influences the health and well-being of marginalized populations. Such understanding is essential for those who wish to promote a more equitable society, including by rectifying health disparities in systemic and meaningful ways.

CHAPTER ONE

Asian, Pacific Islander, and Desi American (APIDA) Populations

The heterogeneous group that includes Asian Americans (AA), Pacific Islanders (including Native Hawaiians), and Desi Americans (DA)—those with Pakistani, Bangladeshi, and Indian ancestry—are commonly referred to using the pan-ethnic acronym APIDA. Those who are members of AA and DA subgroups have ancestry that connects them to populations that historically inhabited more than sixty countries and territories that are currently part of eastern Asia, southeastern Asia, and the Indian subcontinent. About 85 percent of all DA and AA subgroups in the United States identify as Chinese, Indian, Japanese, Filipino, Vietnamese, or Korean. Less-populous subgroups include Pakistani, Taiwanese, Thai, Cambodian, Hmong, Laotian, Bangladeshi, Nepalese, Indonesian, and others. Individuals who are descendants of Indigenous peoples that inhabited and exercised sovereignty over islands in Melanesia, Micronesia, and Polynesia prior to colonization are often called Native Hawaiians (NH), Pacific Islanders (PI), or Native Hawaiians and Other Pacific Islanders (NHOPI). They hail from islands including American Samoa, Fiji, Guam, the Hawaiian Islands, the Mariana Islands, the Marshall Islands, Papua New Guinea, Samoa, the Solomon Islands, Tonga, Tahiti, and others. Collectively, AA and NHOPI populations are sometimes referred to Asian Americans and Pacific Islanders (AAPI); however, in contemporary practice, the acronym APIDA is increasingly used to be more inclusive of Desi people.

At present, APIDA people collectively represent about 7 percent of the total US population; their numbers have increased by over 80 percent since the start of the twenty-first century. Roughly two-thirds are native born while the remaining one-third immigrated to the United States. Over 85 percent of NHOPI populations and three-fourths of AA and DA populations are US citizens. Together, AA and DA people are the fastest-growing ethnic/racial demographic subgroup in the United States. Over 23 million individuals living in the United States currently identify as AA or DA, including those who are multiethnic or multiracial. It is anticipated that their numbers will surpass 35 million by 2060. Another 1.5 million people identify as NHOPI; they represent about one-half of 1 percent of the total US population and many are also multiracial or multiethnic. Since 2000, the total NHOPI population has increased by 60 percent. Among APIDA subgroups, there are significant variations of language, religion, health practices, food preferences, rituals, and other cultural beliefs. Yet they share some similarities as due to their historical and contemporary marginalization within US society. Evidence of such marginalization can be found in various social institutions, including those related to economics, employment, education, health care, and politics. Yet it is also evident in the health issues common among them.

CURRENT STATE OF HEALTH

APIDA populations typically rank higher in terms of overall wellness when compared to Black, Indigenous, and Hispanic/Latinx/Chicanx (HLC) groups; by some measures, they also rank higher than non-HLC whites. Average life expectancy (ALE) among APIDA groups is higher than the US average and highest among all racial and ethnic groups. On average, APIDA people live about 81 years; the average for cisgender women is 82.5 years while it is 78 years for cisgender men. They have the lowest rates of infant and child mortality of all racial and ethnic groups. Fertility rates vary greatly. AA and DA subgroups average fewer children and have lower adolescent birth rates than Black, HLC, and non-HLC white populations. In contrast, fertility rates and teen birth rates among NHOPI are at least 30 percent higher than national averages. Common chronic diseases among APIDA populations include cardiovascular diseases, diabetes, lupus, osteoporosis, and cancer. Heart disease remains the second-leading cause of death among adults. DA and AA populations have lower rates of cardiovascular diseases (e.g., coronary heart disease, stroke, coronary artery disease, and hypertension) than HLC, Black, and non-HLC whites. Yet rates of such diseases are disproportionately high among NHOPI people, especially Chamorro populations (those with ancestry in Guam or the Northern Mariana Islands).

APIDA populations have the highest rates of the osteoporosis among all racial and ethnic groups; rates are highest among cisgender women over the age of 50. Osteoporosis among APIDA people has been linked to biogenetic factors (e.g., hormones and smaller-than-average skeletal frame); however, diet may also play a role, particularly as dairy products are not common in the diets of many AA, DA, and NHOPI cultures. This may be due to traditional norms; however, over 70 percent of APIDA people are lactose intolerant. Disability rates among APIDA groups are lower than among other racial and ethnic groups. About 15 percent of NHOPI and 10 percent of AA and DA populations have a diagnosed disability. There is often shame associated with disabilities among subgroups. Some PI subgroups believe that an individual with a disability is being penalized for offenses committed by an ancestor; similarly, Filipino populations often regard disabilities as punishments inflicted by God. Among Bangladeshi populations, spirit possession is often used to explain cognitive disabilities. Due to the dishonor associated with disabilities, many APIDA people are reluctant to acknowledge them or seek disability-related care.

Rates of certain types of cancer (e.g., breast, prostate, lung, cervical, colorectal, and pancreatic) are lower among APIDA populations compared to other racial and ethnic groups. Yet cancer (of all types) is the leading cause of death among APIDA people. They have higher rates of liver and stomach cancer and are more likely to die from liver, stomach, and throat cancers than non-HLC whites. Cancer rates are lowest among DA but higher among certain AA subgroups including Cambodian, Thai, Laotian, and Hmong communities. Additionally, and although rates of breast cancer and cervical cancer are relatively low among APIDA people, there are disparities. Cisgender APIDA women who immigrate to the United States are five to six times more likely to develop breast cancer than those born in the United States; when compared to US averages, rates of cervical cancer are at least four times higher among Vietnamese, Cambodian, and Laotian people. Combined rates of all types of cancers are highest among Samoan, Japanese, and NH subgroups. Rates of lupus are also disproportionately high among APIDA people. They are more likely than Black, HLC, and non-HLC white groups to get diagnosed in early adulthood; they are also more likely to develop kidney disease and to die prematurely due to lupus than non-HLC whites.

There are also disparities in respiratory health, body weight, and diabetes. Among Chinese, Vietnamese, and Korean populations, rates of asthma are one-third as high as among all other racial and ethnic groups. Yet asthma is more common among Filipinos and NHOPI. Lung cancer is most common among Southeast Asian subgroups; however, mortality rates due to lung cancer are highest among Chinese populations. Among cisgender women who have never smoked, risk of lung cancer is higher for APIDA people than for cisgender women of all other racial and ethnic groups; research suggests this may be linked to genetic factors. Obesity rates are higher than average among some APIDA populations. One-fourth of all NHOPI people are overweight while another 50 percent meet medical guidelines for obesity. Among NHOPI children, one in five is overweight while one in four is obese. NHOPI people are two and a half times more likely to develop diabetes than non-HLC whites. While only one in nine AA and DA over the age of 18 meets medical guidelines for obesity, nearly 20 percent have diabetes; an additional one-third have high blood sugar levels and, thus, are at increased risk for diabetes.

Rates of certain infectious diseases are disproportionately high among APIDA populations. They have the highest rates of chronic hepatitis B (HB) infections among all racial and ethnic groups in the United States. Approximately 1 in 12 APIDA adults are infected with HB; they comprise over half of the nearly two-and-a-half million individuals in the United States with the disease. However, over half are unaware they are infected; thus, they may unknowingly transmit the disease to others. Additionally, rates of liver cancer are 60 percent higher among APIDA populations than non-HLC whites; rates of disability and premature death due to liver diseases and liver cancer are also disproportionately high among APIDA people. However, there are variations among APIDA subgroups. Rates of chronic HB, liver disease, and related mortality are highest among those born outside of the United States, especially cisgender men from Vietnam, Laos, Cambodia, China, and the Philippines. The COVID-19 pandemic also revealed some health disparities that diminish well-being among APIDA populations. During the first two years of the pandemic, they were the least likely of all racial and ethnic groups to get tested for the virus. When compared to non-HLC whites, they were twice as likely to test positive, require hospitalization, and die from the virus.

Over the past two decades, cases of tuberculosis (TB) and sexually transmitted diseases (STDs) have increased among APIDA people. Such populations constitute one-third of all TB-positive populations in the United States. Rates of infection are highest among immigrants from and/or those who travel regularly to the Philippines, China, Vietnam, and India. Additionally, among cisgender NH, rates of HIV infection are 25 percent higher among women and nearly 300 percent higher among men when compared to non-APIDA adults. Yet rates are much lower among AA and DA; such populations represent less than 2 percent of new HIV diagnoses in the past decade. Rates of syphilis, chlamydia, and gonorrhea are also lower among AA and DA groups than national averages. Among NHOPI populations, rates of gonorrhea, chlamydia, and syphilis infections are three to five times higher than among other APIDA groups.

Attention to mental health within APIDA communities has increased in recent years. Yet the shame and social stigma associated with mental illness discourage many from seeking professional support for such issues or discussing them with family and friends. Some subgroups believe that mental illnesses are caused by spirits, demons, or other supernatural forces; others believe those with mental illnesses are being punished by God. Beliefs about appropriate treatments for mental illness also vary and may include prayer, meditation, physical restraint, and/or using physical force to drive evil spirits from the afflicted individual. Many APIDA people lack awareness about mental health resources. Less than 10 percent of those with a mental illness seek treatment. However, rates of health-seeking behaviors for mental illness do vary; they are lowest among immigrants and first-generation US-born APIDA populations. Due to the importance placed on extended kin and cultural networks in many APIDA cultures, those who are geographically isolated and/or who lack access to culturally appropriate resources (e.g., religious facilities, social groups, and health-care providers) are at increased risk of poor mental health.

Nearly one in four AA, NHOPI, and DA individuals will experience a mental illness during their lifetime; some of the most common include anxiety disorders, major depressive disorders, and substance use and abuse disorders (SUAD). Post-traumatic stress disorder (PTSD) has also been identified as a critical concern, especially among immigrants and refugees who experienced armed conflict, natural disasters, and/or political persecution. For many foreign-born populations, the immigration process and resettlement in the United States can contribute to poor mental health. Such experiences can be traumatic, particularly due to culture shock as well as the xenophobic and/or racist attitudes they may encounter. While trauma most directly impacts the affected individual, it may also be passed on to children. This is known as intergenerational trauma. For example, among Japanese American populations, incarceration at US camps during the Second World War caused both individual and intergenerational trauma. Similarly, the systemic suppression and resulting cultural upheaval of NHOPI cultures have been identified as a key factor in intergenerational trauma. More recently, the anti-Asian sentiment and related violence that has occurred during the COVID-19 pandemic has caused PTSD for survivors and their communities; it is anticipated that it will also contribute to intergenerational trauma. Trauma and PTSD are associated with increased risk and severity of anxiety, emotional dysregulation, depression, sleep disorders, poor self-esteem, SUAD, and suicidal ideation. Official reports indicate that rates of suicidal ideation and attempts among APIDA people are 50 percent lower than US averages; yet it is likely that cultural norms that discourage those at risk to seek care have led to underreporting.

Among APIDA adolescents aged 12–18, suicide is the leading cause of death. Many have linked such rates to intergenerational trauma as well as the model minority myth

(MMM). Rooted in US racial/racist hierarchies, the MMM is a stereotype that denies the cultural diversity that exists among APIDA populations while simultaneously advancing the notions that such populations are more intelligent and diligent than other racial and ethnic minority groups (e.g., Black, HLC, and Indigenous people). Internalization of the MMM can lead to increased pressure to excel both academically and financially. Such pressure, in turn, is associated with increased risk of suicide among APIDA teens. It has also been linked to certain high-risk behaviors, including SUAD and risky sexual practices. While APIDA adolescents are somewhat less likely than their non-APIDA peers to regularly engage in sexual activity, those who are sexually active are less likely to follow safe-sex practices. This is especially true of APIDA cisgender young men. Additionally, APIDA teens are only about half as likely as their peers to get tested for STDs or to receive counseling about safe-sex practices from a health-care professional.

ECONOMIC FACTORS

Income, rates of labor force participation, home ownership, and job stability vary considerably among APIDA subgroups. However, such populations tend to have rates of labor force participation that are comparable to and, in some cases, higher than national averages. Yet APIDA people continue to be underrepresented in management and leadership positions. There are multiple factors that affect employment among APIDA populations, including both contemporary and historical inequalities. Although such populations tend to fare better economically than most other racial and ethnic groups, some subgroups are at increased risk for poverty.

Employment and Income

Three-fourths of NHOPI households have at least one adult who is employed full-time and, since 2000, their rates of employment have been consistently higher than US averages. However, average household income among NHOPI populations is around $66,000; this is $5,000 lower than the national average. In contrast, AA and DA populations have the highest average household incomes of all racial and ethnic groups. Over 80 percent of AA and DA households have at least one adult who is employed full-time. In 2019, AA and DA households averaged an annual income of just under $100,000; this was nearly $30,000 more than the average among all US households. Employment rates are highest among APIDA people aged 25–54; nearly 40 percent of those aged 55 and older are also employed. Rates of workforce participation are somewhat higher among cisgender APIDA men than women yet similar among those born outside of the United States and native-born populations.

Roughly one-fourth NHOPI are employed in white-collar jobs (e.g., managerial and administrative) while another 20 percent are engaged in construction, manufacturing, agriculture, or other types of manual labor. Additionally, 17 percent are employed in the service industry, especially in roles related to hospitality and tourism. Since the mid-twentieth century, representation of AA and DA populations in professional positions that require advanced training and credentials (e.g., health-care professionals, upper-level administrators and managers, and attorneys) has increased steadily. They are overrepresented in industries such as finance, insurance, retail, research, service related to computing and technology, computer manufacturing, internet and software publishing, hospitality services (e.g., restaurants, accommodations, and bars), apparel and shoe manufacturing, and personal services such as dry cleaning, laundry, taxi/limousine services, and nail salons. Yet AA and DA people are underrepresented in construction, agriculture, and industries related to natural resources (e.g., oil and gas, fishing, hunting, and logging). Variations in employment are even clearer when examining subgroups. The construction industry employs the greatest number of NH, Samoan, and Tongan people, while the restaurant industry employs the greatest number of Bangladeshi, Cambodian, Chinese, Korean, Laotian, Malaysian, and Thai individuals. Vietnamese populations represent over 25 percent of those employed in nail salons. Within STEM (science, technology, engineering, and math) fields, employment of Indian, Sri Lankan, Chinese, Filipino, Pakistani, and Malaysian populations is twice as high as the national average for all racial and ethnic groups. STEM employment is least common among Cambodian, Hmong, and NHOPI people.

Factors Affecting Employment

Workforce participation among APIDA people is impacted by numerous factors, including the so-called bamboo ceiling. This concept refers to the underrepresentation of such populations in upper-level leadership and executive positions, something that is evident among Fortune 500 companies as well as nonprofit organizations. The bamboo ceiling has also been documented in health care, technology, finance, and postsecondary education (including undergraduate, graduate, and professional programs) as well as in local, state, and federal governments. Such underrepresentation is most pronounced for cisgender women, individuals with disabilities, and members of the LGBTQ+ community. The bamboo ceiling is most often associated with the MMM and accompanying assumptions regarding the supposed assimilationist mentality and accompanying high achieving tendencies of certain APIDA populations, especially AA and DA subgroups. The MMM both facilitates and reinforces structural racism within employment settings. It is often exhibited through unconscious biases that deem APIDA people excellent workers yet simultaneously suggest they lack the skills to be effective leaders. However, overt discrimination (e.g., bullying, social exclusion, verbal abuse, unequal pay, physical violence, harassment, and sexual violence) directed at APIDA populations also occurs in employment settings. Historically, discrimination against APIDA workers has been linked to federal policies such as the Chinese Exclusion Act of 1882, the annexation of Hawaii and the Philippines following the Spanish-American War, and incarceration of individuals of Japanese descent during the Second World War. More recently, anti-APIDA discrimination in the workplace increased during the COVID-19 pandemic.

The economic well-being of NHOPI populations continues to be impacted by the history of colonialism and forced acculturation. Historically, ancestral territories supported subsistence agriculture, fishing, hunting, and small-scale trade/barter. Yet as a principal component of colonization, such territories were annexed by external governments and investors who established large-scale agricultural, husbandry, and fishing enterprises and then exported sugar, pineapple, coffee, meat, fish, seafood, and other products. Loss of ancestral territory due to colonization has been identified as a key contributor to intergenerational trauma among NHOPI people. It not only displaced them but also altered their diets, customs, and lifeways. In addition, it diminished the natural environment in ways that continue to harm the health of NHOPI populations. Loss of territory also devastated traditional economic systems of NHOPI people. In the short term, this prompted the class divides that are common under capitalism. In the long term, it has aggravated economic inequities and reduced financial stability among NHOPI people.

Furthermore, the dual forces of colonization and technology promoted the establishment of many Pacific Island territories as global tourism destinations beginning in the 1880s. At present, tourism/leisure remains one of the primary industries for Samoa, Tonga, Fiji, Hawaii, and the Solomon Islands. Yet tourism is a notoriously fragile industry. Due to the economic changes that resulted from the Great Recession (2007–9), for example, tourism decreased substantially around the world, including to Hawaii and other Pacific Islands. Consequently, unemployment rates in Hawaii nearly tripled, eventually reaching 7 percent overall. However, such rates were 10 percent among Native Hawaiians and 17 percent among Pacific Islanders in the state. Natural disasters and extreme weather events (e.g., tsunamis, flooding, extreme heat, volcanic eruptions, hurricanes, and tornadoes) also have a negative impact on tourism, thereby contributing to the economic vulnerability of NHOPI populations employed in such industries.

During the first two decades of the twenty-first century, unemployment rates were consistently lower among AA and DA populations when compared to other racial and ethnics groups. Yet there was a disproportionate increase in job losses among AA and DA populations during the first year of the COVID-19 pandemic; unemployment rates increased from 2.5 percent at the end of 2019 to nearly 15 percent by May 2020. Additionally, and when compared to pre-pandemic rates, increases in unemployment rates for AA and DA groups were higher than national averages. As the pandemic progressed, rates of labor force participation among such populations were slower to recover than among non-HLC whites. AA and DA groups also had longer-than-average periods of unemployment during the pandemic. Similarly, rates of COVID-related job loss were disproportionately high among NHOPI populations. In Hawaii, for example—the state with the largest NHOPI population in the country—unemployment rates were less than 3 percent in January 2020 but increased to nearly 22 percent only 3 months later. Throughout 2020, Hawaii had the second highest unemployment rate in the nation; in parts of the state, unemployment was over 30 percent. Pandemic-related job losses in Hawaii disproportionately impacted non-Hawaiian Pacific Islanders and Filipinos, especially cisgender women and those with limited English proficiency (LEP). Employment rates among NHOPI people were slower to recover than among HLC, Black, non-HLC white, AA, and DA people. As of mid-2022, rates of labor force participation among all NHOPI populations remained lower than prior to the pandemic.

Poverty Rates and Impacts

Aggregate data suggest APIDA households fare better economically than most other racial and ethnic groups. Yet some APIDA subgroups have high rates of poverty. Among AA and DA populations, poverty rates are comparable to those among non-HLC whites. Yet AA and DA people born in the United States are approximately two-and-a-half times more likely to be poor than their foreign-born peers. In 2019, roughly one in ten AA and DA households had incomes below the federal poverty level (FPL). However, during the same year, 15 to 25 percent of households among Mongolian, Burmese, Bangladeshi, Nepalese, and Pakistani subgroups were below the FPL. Household income is consistently lower among NHOPI people than national averages; it is estimated that one-fifth of such populations live in poverty. On average, APIDA cisgender women earn lower wages than their cisgender male counterparts. However, there is substantial variation. Chinese, Taiwanese, Indian, Japanese, and Malaysian cisgender women earn slightly higher average salaries than their cisgender, non-HLC white male counterparts. In contrast, NHOPI, Hmong, Burmese, Laotian, Vietnamese, Cambodian, Nepali, and Thai cisgender women earn 66 cents or less for each $1 earned by non-HLC white, cisgender men. The COVID-19 pandemic exacerbated economic insecurity for APIDA cisgender women; their employment rates dropped to just over 55 percent—a 20-year low—in the first 6 months of the pandemic.

Rates of home ownership increased from the 1980s through the first two decades of the twenty-first century for APIDA people. However, subgroups with higher average incomes continue to be more likely to own their homes rather than to rent; they are also somewhat less likely to live in multigenerational households (with three or more generations). Rates of home ownership have increased among AA and DA populations since the late twentieth century. Such rates range from 50 to 65 percent among Chinese, Indian, Filipino, and Japanese populations. In contrast, home ownership is less common among NHOPI people; only about 44 percent own their homes. Even though average household income among Vietnamese families is lower than most other subgroups, they have the highest rates of home ownership among all APIDA subgroups; nearly 70 percent own their homes. The COVID-19 pandemic diminished housing security for many APIDA populations. During the first two years of the pandemic, NHOPI, AA, and DA people were more likely than non-HLC whites to be behind on mortgage and rent payments. This was especially common in urban areas with a high cost of living (e.g., New York, Boston, and San Francisco) but also widespread throughout the states of Hawaii, California, New York, and Massachusetts.

At present, approximately half of APIDA populations live in areas with higher-than-average housing costs. Thus, they are at increased risk of housing insecurity. AA and DA populations currently have the lowest rates of homelessness among all racial and ethnic groups; they represent less than 1 percent of those who are housing insecure in the United States. However, it is widely recognized that underreporting and flawed data collection methods contribute to inaccurate information about housing insecurity among such populations. NHOPI people have highest rates of homelessness among all racial and ethnic groups in the United States. In the state of Hawaii, they constitute half of all homeless individuals. Although they represent less than one half of 1 percent of the total US population, NHOPI people constitute 1.5 percent of all those who are housing insecure and, thus, who encounter increased risk of physical and mental health risks due to lack of stable housing arrangements. Food insecurity is also an issue among low-income APIDA populations, yet limited availability of data makes it difficult to assess the scope and severity of the problem. A relatively small percent of all APIDA populations participate in government-sponsored nutrition programs for low-income populations. However, this is likely due to the shame and stigma associated with reliance on such programs within APIDA subgroups. Consequently, risk of nutritional imbalances and related health conditions (e.g., anemia, osteoporosis, being underweight, or overweight) are increased among such populations.

EDUCATIONAL ACCESS AND QUALITY

APIDA populations overall tend to have higher rates of educational attainment than other racial and ethnic groups. Yet there are significant differences in academic performance, degree-completion rates, and learning needs among APIDA subgroups. In addition, APIDA students face some unique challenges within educational settings. Some of these challenges stem from the ongoing influence of the MMM stereotype, yet others are connected to violence and social marginalization.

Educational Enrollment and Attainment

APIDA students represent slightly more than 5 percent of all those enrolled in pre-K, primary, and secondary educational settings—including both public and private—in the United States. AA and DA students outnumber NHOPI students 5 to 1 in public schools. When compared to the total US population, APIDA students in grades pre-K through 12—including one-third of NHOPI students and two-thirds of AA and DA students—are more likely to speak a language other than English at home. Many are also fluent in English. Yet others are English language learners (ELLs) and, therefore, require academic support services and instruction via English as a second language (ESL) programs. English fluency rates are lowest among first-generation US-born students and those who have recently entered the United States, especially those who have fled their home countries due to armed conflict or persecution.

AA and DA student populations overall tend to perform well academically throughout elementary, middle, and high school. They have higher average GPAs; they are more likely than students from other racial and ethnic groups to meet grade-level and college readiness benchmarks for math, reading, and writing; and they tend to score higher on college admissions exams. Although there is scant research concerning variations in average SAT and ACT scores among AA and DA subgroups, existing data indicates there are some differences based on country of birth, socioeconomic status, and sex. For example, cisgender girls tend to score higher on verbal portions of such exams while cisgender boys tend to score higher on the math portion. However, NHOPI students score lower than average than other APIDA subgroups on reading, writing, and math exams throughout their K-12 educational career. By the time they reach eleventh grade, half of NHOPI students do not meet grade-level expectations for reading and writing. Similarly, three-fourths of NHOPI students in eleventh grade do not meet grade-level expectations for math; test scores are lowest among NHOPI students whose total household income is below the FPL. When compared to AA and DA students as well as national averages, NHOPI students have disproportionately high rates of chronic absenteeism and unexcused absences. Additionally, NHOPI cisgender boys are nearly twice as likely as their non-HLC white peers to be suspended, expelled, or otherwise punished in academic settings. In contrast, AA and DA students are least likely to be punished. Disproportionate rates of punishment in academic settings have been linked to diminished mental health of NHOPI students and may impair their academic performance and contribute to rates of absenteeism. When compared to other racial and ethnic groups, APIDA populations are more likely to complete high school and to attend college.

Ninety percent of NHOPI people complete high school; comparatively, 93 percent of AA and DA students earn a high school diploma. The number of APIDA individuals who enroll in and complete postsecondary degrees—including associate's, bachelor's, master's, professional (e.g., MBA, law degree, and medical degree), and doctoral degrees—has increased substantially over the past two-and-a-half decades. Whereas less than 800,000 APIDA students were enrolled in postsecondary institutions in the mid-1990s, their numbers have nearly doubled; in 2020, nearly 1.5 million APIDA individuals were pursuing some type of postsecondary education or training. However, they currently constitute only 3 percent of all those enrolled at four-year colleges and universities and, thus, remain underrepresented among the total US postsecondary student population. Seventy percent of AA and DA people attend college compared to 55 percent of NHOPI populations. Nearly 55 percent of all APIDA adults over the age of 25 have earned a college degree; this exceeds the national average of 40 percent among adults of all racial and ethnic groups. Among foreign-born APIDA adults who have lived in the United States for less than 5 years, two-thirds have earned a college degree. Taiwanese and Indian subgroups have the highest rates of postsecondary attainment and over 75 percent have completed a college degree. In contrast, rates of postsecondary degree attainment are less than 25 percent among Hmong, Cambodian, and Laotian subgroups. Only about one-fifth of NHOPI people currently hold a postsecondary degree; rates of degree attainment are lowest among Samoan, Tongan, Palauan, Chuukese, and Guamanian populations. NHOPI people are more likely to drop out of college, less likely to complete an undergraduate degree in 6 years, and less likely to pursue graduate and professional degrees than AA and DA subgroups.

Challenges in Educational Settings

Within educational contexts, APIDA populations continue to be marginalized. They are underrepresented among teachers in elementary, middle school, high school, and postsecondary contexts. Additionally, they are underrepresentation among educational leadership including K-12 principals as well as deans, vice presidents, and presidents of colleges and universities. Such representation matters in terms of providing diverse perspectives and leadership within educational settings; it also matters in terms of shaping social norms and expectations regarding who is qualified and suited to hold such professional positions.

The MMM also influences the educational experiences of APIDA students. This stereotype promotes the assumption that such students are naturally smarter and more capable of performing well academically than other students. As a result, educators, administrators, and even non-APIDA students and their parents may have higher expectations for academic performance among APIDA students compared to other student populations; this is especially true in STEM subjects. Additionally, the MMM is often internalized by APIDA populations, including both parents and students; it has been linked to increased feelings of shame and stigma when APIDA students encounter academic struggles and has been shown to diminish their likelihood of asking for help when they encounter academic challenges. Those who struggle academically are also at increased risk of diminished mental health, increased anxiety, and lower self-esteem due to such shame and stigma. The MMM has also been identified as a key factor in the promotion of ableism by teachers as well as APIDA parents. Quite simply, when APIDA students encounter the types of memory, language, visual, auditory, and cognitive challenges that are hallmarks of diverse types of learning disorders (e.g., dyslexia, dyscalculia, dysgraphia, and auditory processing disorders), such challenges are typically interpreted as consequences of a lack of commitment and motivation. Thus, APIDA students who encounter such challenges are often told to study more and work harder in school. The same is true for APIDA students with learning difficulties related to certain emotional, developmental, and behavioral disorders (e.g., attention-deficit/hyperactivity disorder, autism spectrum disorders, and anxiety disorders). Such responses are a key contributor to the under-diagnosis of learning disabilities among APIDA students. They also force students to mask learning disabilities and other disorders to avoid stigma and shame. Such masking, in turn, has been shown to diminish mental health and increase anxiety about academic pursuits.

Ongoing harassment, intimidation, bullying, and interpersonal violence also impact APIDA students in educational settings. Some reports indicate that prior to the COVID-19 pandemic, APIDA students were less likely to be victimized in school settings than students from other racial and ethnic groups. However, critics assert that such reports were inaccurate and failed to account for the fact that APIDA students are only about half as less likely to report such victimization to a teacher, school administrator, or law enforcement—this is especially common among those who are foreign-born, have limited English fluency, and/or who fear that reporting such victimization will bring shame to themselves and their family. Recent data confirms that APIDA students are as likely and, in some contexts, more likely than other student populations to be victimized in academic contexts, including in person and online. Some of the most common forms of bullying and harassment experienced by APIDA students include racial slurs, name-calling, making fun of their appearance, ridiculing their culture or religious practices, threatening physical harm, spreading rumors, destruction of property, physical violence (e.g., hitting, pushing, and kicking), and sexual violence. APIDA cisgender girls and LGBTQ+ students are disproportionately targets of sexual violence. Due to the increase in anti-Asian sentiment during the COVID-19 pandemic, bullying and harassment of APIDA students has increased in recent years and nearly three-fourths report being victimized by their peers. Such victimization is associated with increased incidence and severity of physical ailments, sleep disorders, and mental health issues (e.g., anxiety, depression, PTSD, and suicidal ideation). Students who are victimized are also more likely to self-isolate, skip school, fail courses, drop out of school, and abuse alcohol or other substances. As the pandemic waned and schools reopened, many APIDA parents chose online options for their children due, in part, to fears related to bullying.

HEALTH-CARE ACCESS AND QUALITY

One of the most significant factors influencing health care among APIDA people is insurance; rates of coverage vary significantly among subgroups. Disparities in medical research and in clinical settings are also important considerations. Research concerning the health needs of APIDA populations remains scarce and tends to rely on aggregate data rather than attending to the specific health conditions, risks, and practices among unique subgroups. This misrepresentation is reinforced via structural features of the US health-care system. Furthermore, both implicit and explicit biases diminish the quality of care provided to APIDA populations and diminish their access to health care.

Health Insurance Coverage

Prior to the passage of the Patient Protection and Affordable Care Act (ACA) of 2010, nearly 20 percent of AA and DA populations lacked health insurance; they were 27 percent less likely to have health insurance than non-HLC white populations. Yet rates of insurance coverage—including via Medicaid, health insurance marketplace, and employer-sponsored coverage—have increased substantially among AA and DA populations since the implementation of ACA. At present, 93 percent of such populations are insured; collectively, they have the highest rates of health insurance coverage among all racial and ethnic groups in the United States. However, and although rates of insurance coverage have increased among all AA and DA subgroups since 2010, disparities remain. Less than 4 percent of Japanese populations are uninsured. In contrast, at least 10 percent of Mongolian, Burmese, Nepalese, Thai, Korean, Cambodian, Indonesian, and Malaysian subgroups lack health insurance. Mongolian populations have the highest uninsured rates of all AA and DA groups; 17 percent of Mongolians who are US citizens and over 40 percent of those who are non-citizens lack health insurance. There are also variations by age; 4 percent of AA and DA populations under the age of 18 are uninsured yet rates are twice as high among adults.

NHOPI populations have lower rates of health insurance coverage than AA and DA populations. Their rates of coverage are also lower than Black and non-HLC white populations; however, they have higher rates of insurance coverage than HLC and Indigenous populations. Approximately 13 percent of all NHOPI peoples are uninsured, including 8 percent of children and 16 percent of adults. They are more likely than AA and DA subgroups to rely on government-sponsored health insurance for low-income populations and less likely to have employer-sponsored health insurance. Among NHOPI populations, NH people are least likely to be uninsured while rates are highest among Marshallese, Samoan, Fijian, and Chamorro subgroups. Health insurance coverage rates among all APIDA people are higher in states with Medicaid expansion programs under the ACA than in states without expansion programs.

Disparities in Research and Clinical Settings

The US health-care system is organized in a manner that continues to marginalize APIDA populations. They remain underrepresented in medical research and corresponding literature. When research does include such populations, there is a tendency to gather and analyze data about them using the broad categories "Asian Americans" or "NHOPI." This is clear in government reports that present health data about APIDA populations in aggregate form. The use of such umbrella-type categories can help promote general understanding of patterns of disease, disability, and health behaviors by prompting comparison of key health issues among APIDA populations with key health issues among other broadly defined racial and ethnic groups (e.g., Black, HLC, Indigenous, and white populations). However, it also denies the diversity of cultures and correspondingly diverse health issues that exist among such populations.

Lack of attention to diversity among APIDA populations is also evident in clinical settings. Patient intake forms typically rely on the broad racial and ethnic categories that mask crucial differences among APIDA populations, including their varying perspectives on health, illness, and treatment options. Some groups favor an allopathic approach that focuses on treating symptoms, yet others prefer traditional approaches (e.g., herbal remedies, mind-body interventions, acupuncture, acupressure, and massage) to prevent illness. Such traditional approaches are often referred to as complementary and alternative medicine (CAM); there are limited options for trained CAM providers within the US health-care system and many insurance plans do not cover such care. Furthermore, at least 20 percent of APIDA populations have LEP. Language access services (LAS) are intended to promote improved access to health care for populations with LEP, yet there is an ongoing shortage of trained medical interpreters. Thus, some facilities rely on clinical staff who are not trained interpreters or, in some cases, ask patients' family members to serve as translators. Such strategies violate federal LAS standards; they are also associated with increased risk of communication errors. Patients who are not provided with appropriate LAS are more likely to be confused about their health conditions and treatment plan and, thus, more likely to experience poor health outcomes. They are also less likely to seek health care in the future.

Even when fully staffed, LAS typically include only the most common languages/dialects. Thus, barriers to access persist for those who communicate in other languages. For example, it is common for health facilities to provide medical interpreters who are fluent in the Mandarin dialect of Chinese; this is the native language for nearly three-fourths of Chinese, Taiwanese, and Singaporean immigrants to the United States. However, there are also seven other major Chinese dialects plus dozens of minor dialects. While there is a degree of overlap between Mandarin and other dialects, this is not true for all dialects, including Cantonese. Thus, an interpreter fluent in Mandarin cannot provide LAS to a Cantonese-speaking patient. Language access lines (LALs) and telemedicine are increasingly used in clinical settings to help facilitate access for populations with LEP. However, problems with audio/video quality, Wi-Fi reliability, confidentiality, and lack of familiarity among patients who do not use internet and other technologies regularly can render such options less desirable and effective than in-person appointments for some APIDA populations. The use of LALs and telemedicine may also feel disrespectful and/or impersonal to those who expect a more direct relationship with their health-care provider, including NH elders.

The Impacts of Biases

Implicit and explicit biases among health-care providers also serve as barriers to care for APIDA peoples. Sometimes, providers are simply unaware of the unique health beliefs and practices among such populations. Thus, they lack the knowledge necessary incorporate such factors when providing care. This is known as implicit bias; it is unintentional and stems largely from the ongoing lack of substantial research on the specific health needs of APIDA populations, both overall and among subgroups. For example, a nurse who is unfamiliar with the practice of coining—wherein a coin or edge of a spoon is rubbed over the skin of the trunk of the body and sometimes the neck to promote healing—that is common among Cambodian populations may mistake the red marks that result from this practice as a sign of physical abuse. Similarly, a physician who is not familiar with Buddhism—a religion common among AA and DA people—and its tenets regarding the importance of mindfulness and the acceptance of suffering may not be aware that it is common for Buddhists to refuse pain medication as part of palliative care. Lack of awareness of the cultural beliefs that influence health practices is also evident in certain health-care policies, including those that govern childbirth. Many Hmong people continue the traditional practice of burying the placenta in their homes following the birth of a child. They do this so that at the time of death, the soul of the individual can retrieve their placental jacket and it can guide them back to the spirit world where they will be reunited with their ancestors. However, hospital administrators and staff who are not knowledgeable about Hmong cultural practices may implement and enforce policies that define the placenta as biomedical waste that must be incinerated.

Implicit bias is also evident in medical practices that rely on stereotypes regarding which populations are the most likely to be afflicted with certain diseases including diabetes and high cholesterol. For example, high body mass index (BMI) has been linked to increased risk of type 2 diabetes. A BMI of 26–30 is classified as overweight while a BMI over 30 is classified as obese. AA and DA people have lower rates of obesity than NHOPI, Black, HLC, and non-HLC white populations. Therefore, and based on prevailing medical guidelines, many health-care providers do not regularly screen AA and DA populations for diabetes. Current data indicates over 40 percent of such populations are pre-diabetic or diabetic, yet due to lack of regular screening most are unaware of their condition. Thus, they are at increased risk for various health complications (e.g., kidney disease, nerve damage, and impaired mental health) and death due to diabetes. At present, diabetes is one of the leading causes of death among AA and DA communities. Similarly, implicit bias may influence providers' beliefs about the risk of heart disease among APIDA populations. Although APIDA people overall have lower rates of heart disease than Black, HLC, and non-HLC white populations, risk varies considerably among subgroups. For example, Japanese, Vietnamese, Filipino, and Indian subgroups have higher rates of high cholesterol. They are, therefore, at increased risk for health problems related to atherosclerosis (buildup of cholesterol in arteries), including stroke, heart attack, and peripheral artery disease. Providers who are unaware of such disparities are less likely to recommend cholesterol screenings for those most at risk and, consequently, are less likely to detect health problems related to high cholesterol until they become more advanced.

Yet there are times when health-care professionals knowingly promote ideas and/or engage in actions that diminish the quality of care they provide to APIDA people. This is known as explicit bias; it is discriminatory and violates both federal and state laws that govern the US health-care system. Examples include name-calling, belittling of cultural health practices, use of racist slurs, failing to provide LAS services to patients with LEP, use of physical force, and making APIDA populations wait longer to receive services. Recent research indicates that explicit biases in health-care settings have increased due to the COVID-19 pandemic, thereby diminishing the quality of care provided to APIDA patients and the treatment of APIDA health-care workers. Although such biases are most obviously influenced by racism and ethnocentrism, they are also impacted by other types of discrimination including sexism, homophobia, classism, ableism, and transphobia. Thus, biases are compounded for APIDA people who are members of the LGBTQ+ community, disabled, poor, and cisgender women. Patients who encounter explicit bias in clinical settings are less likely to seek health care in the future. They are also at increased risk for misdiagnosis, communication errors, and poor health outcomes. Health-care providers who encounter anti-APIDA sentiment from co-workers or patients are at increased risk of social isolation in the workplace. They also have lower rates of job satisfaction and higher rates of anxiety and depression.

LIVING ENVIRONMENT AND SOCIAL CONTEXT

The social marginalization of APIDA populations continues to shape their experiences and impact their well-being. Such marginalization is evident in stereotypes that are found in both political discourse and popular media. Community context also has a profound influence on the well-being of APIDA populations. While the urban environments where most APIDA populations live can increase risk of exposure to certain types of pollutants and stressors, the ethnic enclaves that are common among some subgroups can also provide important forms of social support and facilitate a sense of connection and belonging.

The Influence of Stereotypes

At present, stereotypes continue to influence attitudes toward and the treatment of APIDA populations, including via the microaggressions they encounter in educational, employment, and social settings. For example, APIDA people are often assumed to be foreigners, regardless of the location of their birth or how long they and their families have lived in the United States. In addition, the MMM remains a prominent stereotype. In addition to obscuring cultural differences among APIDA subgroups, it posits that APIDA populations—especially AA and DA subgroups—are uniformly high achieving to the point that they are deemed a threat to non-HLC whites in educational and employment contexts. This is clear in discourses that criticize the achievements of APIDA people by asserting that they are "taking away" jobs, scholarships, awards, and other types of opportunities from non-HLC whites.

Yet such ideas are not new. On the contrary, similar notions influenced the treatment of APIDA people in the late nineteenth century when critics of immigration policies argued that Chinese populations would displace non-HLC whites in the workforce, bring disease to the United States, and weaken American cultural values by refusing to assimilate. This was known as the yellow peril stereotype, and it prompted the passage of the Chinese Exclusion Act of 1882. Interestingly, NHOPI populations were also regarded as a threat to American society in the late nineteenth century; they were deemed unable to make rational choices or to conform to Western norms and values. Additionally, they were regarded as intellectually inferior, sexually promiscuous, and even dangerous. This was clear in stereotypes prominent in various forms of popular culture of the period. In such sources, NHOPI cisgender men were often depicted as fierce warriors who engaged in cannibalism and had insatiable sexual appetites. For NHOPI cisgender women, the most common stereotypes were embodied in the caricature of the dancing island girl. She was portrayed as young and attractive, dancing in a sensual manner that violated rigid gender and sexual norms of the Victorian era. She wore little clothing but was adorned with leaves, flowers, and seashells. Both her dance movements and her appearance were deemed evidence of the supposed primitive nature of NHOPI populations. Although such depictions were used to promote travel and the purchase of goods, they also served to justify the political, economic, and social control of NHOPI populations. Stereotypical representations that depict NHOPI populations as exotic, primitive, and sexually available remain prominent in contemporary tourism brochures and advertisements.

Similar stereotypes are found in contemporary popular media. APIDA populations remain underrepresented in film and television, accounting for less than 10 percent of all characters with speaking roles and only 6 percent of all characters overall (including those with nonspeaking roles) in mainstream films during the twenty-first century. When such populations are included, they are often depicted in stereotypical ways. Common tropes include the objectification and sexual fetishization of APIDA cisgender women; APIDA cisgender males as violent and aggressive (e.g., engaged in martial arts and members of gangs); AA and DA individuals as inept drivers; AA and DA cisgender male teens and young adults as nerdy, socially awkward, and asexual; NHOPI youth and young adults as unemployed and obsessed with surfing and marijuana; AA and DA people as fixated on wealth and possessions. Less than 5 percent of US films have an APIDA character in a leading or co-leading role. Of those APIDA leads and co-leads, only 12 percent are cisgender women and girls. APIDA cisgender men and boys appear in films at nearly twice the rate of APIDA cisgender women and girls. APIDA people who are members of the LGBTQ+ community or who have disabilities are virtually absent from mainstream film and television; the same is true for elderly APIDA populations. Additionally, APIDA populations are typically presented as foreigners, something that is emphasized via characters who have exaggerated accents and/or lack English fluency. Such representations reinforce the social marginalization of APIDA people and have been identified as contributors to stress and anxiety among such populations. It is also common for NHOPI populations to be portrayed by non-HLC white actors. This practice is referred to as whitewashing; in addition to diminishing employment opportunities for APIDA actors in film and television industries, it reinforces euro-centric notions of beauty, behavior, and culture. Thus, whitewashing has been linked to low self-esteem, body dysmorphia, eating disorders, and suicidal ideation. In addition, stereotypes of APIDA populations have been linked to various forms of victimization of such populations. For example, the fetishization of APIDA cisgender women in media is associated with increased risk of sexual violence for such populations. Furthermore, the yellow peril stereotype resurfaced during the COVID-19 pandemic as AA populations were blamed for the virus and became targets of various forms of hate crimes, including homicide.

Community and Environmental Considerations

Throughout the United States, APIDA populations tend to be concentrated in urban areas; only about 5 percent of such populations reside in rural areas. The states with the highest APIDA populations include New York, Texas, California, New Jersey, Illinois, and Washington. Walkability is often better in urban than rural areas due to availability of sidewalks and public transportation. However, APIDA populations tend to live in urban ethnic enclaves; this is especially common among those who are recent immigrants to the United States. Recent research indicates that such communities tend to be more disadvantaged when compared to more racially and ethnically diverse communities and especially when compared to communities with a higher percentage of non-HLC white residents. Ethnic enclaves typically have higher rates of unemployment and household incomes tend to be lower than national averages. Additionally, they are typically located in older areas of urban environments and/or those areas that suffered from economic disinvestment by local governments and developers. Thus, residents often suffer from substandard living conditions due to aging housing, inadequate green spaces and playgrounds, and outdated transportation infrastructure. The environmental conditions of ethnic enclaves have also been linked to disproportionately high rates of exposure to environmental hazards among APIDA populations, including cancer-causing air pollution. Such factors, combined with common urban problems such as overcrowding, traffic, and noise pollution contribute to increased stress and diminished mental health among APIDA populations. Critics argue that enclaves perpetuate the social marginalization of APIDA people by separating them from non-APIDA populations. Furthermore, the relative isolation of some ethnic enclaves may encourage underreporting of certain types of violence—especially intimate partner violence, child abuse, elder abuse, and sexual abuse—committed by community members.

Yet there are some health benefits associated with living in ethnic enclaves. For many APIDA populations, these communities provide a crucial form of support and facilitate social interactions with others who share their cultural background. Such support may be especially important for those immigrant populations who have limited English fluency and/or who encounter difficulties navigating the social norms and political, educational, and economic institutions of the United States. Although it is common among some APIDA subgroups to live in multigenerational households and/or to live near other family members, not everyone is able to do so. Consequently, ethnic enclaves often function as a type of extended kin network wherein individuals who share common ancestry support one another by providing information about the community, sharing resources, and celebrating holidays and other momentous events or achievements. Thus, there are psychological and social benefits associated with living in an ethnic enclave. Additionally, living in such areas has been found to confer. Certain physical health benefits. For example, pregnancy outcomes are better among APIDA women who live in ethnic enclaves. Living in such areas typically promotes an increased overall sense of physical well-being among residents, something that has been linked to the sense of social belonging that comes from living in a community of individuals with a shared cultural background. APIDA residents of ethnic enclaves are also more likely to have access to health services that meet standards for culturally and linguistically appropriate care.

CHAPTER TWO

Black Populations

The Black population in the United States is heterogeneous and ever changing. It includes those who are descendants of the more than 10 million individuals who were forcibly relocated as part of the trans-Atlantic slave trade that persisted from the sixteenth through nineteenth centuries. It also includes recent immigrants and refugees from various countries in Africa as well as the Caribbean; at present, immigrant and refugee populations represent one-tenth of all Black people who reside in the United States. Collectively, such populations have increased by nearly one-third since 2000. Black people are sometimes referred to as members of African Diasporic communities, African Americans, or Black Americans. In addition, some subgroups may refer to themselves or be referred to by others using hybridized terms that reflect their ancestry and/or country of origin (e.g., Ghanaian American, Haitian American, and Ethiopian American). An increasing number identify as biracial, multiracial, bi-ethnic, or multiethnic; over the past two decades, the number of Americans who identify as Black and as belonging to at least one other racial and/or ethnic group has increased by over 150 percent; such individuals currently represent about 15 percent of the nearly 48 million Black Americans. Those born after 1965 (e.g., members of so-called Generation X, Millennials, and subsequent generations) are significantly more likely than older generations to identify as Black biracial/ethnic or Black multiracial/ethnic.

This chapter focuses on various factors that contribute to health inequities for non-Hispanic/Latinx/Chicanx (non-HLC) Black populations in the United States in the twenty-first century. It focuses on social determinants of health to explore the various factors that both preserve and compound such inequities. The following discussion is grounded in research that recognizes race as a socially constructed concept that is used to categorize groups of people based on shared ancestry and/or perceived similarities in physical traits (e.g., skin color and tone; hair color, texture, and thickness; height; eye color and shape; body composition and weight distribution; and shape and prominence of jaw, forehead, and brow ridge). It posits that the inherent emphasis on racial/ethnic differences that is central to such categorization is a key component of the racial/ethnic hierarchies that continue to dominate US culture and that permeate social institutions. Such hierarchies contribute to the economic, political, educational, and social marginalization of Black people and, by extension, to the health inequities they continue to experience. Such inequities are evident in the high rates of disability, unduly high burden of certain diseases and injuries, and premature death rates that are found among Black populations. They are also evident in the barriers that diminish their access to health care.

CURRENT STATE OF HEALTH

Black populations bear a disproportionate burden regarding certain types of illnesses, diseases, and disorders. This burden contributes to a lower average life expectancy (ALE) for such populations: at the end of 2022, it was just under 71 years. This represents an increase of 7 years since 1970; additionally, from 2000 to 2019, life expectancy among Black populations increased more than among other racial and ethnic groups in the United States. However, the ALE racial gap persists. It remains 5 years lower among Black populations when compared to the national average; furthermore, the ALE among Black people remains markedly lower than ALE among HLC, non-HLC white, and non-HLC Asian, Pacific Islander, and Desi-American (APIDA) populations. Whereas ALE for cisgender Black female populations is approximately 75 years, it is only 67 years for cisgender Black males. During the first year of the pandemic, ALE among Black populations decreased by nearly 3 years. Lack of reliable data makes it difficult to accurately assess ALE among transgender and gender nonbinary Black populations. However, such populations have a substantially lower ALE and are three times more likely to die prematurely than cisgender Black people.

Morbidity and mortality rates related to chronic diseases have steadily decreased among Black populations since the 1960s. However, they continue to disproportionately experience not only early onset but also more severe or complicated manifestation of chronic diseases, greater incidence and severity of comorbidities, and greater mortality rates due to chronic diseases. When compared to national averages, Black people suffer from disproportionately high rates of type 2 diabetes, coronary heart disease, stroke, high blood pressure, some cancers (especially breast, lung, prostate, colorectal, uterine, and kidney cancers), and certain types of respiratory illnesses including asthma as well as chronic obstructive pulmonary disease (COPD). Rates of HIV infection are also disproportionately high among such populations; they represent approximately two-fifths of new HIV diagnoses each year. Prior to the pandemic, leading causes of death among Black adults included heart disease, cancers, stroke, diabetes and related complications, and unintentional injuries (e.g., falls, vehicle accidents, and drowning). Yet in 2020, COVID-19 emerged as the third most common cause of death (after heart disease and cancers) among Black people aged 20 and older; rates were especially high among low-income, incarcerated, housing insecure, and chronically ill populations. At present, unintentional injuries are the leading cause of death for Black cisgender women aged 20–44; for those 45–84, it is cancer; and for those aged 85 and older, it is heart disease. Leading causes of death are dramatically different among Black cisgender adult men: nearly half of those aged 20–44 die via homicide or unintentional injuries; for those aged 45 and above, leading causes of death are heart disease and cancer. There is little comprehensive data related to Black transgender and gender nonbinary (GNB) populations; however, it is clear they are significantly more likely than cisgender Black people to be victims of homicide and suicide.

Traumatic brain injuries (TBI) have a disparate impact on Black populations. Cisgender Black males (including minors as well as adults) have the highest rates of TBI among all racial and ethnic subgroups. Black people who sustain TBI also have disproportionately high rates of TBI-related death. Acts of violence are the most common cause of TBI among Black populations; when such acts include a firearm, the risk of TBI that leads to death increases dramatically. Gun violence also disproportionately impacts Black communities in other ways; indeed, such violence has been identified as a racial justice issue. Black people comprise 60 percent of all victims of US homicides that involve a firearm, and they are ten times more likely than non-HLC whites to die from gun violence. Rates of gun-related homicide are highest among cisgender Black boys and men aged 15–34. But gun violence also has a significant impact on the lives of Black lesbian, gay, bisexual, transgender, queer, intersex, and asexual (LGBTQIA) people, GNB individuals, and cisgender women and girls. In recent years, violent victimization of Black people by the police has been deemed an epidemic. They are nearly three times more likely than non-HLC whites to be shot by police and represent one-third of all fatalities that result from shootings by law enforcement.

When compared to national averages, Black people are more likely to meet clinical guidelines for being overweight (having a body mass index of 25.0 to 29.9) or obese (having a body mass index of 30.0 or more); approximately 70 percent of cisgender males and 80 percent of cisgender females are overweight or obese. Black cisgender women have the highest rates of obesity of all demographic subgroups in the United States. Additionally, Black people born in the United States are significantly more likely to be overweight or obese than those who are foreign-born. However, for many Black people, disparities in body weight and related health status begin during childhood and persist throughout adolescence and adulthood. During infancy and early childhood (up to age 5), one-fifth of Black children meet clinical guidelines for obesity; such rates increase slightly for those aged 6–11; among adolescents, nearly one-third meet clinical guidelines for obesity. Such rates are decidedly higher than national averages among children of all racial/ethnic groups. Black people who are obese have higher comorbidity rates—including due to diabetes, heart diseases, certain types of cancer, and hypertension—than their non-HLC white counterparts. Rates of comorbidities are especially high among those with household incomes below the Federal Poverty Level (FPL), who are uninsured, and/or who rely on government-sponsored health insurance.

Some autoimmune diseases and cognitive decline disorders are also more common among Black populations. Examples of such autoimmune diseases include systematic lupus erythematosus, systemic sclerosis (also known as scleroderma), sarcoidosis, and myasthenia gravis. The same is true for certain genetic diseases and disorders. Most common among these are sickle cell trait (SCT) and sickle cell disease (SCD); these are disorders of the red blood cells and are associated with pain, anemia, organ damage, pulmonary hypertension, increased risk of infection, stroke, liver problems, disability, and premature death. Additionally, memory loss disorders such as Alzheimer's disease and dementia are more prevalent among Black populations when compared to other racial and ethnic groups.

Disabilities are also a significant health concern. Among school-aged children between the ages of 5 and 19, Black people are more likely to be diagnosed with some type of disability related to physical, emotional, and/or cognitive function. Yet there are differences by age. At age 5, Black children are 20 percent less likely to be diagnosed with a disability than their non-HLC white peers and but 20 percent more likely to receive such a diagnosis than their HLC peers. However, by the time they enter fourth grade, Black children have higher disability rates than both HLC and non-HLC white children; they are also more likely to be identified as having a specific learning disability (e.g., dyslexia) or a developmental or behavioral disorder that impedes learning (e.g., attention-deficit hyperactivity disorder (ADHD), oppositional defiant disorder (ODD), and conduct disorder (CD)). Such disparities persist throughout adolescence and into adulthood. Approximately one quarter of all Black adults aged 19 or over have a diagnosed disability; nearly half of those individuals have two or more disabilities. The most common among such disabilities include mobility impairments (e.g., arthritis, neuromuscular disorders, skeletal anomalies or disorders, and severe damage to or loss of limb), cognitive impairments (e.g., due to stroke, developmental disorders, memory loss disorders, or TBI), and loss of vision or hearing. Among all age groups, disability rates are highest among Black people with incomes below 200 percent of the FPL.

Rates of certain acute illnesses, infectious diseases, and injuries are also unduly high among such populations. Examples include respiratory illnesses such as influenza, pneumonia, the common cold, and bronchitis. Although they comprise only about 13 percent of the total US population, Black people represent one-fourth of those who have contracted COVID-19; during the first two years of the pandemic, Black adults were three times more likely to die due to the virus and related complications than non-HLC whites. Rates of viral hepatitis, congenital hepatitis, and tuberculosis (TB) are also disproportionately high. Unintentional injuries such as falls, automobile accidents, exposure to smoke and fire, contact with plants or animals, and exposure to extreme temperatures or weather conditions (e.g., heat wave, tornado, drought, and flooding) are more common as well. Since 2019, work-related injuries and fatalities due to transportation, interpersonal or animal-related violence, exposure to harmful substances, and equipment have decreased among Black workers, yet they remain more common among Black employees when compared to national averages.

Black populations continue to experience disparities in the realm of sexual and reproductive health. On average, the age of sexual debut is slightly lower among Black adolescents than among most other racial and ethnic groups. However, timing varies significantly based on geographic location as well as sex and gender identities. Black people residing in more urban areas tend to have their first experience at a younger age than those residing in rural areas; cisgender boys typical have sex at a younger age than cisgender girls; cisgender heterosexual (cishet) populations generally have their first sexual experience at a younger age than LGBTQIA populations. Additionally, Black populations have the highest rates of sexually transmitted infections (STIs)—including chlamydia, syphilis, gonorrhea, and HIV—among all racial and ethnic subgroups. Since the start of the twentieth century, rates of unintended pregnancy and adolescent childbearing have decreased among Black populations. However, such rates remain higher than national averages—approximately three-fifths of births to Black adolescents and adults are unintended; birth rates among Black teens are 50 percent higher than national averages. Overall, the fertility rate has steadily declined among Black populations over the past two decades, particularly among those with a college education. However, poor pregnancy outcomes remain a pressing concern. Black pregnant individuals have disproportionately high rates of complications during pregnancy, labor, delivery, and the post-partum period; examples include preeclampsia and eclampsia (related to high blood pressure), obstetric embolism, heart failure, and hemorrhage. They are also more likely to experience a miscarriage, stillbirth, and emergency surgical delivery. Rates of obstetric death among Black people are higher than among all other racial and ethnic groups and three times higher than among non-HLC whites.

Rates of premature birth of Black infants are 60 percent higher than national averages; such rates are particularly high among those who experience the most significant disparities in relation to income, educational attainment, and access to health care. Black populations are more likely than HLC, APIDA, and non-HLC white populations to receive no prenatal care or to only receive such care during the later stages of pregnancy. Preexisting health conditions (e.g., diabetes and high blood pressure) and age of the pregnant individual (e.g., being under age 20 or being over age 35) have been identified as contributing factors in poor pregnancy outcomes among Black populations. Yet the chronic stress that results from racism is also a significant factor. Premature birth has been linked to increased incidence of respiratory issues, difficulties maintaining body temperature, and feeding difficulties for Black infants in the weeks and months immediately following birth. Such infants are also at increased risk of developing hearing and vision problems, cerebral palsy, developmental delays, and intellectual/learning disabilities. The leading causes of death among Black infants include complications related to premature birth and low birthweight, congenital malformations, birth injuries (e.g., brain injury due to oxygen deprivation during labor and/or delivery), and sudden infant death syndrome (SIDS). Mortality rates are more than twice as high among Black infants when compared to their APIDA, HLC, and non-HLC counterparts.

Black children also experience disproportionately high rates of what are collectively referred to as adverse childhood experiences (ACEs). These experiences undermine an individual's sense of stability and safety. Rates of abuse, neglect, and violent victimization are unduly high among Black children. They also experience higher-than-average rates of food insecurity and housing insecurity, poverty, incarceration of a parent, death of a close family member, and exposure to substance use and abuse. Racism is a common ACE that impacts Black children. They are also more likely than their HLC, APIDA, and non-HLC white peers to experience multiple ACEs. While ACEs can cause immediate psychological trauma, they also contribute to toxic stress; such stress negatively influences brain development as well as physical health and social interactions. Thus, ACEs can impact an individual throughout their lifespan. During childhood, ACEs increase Black children's risk of academic challenges; behavioral problems and developmental delays; diminished decision-making skills; interpersonal challenges; non-suicidal self-harming behaviors; suicidal ideation and suicide attempts; and high-risk behaviors related to sex, drug and alcohol use, violence, and illicit activities. Among Black adults, ACEs have been linked to increased risk of stroke, cancer, depression, substance use and abuse disorders (SUAD), autoimmune diseases, certain types of cancer, and cardiovascular diseases, among others.

Black populations experience significant challenges to their psychological health and well-being. Among adults, nearly 30 percent meet the criteria for a diagnosable, chronic mental illness or disorder such as anxiety, depression, schizophrenia, PTSD, or SUAD. Rates of mental illness among Black populations have increased by more than 50 percent over the past three decades. Yet they are less likely than APIDA and non-HLC white populations to receive treatment for a mental or psychological health issue. Anxiety, depression, and other mood disorders are diagnosed more often among Black cisgender women than Black cisgender men; such disorders are nearly twice as common among those living below the FPL than those with higher incomes. They are also disproportionately high among LGBTQIA populations. Black people of all ages are less likely than non-HLC white populations to die from suicide; however, Black adolescents are at least 50 percent more likely to attempt suicides than their non-HLC white peers. Additionally, suicide rates are four times higher among Black cisgender men than cisgender women. Since the start of the COVID-19 pandemic, suicide attempts and related deaths increased by over 40 percent among Black people of all ages; among adolescents, such rates nearly doubled. Rates of suicidal ideation and attempts are nearly 50 percent higher among Black transgender and GNB adolescents than among Black cisgender teens. Deaths due to drug overdoses are also disproportionately high among Black populations.

In recent years, the concept of weathering has been used to acknowledge the cumulative impact of stress caused by systemic, institutional, and interpersonal discrimination. This concept refers to a faster-than-average decline in physical and/or mental well-being throughout the lifespan. Thus, it offers a way to acknowledge and discuss how racism contributes to exacerbated health inequities among Black populations. The weathering hypothesis also asserts that such inequities are most pronounced at the intersection of various types of oppression, including racism, ableism, sexism, homophobia, transphobia, and economic marginalization, among others. Additionally, those who are descendants of enslaved populations continue to contend with the realities of intergenerational trauma. Such trauma diminishes both physical and mental health and is associated with internalized oppression, including diminished self-esteem and self-concept. Furthermore, and like ACEs and other forms of trauma, intergenerational trauma can alter epigenetic expression (that is, how particular genes are activated). Thus, such trauma not only increases allostatic load and contributes to weathering but can also alter brain chemistry, diminish immune response, contribute to emotional dysregulation and sleep disorders, increase risk of certain types of chronic conditions (e.g., diabetes, heart disease, high blood pressure, PTSD, depression, and SUAD), make it difficult to form and maintain healthy relationships, and foster feelings of insecurity and fear.

ECONOMIC FACTORS

Black Americans remain economically vulnerable. This is evident in patterns of income, wealth, and debt. However, there are differences by age, sex, gender, and country of origin as well as household composition. Although Black populations participate in the workforce at a rate that is consistent with national averages among all racial and ethnic sub-groups, the racial wage gap and ongoing racial segregation in the workplace continue to diminish not only their earnings and access to benefits but also their opportunities for promotion and leadership. Thus, economic factors have both immediate and long-term impacts on their financial stability as well as their health.

Income, Wealth, and Debt

Patterns in average household income and employment are key to understanding the economic status of Black populations and provide insight into the various health disparities and inequities they experience. At present, Black populations have the lowest average household income of all racial and ethnic groups in the United States. This pattern has remained consistent throughout the first two decades of the twenty-first century; since the mid-twentieth century, median income among households headed by Black people has remained consistently lower than among households headed by APIDA, non-HLC white, and HLC people. In 2021, the household income for Black Americans averaged $48,000; this was approximately $22,000 less than the national average among all households. Over half of all households headed by a Black adult earn less than $50,000 annually. Average household income is higher among those who identify as Black multiethnic, multiracial, or HLC. When compared to other immigrant groups, Black immigrants have lower average incomes. However, Black people born in the United States are nearly 50 percent more likely than Black immigrants to have household incomes below $25,000. At least two-fifths of Black LGBTQIA populations live in households with incomes below the FPL. Household income varies considerably by family composition. Among Black families with minor children, median income is $35,000 for cisgender female-headed households with no spouse or partner present; however, it is nearly $20,000 higher for cisgender male-headed households with no spouse or partner. For two-parent households, median income is more than two times higher than among those headed by unpartnered cisgender women and 20 percent higher than among those headed by unpartnered cisgender men.

When compared to national averages, Black Americans have significantly less wealth. Their total household wealth is approximately 70 percent lower than among non-Black households. Additionally, they tend to have fewer assets and those assets are less diversified. Among all black-headed households, less than 10 percent have stocks, bonds, or securities; only one-third have retirement accounts; less than 5 percent have business assets; 2 percent have nonfinancial assets (e.g., art, jewelry, and antiques) valued at more than $5,000; and just under 10 percent own real estate that is not their primary residence (e.g., rental property, farm land, and business property). While their rates of asset ownership are much higher regarding bank accounts, vehicles, and primary residence, the relative values of such assets are markedly lower than national averages. For example, nearly 97 percent of Black households have a checking or savings account; however, the average value of such accounts is less than $2,000; this is less than one-fourth the value of similar accounts among non-HLC white households. Roughly 45 percent of Black households own their homes; the average value of such homes is just over $150,000. In contrast, home ownership averages 65 percent and average home values are nearly $350,000 among all Americans. Additionally, Black populations tend to have a disproportionately high debt-to-income ratio. They also tend to have riskier debt (e.g., credit card debt and payday loans) that includes higher interest rates and penalties for late payment as well as greater risk of default. The combination of fewer economic assets plus greater debt jeopardizes their financial stability. It also diminishes their health. In addition to contributing to stress and anxiety, financial insecurity limits access to timely, high-quality health care. In the past year alone, one in three Black Americans has not gotten care that was recommended by their health-care provider because they could not afford it; another 45 percent postponed health care due to cost.

Employment

At present, Black populations represent roughly 13 percent of all those employed in the formal labor economy in the United States. Their labor force participation rate is 63 percent; this is on par with national averages. Yet the unemployment rate among Black people aged 16 and over is nearly twice as high as national averages; this is a pattern that has persisted since at least 1954 when the US Bureau of Labor Statistics first began to report employment data among various racial and ethnic groups. The wage gap is a significant factor among Black employees. On average, Black cisgender men earn only 87 cents and Black cisgender women earn only 64 cents for each $1.00 that is earned by cisgender white men. Among Black cisgender men employed full-time, average weekly earnings are $950; such earnings are $100 less for Black cisgender women. The wage gap is even more pronounced for Black LGBTQIA populations; on average, their earnings are about 20 percent less than their Black cisgender counterparts. The wage gap is largely a reflection of occupational segregation. Black workers are overrepresented in low-wage jobs, many of which do not require specialized education, training, or certification prior to employment. Examples include food preparation and service, cashiers, retail sales, personal care assistants, home health aides, social service workers, warehouse workers (e.g., stocking, moving, handling, and shipping freight), custodial and maintenance staff, and entry-level office staff. They also remain marginalized in higher-paying professions such as architecture, data analysis, health specialties (e.g., researchers, administrators, and surgeons), business and finance, management, STEM fields, and legal occupations (e.g., lawyers and judges). While there has been an increase in Black elected officials since the mid-twentieth century, Black populations remain underrepresented among elected officials, including in federal, state, and local contexts. Black cisgender women and Black LGBTQIA populations remain especially scarce among those serving as senators, representatives, mayors, judges, members of city councils, and in other elected positions. However, the racial wage gap also reflects the systemic discrimination that continues to impact Black workers. Such discrimination diminishes not only employment opportunities but also the likelihood of promotions, raises, and earning a living wage. It also reduces access to employment benefits such as health insurance, sick leave, paid vacation, flexible spending accounts for expenses related to health care and childcare, and retirement savings. Thus, while the wage gap has an immediate impact on Black workers and their families and can make it more difficult for them to afford housing, food, health care, and other necessities, it also has long-term implications for their financial well-being.

At least one in four Black workers has reported experiencing race-based discrimination; many more do not report such discrimination out of fear that they will lose their job or otherwise be punished. Data indicates that Black cisgender women, LGBTQIA populations, and those under age 40 encounter disproportionately high rates of discrimination while working. Such discrimination is reflected in the persistent wage gap and ongoing patterns of labor force segregation. Yet it also contributes to disproportionately low rates of promotions and raises as well as disproportionately high rates of warnings, demotion, and job loss. Workplace discrimination has also been linked with negative health outcomes among Black workers. Those who encounter such discrimination often experience decreased self-esteem and feelings of self-worth. Increased incidence and severity of stress, anxiety, and depressive disorders as well as headaches, musculoskeletal complaints, high blood pressure, heart disease are also common. Many Black people also participate in the informal economy, providing services or work that is paid for in cash or via a barter system. Examples include home repairs, auto service, hair services, and babysitting. Many engage in such activities to avoid the discrimination they encounter in the workplace; others do so to help balance income-earning activities with family-related responsibilities. Yet informal sector activities often provide inconsistent income and do not include health insurance or other benefits.

Poverty

Poverty rates among Black Americans reached their lowest point ever in 2019 yet remained disproportionately high. At present, half of all Black-headed households have incomes below 200 percent of the FPL. Furthermore, one-fifth percent of Black people live below the FPL; this is nearly approximately 70 percent higher than the national average and more than twice as high as the poverty rate among APIDA and non-HLC white populations. There are variations in poverty rates among different subgroups. For example, poverty rates are at least 20 percent higher among Black LGTBQIA adults than among Black cishet adults. When compared to working-age adults (ages 18–64), Black children under the age of 18 and Black adults aged 65 and over are more likely to live in poverty. Rates of poverty are nearly 20 percent higher among Black cisgender women than among Black cisgender men. Households that include minor children and that are headed by unmarried or unpartnered cisgender women comprise nearly three-fourths of all Black households living at or below the FPL. Households headed by foreign-born Black populations tend to have higher incomes and, thus, are less likely to live in poverty than Black people born in the United States. However, those born in South America or in the Caribbean tend to have lower poverty rates than those born in Mexico or in countries in Central America and Mexico.

Economically, many Black Americans remain vulnerable in times of economic crisis. Thus, even those households who are above the FPL may find themselves pushed into poverty. During the Great Recession, for example, decreases in employment rates and average household income were disproportionately high among such populations. As a result, poverty rates among Black households increased by one-fifth between 2008 and 2010. Similarly, during the COVID-19 pandemic, Black workers lost their jobs at a much higher rate than HLC, APIDA, and non-HLC whites, with rates of job loss more pronounced among cisgender women than cisgender men. Consequently, the pandemic both reinforced and expanded the racial income gap. Average household income among Black populations declined during the pandemic and, as a result, poverty rates increased. Thus, such populations increasingly sought assistance through government-sponsored programs for low-income populations. Some states did expand assistance to low-income households during the pandemic; in other states, however, the decline in social welfare assistance that began in 1996 with the passage of the Personal Responsibility and Work Opportunities Reconciliation Act (more commonly known as welfare reform) continued even during the pandemic. For example, in 2020, at least fourteen states (e.g., Texas, Louisiana, Indiana, Alabama, Wyoming, and others) provided TANF grants to less than 10 percent of all families who were living in poverty. Given the racism that was the driving force behind welfare reform in 1996 and that continues to shape American attitudes and policies related to social welfare programs, it is not surprising that Black people were among those most affected by policies and practices that limited access to social welfare programs during the pandemic. Thus, although the pandemic altered the economic landscape for many Americans, it disproportionately affected Black populations and pushed many even further into poverty.

Poverty has immediate impacts on the health and well-being of Black people. It limits their access to adequate amounts of healthy food as well as their access to safe, affordable housing. Nearly one-fifth of Black Americans are food insecure; rates of food insecurity are three times higher among Black children when compared to their non-HLC white counterparts. They are also overrepresented among housing insecure populations in the United States and currently comprise over 40 percent of homeless Americans. While food and housing insecurity have immediate detrimental impacts on health and well-being, it is equally important to recognize the influence that long-term exposure to the realities of economic scarcity has on health. Poverty is a traumatic experience and a unique type of ACE, particularly as it explicitly increases likelihood of experiencing other ACEs (e.g., food insecurity and housing insecurity). Thus, poverty diminishes both physical and mental health. Furthermore, research demonstrates that the stress associated with poverty can alter epigenetic expression, specifically DNA methylation and structure. Thus, the health-related consequences of poverty are passed on genetically to future generations. Poverty-related epigenetic alterations are associated with increased risk and severity of depression, anxiety, and other types of mental illness; they have also been linked with increased risk of certain physical health conditions including high blood pressure, diabetes, chronic pain, and immune system dysfunction.

EDUCATIONAL ACCESS AND QUALITY

Disparities in academic performance, persistence, and degree completion rates among Black students have been linked to economic factors as well as de facto racial segregation in the US educational system. Other key considerations include the ongoing marginalization of the experiences of Black populations in the curriculum, underrepresentation of Black people among educational professionals, and disciplinary practices that disproportionately target Black students and that have been identified as a key contributor to the school-to-prison pipeline. Consequently, ongoing issues related to educational access and quality contribute to economic barriers as well as informational barriers to health care among Black populations.

Preschool, Primary, and Secondary Education

Black students represent 15 percent of those enrolled in pre-K-12 public education programs. Their rate of enrollment in pre-K programs is on par with national averages; however, they are far more likely to enroll in public than private programs. Only one in seven is enrolled in high-quality preschool programs that offer developmentally appropriate instruction by highly qualified teachers and in a manner that recognizes and responds to the unique social and educational needs of each child. In recent decades, the racial gap in school readiness among children preparing to start kindergarten has narrowed considerably, including in relation to language skills, numeracy, cognitive development, and social-emotional skills. Yet disparities remain. Although their average scores on academic and behavioral measures have increased over the past two decades, Black children continue to receive disproportionately low scores on kindergarten readiness measures. However, Black girls are more likely than Black boys to meet school readiness measures. Throughout elementary and middle school, Black children are underrepresented in programs for gifted and talented students. By fourth grade, their scores on standardized math and reading tests are significantly lower than national averages. And by eighth grade, their average scores on standardized reading and math tests are the lowest among all racial and ethnic subgroups. Throughout elementary and middle school, Black children attending public schools are disproportionately represented among those diagnosed with disabilities that impact learning, emotional regulation, social interactions, and behavior. However, a growing body of research demonstrates that bias is a key contributor to such diagnoses and the resulting misplacement of Black pupils in special education classes.

At the secondary level, patterns related to academic achievement among Black students persist. In grades 9–12, they tend to have lower grades and earn lower scores on standardized exams in core subjects (e.g., government, natural sciences, math, English, and social sciences). By the time they reach twelfth grade, under 20 percent meet national proficiency standards for reading and only 8 percent meet national proficiency standards for math. They also tend to earn disproportionately low scores on college entrance exams. Whereas the average total SAT score among all students in 2021 was 1,060, the average among Black students was 126 points lower. On the ACT, Black students earned scores that were 20 percent lower than national averages. Three-fifths of Black students complete high school without the full range of analytical skills, learning strategies, and knowledge—especially in areas such as math and science—that have been deemed central to college readiness. Enrollment is especially low among those from low-income families and those attending schools that receive Title I financial support. Such schools tend to be concentrated in geographic areas with high poverty and low tax revenues. Although Title I can improve access to and quality of education, the reality is that that such funding is inadequate to fully compensate for economic disparities. Consequently, Black students attending low-income schools do not have adequate access to special education services, tutoring, and experiential learning opportunities. They also lack adequate access to advanced placement (AP) courses and International Baccalaureate (IB) programs. Black high school students represent only one-tenth of all students who enroll in all AP courses; they comprise less than 3 percent of students in AP science, technology, engineering, and math (STEM) courses. They represent less than 10 percent of students enrolled in IB programs and dual-enrollment courses. Such limitations diminish the educational experience and academic achievement of Black students. Yet even those who have access to advanced educational options often feel they don't belong in such courses, aren't aware of the importance of pursuing such courses, and are not represented in the content of such courses. Such factors not only discourage them from enrolling in such courses but also impede engagement with course content among those who do enroll. Limited access to advanced courses and educational programs diminishes the likelihood that Black students will secure admission and merit-based scholarships to highly competitive college and universities. Such limitations have also been linked to the underrepresentation of Black students in college STEM courses and, consequently, in STEM careers.

School climate is also an important consideration. Black students are disproportionately subject to school discipline. They are twice as likely as their peers to be suspended or expelled for minor infractions such as using a cell phone in school or dress code violations. School officials are also more likely to involve police for discipline cases involving Black students. Such students represent one-third of all referrals to and arrests by law enforcement officers; rates of such referrals and arrests are highest among Black cisgender male students. Excessive discipline has been linked to academic underperformance as well as increased risk of dropping out of school. While the dropout rate among Black students has declined since 2000, it remains 10 percent higher than the national average. However, in cases where Black students are victimized (e.g., bullying, harassment, assault, sexual or relationship violence), school officials are much less likely to intervene, to implement disciplinary measures against the perpetrator, or to involve law enforcement. School climate is also shaped by ongoing patterns of segregation. Although the decision of the US Supreme Court in the case of *Brown v. Board of Education (1954)* declared racial segregation in public schools unconstitutional, the reality is that de facto separation of Black students persists. Three-fifths of Black students attend high-poverty schools—those where more than 50 percent of students qualify for free or reduced-price lunch—where most of their classmates identify as Black, AI/AN, or HLC. Students attending such schools tend to have lower grades and are more likely to drop out of school than those attending more affluent schools. In public schools, only 6 percent of teachers and 10 percent of principals are Black; rates are even lower in private schools. Furthermore, Black people remain marginalized in the curriculum, particularly as courses in history, art, STEM fields, sciences, and other fields continue to prioritize a Eurocentric perspective. While critical race theory (CRT) offers an avenue for combatting racism and promoting diversity in education, political backlash has led to legislation that bans CRT in some states. By the end of 2021, nine states had passed such legislation; at least twenty more had introduced similar legislation. Some educators practice more inclusive pedagogy that not only includes attention to the experiences and accomplishments of Black people but also incorporates anti-racism content and teaching methods. Yet some teachers who have introduced concepts related to racial oppression and systemic discrimination in the classroom have been sanctioned and sometimes fired.

Postsecondary Education and Training

Within the context of postsecondary settings, enrollment rates among Black students have increased since 2000. At present, just over one-third of Black students pursue a postsecondary degree, certificate, or other type of training after completing high school. However, less than half earn a degree within 6 years of starting college; more than half drop out without ever earning a 2-year (associate's) or 4-year (bachelor's) degree. Rates of successful degree completion are even lower among Black cisgender men—only 2 in 5 of those who enroll in college earn a degree. Black populations remain underrepresented in postsecondary institutions, including in undergraduate, graduate, and professional programs. In total, they represent 13 percent of all postsecondary students. Black students earn approximately 12 percent of associate's degrees awarded in the United States. They also earn one-tenth of bachelor's degrees, 13 percent of master's degrees, and 9 percent of doctoral or professional degrees (e.g., law, medicine, and architecture). Rates of degree attainment are higher among Black cisgender women than Black cisgender men. Black LGBTQIA populations have lower postsecondary enrollment and degree completion rates than their cishet counterparts. Among foreign-born Black adults, one-third have at least a bachelor's degree; 12 percent have earned a master's degree or other advanced degree. Black students remain underrepresented in STEM majors, law, finance, marketing, architecture, advanced health care (e.g., medical school and dental school), and other fields associated with high-paying careers. At most highly selective colleges and universities, enrollment among Black students has decreased in recent years. In some states, there has been an increase in efforts to promote postsecondary vocational and technical training programs (e.g., hospitality, medical coding, cosmetology, and automotive repair) for Black students. Such programs typically take a short time to complete, are less expensive than 4-year institutions, and can provide a more direct pathway to employment. Yet they also tend to lead to relatively low-wage jobs. Thus, some have criticized the promotion of such programs as a measure that reinforces racial economic inequities.

The type of climate-related issues found in K-12 settings is also evident in postsecondary institutions. Black college students tend to be punished more harshly for academic and conduct-related infractions than non-HLC white students; they are more likely to face academic probation or academic dismissal for such matters. Both explicit and implicit biases persist in postsecondary contexts. Such bias is evident in what are known as microaggressions; these are typically unintentional, subtle comments or actions that demonstrate a negative attitude toward or belief about a particular group of people. However, blatant verbal and/or physical attacks, including hate crimes against Black populations, have increased over the past decade on college and university campuses. Some schools maintain Black Studies or African American Studies programs that promote attention to the religious, social, historical, economic, and political dimensions of Black communities, both in the United States and globally. Additionally, many institutions have cultural centers and/or diversity, equity, and inclusion (DEI) programs. However, Black studies programs tend to be small; collectively they graduate just over 1,200 majors per year. Additionally, Black studies programs and DEI initiatives remain underfunded; thus, when budgetary concerns arise, such programs and initiatives may be jeopardized. Some Black students opt to attend historically Black colleges and universities (HBCU); such institutions provide a more supportive educational environment that both acknowledges and celebrates Black culture, traditions, and identities. Yet HBCUs represent under 3 percent of all postsecondary institutions in the United States.

The composition of the workforce in postsecondary institutions also reflects campus climate. Black people comprise less than 6 percent of full-time faculty overall; they are concentrated in nontenure track (e.g., instructors and lecturers) and part-time positions but hold a relatively small percent of all associate professor and full professor positions. They currently hold less than 5 percent of all positions as academic department heads. Black populations are more represented in staff positions in postsecondary institutions, yet they are overrepresented in service, clerical, and maintenance positions and remain marginalized in higher-paying positions in student affairs, information technology, and institutional affairs. They also remain marginalized in campus-wide leadership positions, including as college and university presidents, provosts, and deans. At all levels of postsecondary employment, Black faculty and staff tend to be paid less than their non-HLC white and APIDA peers. Inequities in professional appointments and salary are greatest for Black cisgender women and Black LGBTQIA populations.

Financial considerations are significant in shaping the experiences of Black students. Over 70 percent of those attending undergraduate programs qualify for need-based Pell Grants. In addition, nine out of ten Black students take out loans to help pay for their undergraduate education. By the time they complete a bachelor's degree, Black students have an average of $30,000 as student loan debt; this is more than the average student loan debt among all other racial and ethnic groups. Those graduating with a bachelor's degree have, on average, $25,000 more in student loan debt than their non-HLC white peers. Black cisgender women carry the most student loan debt among all demographic subgroups. In the years after completing their undergraduate education, Black people are more likely to have difficulty making on-time student loan payments and to default on their loans. This is due, in part, to the reality that average student loans payments consume a sizeable portion of total household income, even for those with incomes well above the FPL. However, due to complex factors including employment discrimination, inflation, and the underrepresentation of Black populations in higher-paying professions, the educational debt Black students incur may diminish their financial well-being for decades after they leave college and, consequently, can exacerbate economic barriers to health care.

Other Considerations

Nearly one-fourth of Black adults have low English literacy skills. Rates of low literacy are higher among those born in the United States than among foreign-born Black populations. Another one-fourth of Black adults have low numeracy skills and, therefore, struggle to make sense of and apply basic mathematical information. Rates of low literacy and low numeracy are particularly high among incarcerated, low-income, and housing insecure populations and among those who did not complete high school.

Those with low literacy and/or low numeracy are at a disadvantage in health-care settings. They may struggle to accurately complete intake and health history forms and to accurately understand health information brochures, discharge paperwork, and medicine labels. Furthermore, over 50 percent of Black adults have basic health literacy or low health literacy; consequently, they may struggle to understand health insurance coverage, follow health written or verbal instructions from health-care professionals, navigate the health-care system, follow recommendations for medication dosage and timing, engage in preventative health screenings, and otherwise obtain information needed to promote their health and well-being. Although it is clear that culturally, educationally, and linguistically appropriate health services—including those that use visual representations and certain types of technologies as well as services offered through Black-centered community centers and religious institutions—can help improve health literacy among Black populations, such approaches remain both underutilized and underfunded.

It is also important to consider the relationship between education and incarceration as a racial justice issue. More specifically, the undue burdens and ongoing marginalization that Black populations encounter in educational settings are associated not only with reduced academic achievement and degree completion rates but also with increased likelihood of incarceration. At present, Black populations represent one-third of all Americans who are in jails and prisons. Nearly two-thirds of Black cisgender young men who drop out of school during adolescence or early adulthood will enter the criminal justice system at some point in their lives. Among incarcerated Black cisgender women, one-third do not have a high school diploma or equivalency (known as the General Educational Development tests or GED). Less than 4 percent of all incarcerated Black populations have a college degree. Promoting access to education for inmates has been shown to dramatically reduce recidivism rates, promote physical as well as mental well-being, and foster social mobility for formerly incarcerated individuals and their families. Yet there are few options for education within the criminal justice system. Some facilities do provide GED programs, life skills training (e.g., classes that focus on budgeting, interpersonal relationships, and stress-reduction techniques), non-credit creative arts programs, job training and certification options, and even college degree options. However, the reality is that inmates encounter significant and often insurmountable barriers that make participation in such programs unaffordable or otherwise unrealistic. Thus, while the marginalization Black populations encounter in educational settings increases their risk of imprisonment, the barriers to education they experience within correctional settings diminishes the likelihood that those who are incarcerated will ever further their education.

HEALTH-CARE ACCESS AND QUALITY

Much of early American scientific research and practice were rooted in the false notion that race is biologically determined rather than socially constructed. This concept served as the foundation for unethical and inhumane medical practices that targeted Black populations well into the twentieth century. Although a variety of laws and professional standards prohibit such discrimination at present, the reality is that both explicit and implicit bias remain core features of the US health-care system and influence not only the care provided to Black patients but also the treatment of Black health-care professionals. Such biases, combined with persistent economic, geographic, cultural, informational, and linguistic barriers to care, continue to diminish the health of Black people as well as their trust in the US health-care system.

The History of Scientific Racism

Historically, the US health-care system has relied on and reinforced the idea that racial identity is rooted in biology and genetics. Ideas that purported the supposed biological origins of race can be traced back to even the earliest years of nation. For example, in early America, a time when notions of freedom and individual rights shaped political ideology, many defended and justified the institution of slavery based on core ideas of the Enlightenment—specifically science, reason, and logic—as they argued that there was an inherent racial hierarchy. Within that hierarchy, Black populations were deemed fundamentally, inherently different from and biologically inferior to white populations. Thus, they were deemed not fully human. While such thinking was used to justify slavery and to prevent Black populations from accessing political rights, it also became the basis for scientific racism in the period. This is clear in the medical experiments that were performed on enslaved populations. Historical records demonstrate that in the 1800s, physicians in southern states regularly conducted amputations, removal of organs and other body parts, repair of broken bones, removal of tumors, examining the brain (e.g., drilling into the skull), and other experiments on Black populations. They did so without consent, without the use of pain relief, and with the use of physical restraint measures such as tying individuals to the exam table. Some of the most well-known of such experiments were those conducted by James Marion Sims. Often referred to as the founder of modern gynecological practice, Sims regularly performed gynecological experiments on cisgender

Black women, often inviting his colleagues to watch. Some medical schools also used slaves in the training of medical students; other medical schools regularly exhumed recently deceased slaves from their graves and used their bodies to teach students about anatomy and physiology.

Ideas about the supposedly inherent biological difference of Black populations were also central to the pseudo-science of eugenics (sometimes referred to as scientific racism) that was popular in the late nineteenth century and throughout the decades of the early twentieth century. Drawing on ideas that had been used to classify plants based on color, shape, size, reproductive patterns, and similar features, prominent scientists used a similar approach to classify human populations. Consequently, certain physical features (e.g., skin tone, skull size and shape, eye color, eye shape, size of nose, jawline, and lips) were presented as supposedly incontrovertible, scientific evidence of inherent biological differences between various populations. This classification system was inherently political and used to divide human populations into three categories they referred to as Caucasoid, Mongoloid, and Negroid. Through their reliance on and application of this classification system, scientists not only reinforced the racial hierarchy that had existed during slavery but also further integrated scientific racism into health-related research and practice. This is most obvious, for example, in the field of eugenics, which relied on Darwin's theory of natural selection to advance the theory that selective reproduction could improve the health of human populations. Consequently, eugenics served as the foundation for medical research and practice that violated the human rights of Black populations. Historical examples of such research and practice include forced sterilization programs, the Tuskegee syphilis study (1932–72), and the creation of the first immortalized stem cell line—such cells can reproduce indefinitely and, thus, are highly valued for medical research—from tissue samples taken from a 31-year-old Henrietta Lacks without her knowledge and without her consent.

At present, there are a variety of laws in place that aim to prevent discrimination and to promote fair and equitable practices in health-care settings. Examples include the Fourteenth Amendment (specifically the equal protection clause), the Civil Rights Act of 1964, the Americans with Disabilities Act (1990), and the Patient Protection and Affordable Care Act (ACA) of 2010. The importance of inclusive, equitable health-care practice is also emphasized in the professional oaths taken by many health-care professionals. This is clear, for example, in the Hippocratic Oath. However, the history of scientific racism continues to influence the attitudes that Black populations have toward the US health-care system. Some have a reasonable amount of trust in health-care researchers and practitioners, yet many remain suspicious of those in the health-care field and cite the historical events described above as central considerations in their suspicions. In addition, nearly two-thirds believe that research misconduct targeting Black populations is as likely now as in previous decades. Only one-third of Black populations believe that there are adequate measures currently in place to prevent discriminatory misconduct in health-care settings or to enforce accountability for medical researchers and practitioners whose actions violate anti-discrimination laws. Black Americans who indicate a low degree of trust in the US health-care system are less likely to engage in health-seeking behaviors. They are less likely to engage in preventative screenings, obtain vaccines, follow medical advice for both acute and chronic conditions, make follow-up appointments, modify behaviors to help alleviate health conditions, fill prescriptions, and take medication as indicated.

Biases in the Health-Care System

Nearly three-fourths of Black populations believe that racial bias remains a significant problem within the US health-care system and indicate that they continue to be treated in unfair and discriminatory ways within that system. This is due to a combination of both explicit and implicit bias among providers as well as structural inequities. Explicit bias is overt discrimination. It is evident in the racial slurs and the demeaning, dehumanizing comments that some providers use when interacting with patients or the assumptions and judgments they sometimes make about patients. For example, research indicates that in emergency rooms, some providers assume that Black patients are drug-seeking. Data also indicates that in the realm of sexual and reproductive health, some providers promote birth-control methods—including long-acting reversible contraceptives (LARCs) as well as permanent sterilization—in an aggressive manner that reflects eugenics ideology and in ways that violate fundamental reproductive rights. Explicit bias is also evident in the fact that some providers refuse to treat Black patients, purposefully provide inferior care to such patients, or knowingly violate medical safety standards and patient rights (e.g., informed consent and confidentiality) when providing care to Black patients. Twenty percent of Black adults who sought medical care in the past year indicate they were overtly discriminated against while doing so.

However, implicit bias also contributes to the substandard treatment that Black populations encounter in health-care settings. This bias stems from negative beliefs and stereotypes that providers have internalized about Black populations. Although providers are not consciously aware of such bias, research demonstrates that implicit bias continues to diminish the quality of care provided to Black patients. For example, research demonstrates that many health-care providers regard Black patients as less intelligent, less cooperative during medical exams and other procedures, and less likely to comply with treatment plans. They also tend to believe that Black patients have a higher tolerance for pain and, therefore, are less likely to provide adequate pain relief to them for injuries or other maladies. Implicit bias has also been linked to disparities in emergency health care. For example, Black populations—including both children and adults—experience longer-than-average wait times when seeking emergency care. Additionally, emergency room physicians are less likely to regard the health-related concerns of Black patients as genuine emergencies, less likely to admit them to the hospital for a medical emergency, and tend to order fewer diagnostic tests (e.g., blood tests, X-rays, urine analysis, electrocardiogram, and computed tomography (CT) scan) as part of the care they provide to such patients. Yet the disparate treatment of Black patients extends beyond the ER and has been documented in all fields of medicine; such treatment stems from both structural components of the health-care systems (e.g., continued closure of hospitals in predominantly Black communities, increasing restrictions of Medicaid in some states, and limited access to culturally competent health care) as well as the behaviors of individual providers. For example, while Black populations have disproportionately high rates of memory loss disorders, they are less likely to receive appropriate medical care related to diagnosis, medical treatment (such as cholinesterase inhibitors to help alleviate behavioral and cognitive symptoms and slow disease progression), and specialty care (e.g., neurology, geriatrics, occupational therapy, and palliative care) for such disorders. Additionally, patterns of racial segregation and disparate treatment have been identified in neonatal intensive care units (NICUs) across the country. Black infants tend to be cared for in lower quality NICUs and to receive both lower-quality care and less timely care. In the realm of sexual and reproductive health, Black populations tend to have worse access to STI screenings and to prenatal care. Among Black cisgender women seeking reproductive and sexual health care, common complaints include providers' giving them inaccurate information (e.g., about risks associated with certain types of contraception), denying their right to informed consent, and having their health complaints and questions about the care provided to them dismissed by health-care professionals. Black LGBTQIA populations are often refused medical treatment; they are also frequently verbally and/or physically abused by health-care providers. Similar patterns of disparate access to care and discriminatory treatment by providers have been identified in preventative care (e.g., access to regular health screenings), use of complementary and alternative medicine (e.g., herbs, prayer, and folk remedies), geriatric care, and palliative care.

Both structural racism and the biases that inform both the beliefs and behaviors of health-care professionals have a significant impact on the health of Black populations. They diminish both access to health care and the quality of care. Such factors are also associated with decreased effectiveness of communication between providers and patients, thereby decreasing safety and increasing risk of misdiagnosis. Additionally, structural racism and provider biases have been identified as key factors in the mistrust that many Black populations continue to harbor toward health-care providers and the US health-care system overall. Those who believe their health-care providers treat them in unfair and discriminatory ways are less likely to engage in future health-seeking behaviors for themselves as well as their family members. Furthermore, Black patients who encounter racial bias within the health-care system often share their experiences with their friends and other members of their communities; thus, bias experienced by a single individual can contribute to mistrust of health-care providers within Black communities more broadly. Medical mistrust, for example, contributed to vaccine hesitancy among Black populations in relation to the COVID-19 vaccine. Additionally, those who experience discriminatory care are less likely to follow through with treatment plans including taking prescribed medication, modifying diet or exercise habits, and attending follow-up appointments. Thus, due to their influence on health-seeking behaviors, trust of health-care professionals, and adherence to treatment plans, structural racism and racial biases have been identified as key factors in the disproportionately high rates of morbidity and mortality rates that persist among Black populations.

However, structural racism and biases also influence the US health-care system in other ways. Black populations remain underrepresented among health-care professionals; such disparities are greatest in higher-paying positions that involve graduate and professional degrees. Within medical schools, and although their numbers have increased since 1990, less than 4 percent of full-time faculty currently identify as Black or African American; the majority are appointed at the rank of assistant professor and, therefore, have not yet been granted tenure. Such professors tend to be concentrated in clinical specialties such as family medicine, obstetrics, and gynecology; their numbers are significantly lower in areas such as neurology, otolaryngology, clinical pathology, radiology, orthopedic surgery, and ophthalmology. Similarly, Black populations comprise only one in twenty physicians who are currently licensed and actively practicing in the United States.

Although their representation is higher among hospital administrators—approximately one in eight administrators identifies as Black or African American—they tend to be paid less than APIDA, HLC, and non-HLC white administrators. Among nurses, and even though they are more likely to have a graduate nursing degree than their non-HLC white counterparts, Black populations represent only 11 percent of licensed nurses; they tend to earn lower wages and are underrepresented in nursing specialties including as nurse midwives, nurse anesthetists, and nursing administrators. However, they currently represent one-third of all home health aides, the majority of whom are cisgender women. The wages associated with such employment fall far below average median income for full-time workers in the United States. Microaggressions and other expressions of bias they encounter in clinical settings also shape the experiences of Black health-care providers. Such bias has been documented in hiring, review and promotion practices, interactions with co-workers, and the relative support and inclusion they experience within the health-care workplace. In addition, they often encounter disparaging statements and even acts of physical aggression from patients. Discriminatory treatment by supervisors, co-workers, and patients has also been linked to lower rates of job satisfaction as well as disproportionately high rates of work-related stress, absenteeism, and workforce turnover among Black health-care workers.

Access to Health Care

Black populations continue to experience barriers to health care, including economic and geographic barriers. Despite the expansion of health insurance programs under the ACA, disparities in coverage remain. Although rates of insurance coverage for nonelderly adult Black populations have increased since passage of the ACA, they remain about 30 percent more likely to lack health insurance coverage than their non-HLC white peers; the racial gap in coverage is most pronounced in states that have not expanded Medicaid coverage. In addition, given factors such as disproportionately low average household income and wealth, the racial wage gap, high debt-to-income ratio, and higher-than-average rates of poverty, food insecurity, and housing insecurity among Black populations, they are more likely to find health care unaffordable. At present, approximately one in six nonelderly Black adults go without medical care due to lack of affordability. Given their economic vulnerability, the elderly, those with chronic health conditions and/or disabilities, and single-mother-headed households are among those Black populations most likely to have difficulty paying for medical care or to go without care due to the cost of such care.

Geographic barriers to care are also a problem for many Black populations. For example, over two hundred hospitals in the United States have closed since 2000; although rural areas have been disproportionately impacted by such closures, some urban communities—including predominantly Black neighborhoods in Chicago, Atlanta, and Philadelphia—have also experienced the loss of such facilities. Yet regardless of whether they live in rural or urban areas, Black populations are among those groups most affected by such closures and, as a result, encounter additional geographic barriers that limit their access to care. Predominantly Black communities tend to have fewer hospitals, clinics, pharmacies, drugstores, and private health practices than areas with a lower concentration of Black people. While some communities offer free health clinics, these offer only a limited range of services and typically cannot facilitate access to secondary- or tertiary-level diagnostic and treatment options. Furthermore, free pop-up clinics and mobile clinics have been used with some degree of success in Black communities. Such clinics are typically situated in a park, shopping center, religious facility, school, or community center. Some of the most common types of care provided via such clinics include immunizations, basic health screenings, basic eye care and dental care, mammograms, and family planning services. However, such clinics tend to operate on a small scale and, therefore, can serve only a limited number of patients. Furthermore, the rather public nature of such clinics may discourage individuals from seeking care at such locations.

In addition, the limited availability of culturally competent care continues to diminish access to health care and the quality of care provided to Black populations. Many health-care providers are simply not aware of the discriminatory experiences that Black patients encounter and their resulting mistrust of health-care providers. Consequently, such providers may not take appropriate time to develop the type of rapport necessary to earn the trust of their Black patients and to facilitate open, effective communication with such patients. Furthermore, many providers are not aware of the various folk remedies (e.g., use of plant, animal, and mineral substances) that Black populations have passed down for generations and that they may continue to use in conjunction with more contemporary biomedical treatments. While many believe that folk remedies are exclusive to Black immigrant communities, the reality is that such remedies are frequently used among Black populations who have been in the United States for generations. Health-care professionals may not fully understand the religious, cultural, or personal reasons why Black patients rely on such remedies and, thus, are not able to effectively incorporate them into treatment plans. In other cases, providers may outright dismiss such remedies as unimportant or ineffective. This may offend the cultural beliefs and values of their patients; such dismissal is also associated with an increase in mistrust of health-care providers and decrease in health-seeking behaviors among Black populations.

Access to educationally and linguistically competent care continues to diminish the care provided to Black populations. Rates of low literacy among US-born Black populations are higher than national averages. Those with low literacy are also at increased risk for low health literacy and, therefore, may struggle to understand medical intake forms, written treatment plans, health insurance statements, and other written communication pertaining to their care. In addition, although rates of English literacy are relatively high among Black immigrant populations, roughly one in ten communicates primarily in a language other than English. Those who speak French, Spanish, and French/Haitian Creole may have an easier time finding a provider who can provide care in their native language. However, those who primarily speak Bantu languages (e.g., Swahili, Zulu, Xhosa, and Kirundi), Cushitic languages (e.g., Kwara, Bilin, Burunge, Beja, and Gorowa), Amharic, Somali, or other less common languages (including many of the more than five hundred languages spoken in Nigeria) typically have a much more difficult time accessing linguistically appropriate health care. While telehealth language lines can help to bridge gaps and promote access to linguistically appropriate care, the use of such options can diminish both efficiency and effectiveness of communication in health-care settings.

LIVING ENVIRONMENT AND SOCIAL CONTEXT

Historically, Black populations were segregated under US law. Despite changes to such laws, social norms contribute to ongoing discrimination and disparate treatment of Black populations. This is clear in the persistence of segregated housing as well as the fact that Black communities tend to have poorer-quality housing with less access to healthy food options, social services, and recreational areas. Such communities are often the target of over-policing, something that contributes to disproportionately high rates of surveillance, arrest, conviction, and incarceration among Black people. Yet the bias that contributes to segregation is also evident in social attitudes toward such populations, including in the various stereotypes that are evident in media and popular culture. Such stereotypes have been linked to the ongoing social marginalization and various forms of violence against Black people.

Persistent Segregation and Its Consequences

In the final months of the US Civil War, the US Congress passed the Thirteenth Amendment to the Constitution, effectively outlawing slavery. While this did expand rights for Black populations, this historic change was met with backlash from policymakers and voters who sought to limit the social inclusion of newly freed Black populations in American society. In the months immediately following the passage of the Thirteenth Amendment, for example, southern states such as South Carolina and Mississippi implemented what were known as Black Codes that attempted to preserve white supremacy and control. They did this by restricting the economic, social, and political activities of Black populations and promoting segregation. For example, such codes forbid marriage between Black and white populations. They also prohibited Black populations from owning certain types of property or operating certain types of businesses, testifying in court against a white defendant, being taught to read or write, and living in certain areas or parishes. Following the ratification of the Reconstruction Act of 1867 as well as the Fourteenth and Fifteenth Amendments, the racism and resulting segregation that had formed the core of the institution of slavery and the Black Codes did not disappear. On the contrary, they remained entrenched in American society via what became known as Jim Crow laws. Such laws were established as early as 1877 and sought to maintain the oppression of Black populations by restricting them to segregated schools, restaurants, theaters, churches, hospitals, parks, and neighborhoods. The US Supreme Court decision in *Plessy v. Ferguson (1896)*, based on the concept of separate but equal, established that such laws did not violate the Fourteenth Amendment and, consequently, provided a legal precedent that permitted the expansion of the Jim Crow system. Yet the marginalization of Black populations was also reinforced socially. This is evident in the activities of the Ku Klux Klan (KKK). Founded by a group of former Confederate soldiers at the end of the Civil War and with the aim of thwarting Reconstruction efforts, the organization relied on tactics such as threats, beatings, rape, murder, and public lynchings to intimidate and terrorize Black populations and non-Black groups who spoke out against segregation or otherwise acted in ways that promoted racial equity and integration.

Throughout the twentieth century, segregation defined American neighborhoods. Although the Federal Housing Administration (FHA) was established in 1934 to promote housing standards and to improve access to affordable housing, the FHA regularly denied mortgage insurance on loans for housing located in or near neighborhoods inhabited primarily by Black populations. This practice, known as redlining, remained part of formal FHA policies for several decades. In the early half of the twentieth century, the FHA also supported the creation of suburban communities, specifically as a means of expanding housing for working-class families and military veterans. However, many of home builders subsidized by the FHA—including Levitt & Sons, creators of the single-family, mass-produced homes that formed the suburban communities that were commonly referred to as Levittowns—explicitly limited sale of the homes they created to white populations. The US Supreme Court decision in *Shelley v. Kraemer (1948)* asserted that restricting home ownership based on race violated the equal protection clause of the Fourteenth Amendment. Additionally, the decision in *Brown v. Board of Education (1954)* overturned the separate but equal precedent that had been established by the *Plessy* decision. Despite these legal changes, however, discriminatory housing practices persisted. Within the Eisenhower administration, for example, various policies both permitted and, in fact, encouraged racially segregated housing. In 1968, passage of the Fair Housing Act (FHA) sought to rectify such segregation by expanding anti-discrimination laws in relation to housing purchases and rentals. The number of incidents of explicit discrimination in housing has decreased somewhat over the past 50 years and, thus, there has been a measurable decline in residential segregation since passage of the FHA. Yet such segregation has not been eliminated. On the contrary, due to the combined influences of economic inequities, increasing urbanization, and gentrification, residential and housing segregation remains the norm rather than the exception. This is true in urban, suburban, and rural communities.

It is estimated that seven out of ten Black people live in communities that are racially and ethnically segregated. Additionally, and regardless of average household income, they are overrepresented among those residing in low-income communities. Such factors diminish their access to a variety of resources. For example, food deserts have been identified as a significant concern. At least 20 percent of all Black populations reside in areas where their access to grocery stores, farmer's markets, and non-fast-food restaurants that provide access to affordable, fresh food options is restricted. Additionally, such communities are often food swamps that are characterized by an abundance of fast-food restaurants and convenience stores. Food swamps typically provide options that are more affordable. However, foods available in such areas tend to be highly processed and calorie dense; they also typically contain high levels of fat, cholesterol, and sodium but relatively low levels of vitamins and minerals. Food deserts and food swamps are associated with impaired nutritional well-being as well as a variety of chronic conditions, including high blood pressure, metabolic syndrome, diabetes, and cardiovascular disease. Additionally, those who reside in predominantly Black communities tend to have access to fewer recreational and leisure facilities (e.g., parks, sports fields, green spaces, community gardens, playgrounds, and swimming pools). Limited access to such options has been linked to impaired physical health as well as increased rates of certain mental health conditions (e.g., depression, certain mood disorders, and anxiety). Such communities also tend to have fewer options for social services, religious centers, schools, shopping, libraries, and emergency services. Environmental factors also impair the health of Black communities. Air pollution, contaminated water, and toxic waste are common concerns. Similarly, many

Black neighborhoods consist of older homes that were created with poor-quality building materials, thereby increasing risk of exposure to a variety of harmful substances, including mold, asbestos, lead, and carcinogens. Health risks associated with such exposure include respiratory ailments, various types of cancer, damage to the nervous system, endocrine disorders, and fertility issues. Yet such issues can also contribute to stress, anxiety, depression, and other mental health challenges.

Structural racism in policing has been identified as a pressing public health issue due to its impact on both physical and mental health. Black populations continue to be disproportionately targeted for policing. For example, police conduct patrols and conduct traffic stops, property searches, bodily searches, social media monitoring, and surveillance (e.g., facial recognition devices, video monitoring, and drones) more frequently in Black communities than in non-HLC white communities. Police brutality and excessive use of force are also more common in Black communities. Thus, officers are also more likely to harass, verbally abuse, commit acts of physical and/or sexual violence, and use excessive force (e.g., use of a taser, baton, pepper spray, teargas, or gun) when interacting with Black populations, including those who are unarmed. They are also more likely to use deadly force; consequently, Black populations are overrepresented among those killed by police officers. In recent years, and in response to police killings of unarmed individuals such as Breonna Taylor, George Floyd, Tamir Rice, Atatiana Jefferson, Botham Jean, Philando Castile, Michael Brown, and many others, police brutality has been identified as a reflection of structural racism and has prompted widespread protests and calls for reform of—and, in some cases, abolishing—law enforcement units across the country. However, such calls have been met with considerable resistance. The over-policing of Black populations also contributes to racial disparities in the criminal justice system. Black populations are overrepresented among those who are arrested, prosecuted, convicted, and incarcerated. They also tend to receive longer average sentences, regardless of the crime. Black populations are incarcerated in state prisons at six times the rate of non-HLC white populations. In some states, Black populations comprise over half of all incarcerated individuals. Nationally, Black populations represent nearly 40 percent of those in jails or prisons. They also represent half of those who are serving life sentences. Within jails and prisons, Black populations are subject to more frequent and harsher discipline (e.g., being placed in solitary confinement or having recreation time or visiting privileges revoked) and to be denied access to medical care. However, they are also subjected to disproportionately high rates of physical, psychological, and sexual abuse from correctional officers and from other inmates.

Social Attitudes, Stereotypes, and Their Consequences

Black populations overwhelmingly indicate that racism continues to impact their lives in significant ways and that there is inadequate attention to race relations and structural racism in the United States. However, non-HLC white populations are only about half as likely to identify racism as a societal problem; those who do regard it is as significant issue are more likely to believe that anti-Black racism is a result of individual actions rather than systemic inequities. Perspectives on racism and its impact on Black populations also vary by political affiliation: while nearly 80 percent of non-HLC white Democratic voters believe there is more work to be done to achieve racial equity in contemporary America, three-fifths of Republican voters and 40 percent of Independent voters believe that racism and its impact on Black populations receive too much attention. However, it is clear that voters who are part of Generation Z (born between 1995 and 2012) tend to be more aware of structural racism and its impacts than previous generations; they are also more likely than those who are part of the Millennial generation (born between 1980 and 1994) and earlier generations to identify racial equity as an important social issue and to volunteer for, donate to, or otherwise take action to support organizations (e.g., Black Lives Matter, Movement for Black Lives, Southern Poverty Law Center, and National Fair Housing Alliance) that promote the rights of Black populations. Despite this, racial bias and anti-Black sentiment persist. For example, although the US Supreme Court decision in *Loving v. Virginia (1967)* found the anti-miscegenation laws that had been part of the Jim Crow era and existed well into the mid-twentieth century were unconstitutional, one-fifth of Americans continue to oppose interracial marriage. Additionally, students and parents tend to provide lower ratings for Black teachers; employees tend to provide lower ratings for Black supervisors and Black employees tend to receive lower job performance ratings. Research suggests that anti-Black bias is learned at a young age; by the time they enter preschool, children are less likely to engage socially and to share toys with their Black peers than with non-HLC white peers. Racial segregation also continues to dominate social settings—the majority of non-HLC white Americans do not have any close friends who are Black and do not frequent social settings where they interact with Black populations. In recent years, racial resentment among non-HLC white, APIDA, and HLC populations has also contributed to increasing opposition to Black-centered social and political movements.

Additionally, recent research demonstrates that nearly half of Americans have internalized stereotypes that demean, dehumanize, or otherwise disparage Black populations. Such stereotypes are sometimes passed down within family networks. Other times, they are learned from peers. However, due to both their accessibility and their pervasiveness in US society, media and popular culture are also key contributors to the perpetuation and dissemination of stereotypes of Black people. Some of the most common among such stereotypes include those that depict Black people as inherently dangerous, unintelligent, uncultured, irresponsible, lazy, and hypersexual. In the late nineteenth and early twentieth centuries, for example, short stories, films, novels, cartoons, postcards, minstrel shows, songs, and other sources depicted Black people as inherently dangerous, simple-minded, uncivilized, irresponsible, lazy, and hypersexual. Additionally, incorporation of simian-like imagery (e.g., elongated fingers, toes, arms and legs; enlarged eyes and lips; a protruding forehead and jawline) was used to portray Black people as subhuman. Yet such stereotypes are not simply a thing of the past; on the contrary, they persisted throughout the twentieth century and are a feature of contemporary US society. For example, from the 1970s onward, explicitly racist statements and imagery have been central to the War on Drugs and have contributed to the targeting of Black populations for increasing surveillance, arrest, prosecution, and incarceration. In the 1990s, stereotypes of Black people as lazy, hypersexual, and scheming—this was epitomized in the caricature of the so-called welfare queen—became a central part of the discourse that propelled welfare reform and state-level welfare experiments, including child exclusion and mandatory birth-control components. Similarly, political cartoons that represented Barack Obama as primate-like appeared during Obama's campaign for the presidency as well as during his two terms in office. Other contemporary stereotypes include Black people as sexually promiscuous, the angry Black woman, the Black man as criminal, and the uncultured Black immigrant. Black LGBTQIA populations remain underrepresented marginalized in media and popular culture; when they are depicted, it is often via stereotypes that focus on drug addiction, sex work, HIV/AIDS, mental illness, or an eccentric lifestyle.

The consequences of such stereotypes are significant. They contribute to internalized racism, diminished mental health, decreased self-confidence, and feelings of exclusion among Black populations. In addition, stereotypes continue to inform and influence the treatment of Black populations in the workplace, health-care settings, educational institutions as well as in stores, restaurants, leisure facilities, and other social settings. Racist stereotypes also continue to pose a threat to the safety and well-being of Black populations and have been identified as a key factor in various types of violence against them. For example, research demonstrates that such stereotypes and related confirmation bias continue to inform and effect police responses to Black suspects and contribute to increased likelihood of shootings and other forms of police brutality against such suspects. The racism perpetuated by stereotypes has also been linked to other forms of violence against Black populations, including the lethal aggression—sometimes referred to as vigilante violence or modern-day lynching—perpetuated by citizens. Recent examples of such aggression include attacks on Black cisgender young men, including Trayvon Martin in 2012, Ahmaud Arbery in 2020, and Ralph Yarl in 2023. So-called stand-your-ground (SYG) laws, which have legalized the use of lethal force as an act of self-defense if an individual believes their life is in danger, have increased homicide rates overall in the United States. Evidence also indicates such laws encourage lethal aggression. Such laws are not racially neutral. When a non-HLC white individual invokes SYG as a defense for the killing of a Black individual, they are five times more likely to be acquitted of any wrongdoing than when the roles are reversed. Stereotypical depictions such as the Mammy, Jezebel, and Sapphire have been identified as significant factors in the disproportionately high rates of police violence, sexual violence, and intimate partner violence perpetuated against Black cisgender women and girls. Dehumanizing and sexually objectifying stereotypes formed at the intersections of race, gender identity, and sexual identity have also been linked to fatal violence against Black LBGTQIA individuals.

CHAPTER THREE

Disabled Populations

Those who experience physical, cognitive, emotional, and/or sensory characteristics that substantially limit one or more major life activities (e.g., eating, movement, breathing, speaking, and working) are collectively referred to as people with disabilities (PWD). The medical model of disability relies on scientific definitions and corresponding medical diagnoses to define disabilities; consequently, this model defines disabilities as stemming from individual limitations and deficiencies. In contrast, the sociopolitical model asserts that disabilities are both socially constructed and highly politicized. This model asserts that disabilities are not inherent in individuals, per se, but are instead a consequence of various social factors, including the way that society is organized, dominant attitudes toward atypical abilities, and the political framing of disabilities. Over 60 million PWD reside in the United States. Twenty-five percent of adults of working age experience some type of disability; one in ten children under the age of 18 experiences a disability. Rates are lowest among infants and young children, somewhat higher among adolescents, and then increase incrementally throughout adulthood. Rates are highest among those aged 65 and older, with approximately one-third of elderly populations experiencing a disability. Regardless of age, PWD are at increased risk for various types of morbidities and for premature death. Despite the parameters of the Americans with Disabilities Act (ADA) of 1990 and other anti-discrimination legislation, PWD remain marginalized and excluded in American society.

This chapter focuses on the health and well-being of PWD in the United States. It begins with the explanation of various types of disabilities and then explores social determinants of health to illustrate how such factors influence the experiences of PWD. However, and in recognition of social change efforts, it also highlights measures that have promoted civil rights, inclusion, and health for PWD. Historically, a variety of terms were used that perpetuated the notion that PWD are flawed, deficient, and inferior; they also tended to focus on the disability rather than the individual. Examples of terms that were used at various points during the nineteenth and twentieth centuries include disabled, handicapped, intellectually deficient, differently abled, crazy, lunatic, invalid, deformed, special, nonverbal, leper, hearing impaired, lame, and feeble-minded. However, in recent decades and due to increasing awareness of the ways in which such terms reinforce ableism, discrimination, biases, and stereotypes, such terms have largely been abandoned in the context of medical care, academic inquiry, politics, and social services. Thus, in accordance with contemporary standards of inclusion and anti-discrimination such as those endorsed by the United Nations, this chapter uses person-first language. Descriptions such as person with a disability, people with disabilities, person who is blind, and people with visual impairments are used throughout.

CURRENT STATE OF HEALTH

There are many different types of disabilities. Some are short term with a duration of only a few weeks or months and others last for years. Still others are intermittent—they may be more significant at certain times but less so at other times. In some cases, individuals experience disabilities throughout their lifespan. Some disabilities are easily detected by others—typically due to reliance on assistive devices, specific forms of communication, or atypical structure and/or function of major body parts—and are often referred to as visible disabilities or apparent disabilities. Examples of visible disabilities include mobility impairments that result in use of a cane, walker, wheelchair, or other assistive device; hearing loss or deafness that necessitates reliance on visual-manual modes of communication (e.g., American sign language); or significant vision loss or blindness that results in use of the tactile system of reading and writing known as braille. However, over 90 percent of disabilities are not easily detected by others in typical social situations; these are known as non-visible or hidden disabilities. Examples include advanced forms of certain chronic health conditions (e.g., diabetes, cancer, chronic obstructive pulmonary disease (COPD), and Crohn's disease), learning disabilities, sensory processing disorders, certain psychiatric disabilities (e.g., post-traumatic stress disorder (PTSD), bipolar disorder, depression, anxiety, schizophrenia, and eating disorders), and some infectious diseases (e.g., Lyme disease, HIV/AIDS, and tuberculosis). Disabilities affect individuals in a variety of ways; therefore, two individuals with the same disability may experience that disability in radically different ways depending on a variety of social and economic factors. Disabilities are typically grouped into the following categories: physical disabilities, cognitive disabilities, and psychological disabilities. Yet some span multiple categories.

Physical disabilities relate to the physical function of various parts of the human body. They are typically organized into sensory, mobility, and brain/neurological disorders. Sensory disabilities are among the most common types of physical disabilities. They involve reduced function or loss of hearing, vision, smell, taste, or touch/sensation; however, some individuals are born without functioning sensory organs (e.g., without the optic nerve needed for vision). Sensory disabilities sometimes occur because of certain health conditions, diseases, or injury; for example, shingles, measles, and hypertension can contribute to reduced auditory function or loss of hearing; diabetes, traumatic head injuries, myasthenia gravis (an autoimmune disorder), and Lyme disease can reduce vision. Other times, sensory disabilities stem from dietary deficiencies or from medical treatments. Chronic vitamin B12 deficiency may lead to vision loss, while chemotherapy treatments may result in long-term reduction in and sometimes permanent loss of olfactory (smell) and gustatory (taste) function. Approximately 8 million individuals in the United States currently experience complete vision loss (often referred to as blindness) or partial loss of visual acuity that cannot be rectified via surgery, medication, or eyeglasses/contact lenses. Rates of vision-related disabilities are three times higher among those over age 65. Auditory disabilities related to partial or complete loss of hearing affect nearly 40 million Americans aged 12 and older. Approximately one in six adults over age 18 requires an auditory assistive device; four out of every 1,000 children in the United States are born with a hearing-related disability. Hearing loss and deafness are most common, however, among elderly populations: one-fourth of those aged 65–74 and half of those over the age of 74 have profound or complete hearing loss. Disabilities related to smell, touch, and taste are less common; however, it is estimated that more than 50 million Americans experience partial or full loss of such senses.

A second major category of physical disabilities are those that affect an individual's mobility of and/or ability to control parts of their body, especially arms, fingers, hands, legs, feet, toes, pelvic muscles, and vertebral column. Such disabilities most often stem from anomalies of or injuries to skeletal, muscular, and/or neurological systems; they are associated with difficulty engaging such activities as walking, standing, climbing stairs, driving, writing, typing, and conducting activities of daily living (e.g., cooking, maintaining hygiene, feeding oneself, taking medication, and using the toilet). Some stem from trauma. Among military personnel, for example, injuries sustained during combat may necessitate partial or complete amputation of one or more limbs. Injuries and health problems sustained in work settings, vehicle accidents, and sports activities (e.g., burns, exposure to toxins, repetitive stress injuries, broken bones, neck and back injuries, and concussions) may also result in short- or long-term movement-related disabilities. Traumatic brain injuries (TBI) sustained due to falls, assault, transportation accidents (including drivers, passengers, and pedestrians), and firearms are another common cause of mobility impairments and can impair balance and coordination. At least 1.5 million in the United States sustain a TBI each year; rates are highest among adolescents and elderly populations. Another common trauma-related cause of changes in mobility is spinal cord injuries (SCI). An SCI that occurs low on the spinal cord may result in paraplegia; an individual with paraplegia typically cannot independently and voluntarily move their legs or control their pelvic organs. In contrast, an SCI that occurs high on the spinal cord is associated with quadriplegia (sometimes referred to as tetraplegia); it causes paralysis from the neck down. An individual with quadriplegia does not have the ability to independently move their legs, arms, or trunk of the body and needs mechanical support to breathe. With intensive rehabilitation and due to the relative plasticity of the nervous system, some individuals with SCI can regain some degree of muscle function and limb movement. Most, however, do not.

While many mobility impairments are a consequence of trauma, others stem from inherited conditions, exposure to teratogens, infections, or diseases. Hereditary movement disorders are inherited and typically associated with muscle spasticity, tremors, stiffness of joints, difficulties with coordination, and loss of balance. Examples of such disorders include Huntington's disease (which causes progressive degeneration of nerve cells) and Wilson's disease (a disorder that results in difficulties with walking and coordination). Congenital anomalies—sometimes referred to as birth defects—are irregularities in structure or function of the body that occur during embryonic or fetal development; while they are sometimes detected during a fetal ultrasound or at time of birth, other times they are not identified for years. Spina bifida, a neural tube defect characterized by incomplete development and closure of the spinal column, is one type of congenital anomaly. It has been linked to inadequate dietary intake of folic acid during pregnancy. Individuals with spina bifida may experience partial or complete paralysis of legs and muscles of the pelvis; thus, they may be unable to control urination and excretion as well as the muscles of the legs and feet. Although spina bifida rates have declined dramatically since the 1980s—due, in large part, to sustained public health campaigns that promote folic acid intake among individuals who are able to become pregnant—nearly 1,500 infants with spina bifida are born in the United States each year. Some congenital anomalies result from exposure to certain types of medication. For example, during the 1950s and 1960s, the drug thalidomide was used to treat hyperemesis gravidarum (more commonly known as morning sickness) in pregnant individuals. The drug was later found to have a teratogenic effect; consequently, children who were exposed to thalidomide in utero were often born with shortened arms and legs or missing fingers, toes, hands, or feet. In some cases, their limbs and digits were missing altogether. Approximately one-tenth of birth defects are a consequence of exposure to medication in utero. Yet congenital anomalies may also result from exposure to toxic substances in home or work environments, typically via air pollution, water pollution, or building materials. Examples of such substances include chlorinated solvents, dioxins, pesticides, polychlorinated biphenyls (PCBs), per- and polyfluoroalkyl substances (PFAS). Still other congenital anomalies that impair movement have been linked to infectious diseases. Exposure to the varicella virus (which causes chickenpox) in utero can result in arrested development of limbs and digits in the fetus, thereby increasing risk of mobility impairments.

Certain types of chronic health conditions and infectious diseases can also impede movement and physical function. Rheumatic diseases involve the autoimmune system and create an inflammatory response; they typically affect the joints, tendons, and ligaments but can also affect muscle, bone tissue, and impair function of internal organs and connective tissue. Such diseases cause inflammation and pain, most commonly in the joints of the hands, feet, knees, shoulders, and fingers; therefore, such diseases can make it difficult to conduct even basic tasks such as buttoning clothing, writing, and attending to personal hygiene. It is estimated that over 50 million Americans have a diagnosed rheumatic disease; examples include gout, bursitis, rheumatoid arthritis, scleroderma, osteoarthritis, systemic lupus erythematosus, polymyalgia rheumatica, and ankylosing spondylitis. Although these are most common among adults, they sometimes occur in children. Other chronic health conditions that can increase risk and severity of physical limitations include COPD, asthma, diabetes, obesity, heart disease, and cancer. The risk of functional decline and physical disability is greater among those who have two or more chronic health conditions. Chronic pain that is not controlled with medication, physical therapy, behavioral modification, or other treatments is another contributor to physical disabilities. However, while chronic pain in and of itself can be disabling, the US government typically requires that an underlying health condition that causes such pain is diagnosed for individuals with chronic pain to be eligible for disability benefits. Some infectious diseases are also associated with increased risk and severity of disability, particularly as they may hinder some physical activities and damage the structure and/or function of internal organs or body systems. For example, some respiratory diseases—including COVID-19, Middle East Respiratory Syndrome (MERS), tuberculosis, severe acute respiratory syndrome (SARS), measles, pertussis (whooping cough), and pneumococcal meningitis—can contribute to chronic breathing difficulties.

Certain sexually transmitted infections (STIs) (e.g., HIV/AIDS, syphilis, and gonorrhea) can impede movement and physical function. There are more than 20 million new cases of STIs each year in the United States. Nearly 70 million Americans have one or more active STIs. Some disabilities that stem from STIs include neurological issues, suppressed immune system function, and blockages of the reproductive tract. STIs have been linked to one in four cases of infertility.

The third subgroup of physical disabilities is those that stem from brain abnormalities and neurological disorders, particularly those that cause death of or atypical function of cells in the nervous system. Given the role of the nervous system in stimulating both voluntary and involuntary movements, related disabilities often result in problems with coordination and balance, muscle weakness, difficulties of the digestive system (e.g., swallowing and defecating), loss of physical sensation, pain, seizures, spasms and shaking, and paralysis. An individual may be born with such conditions; this is the case with what are commonly referred to as neural tube defects, including anencephaly (in which part of the skull and/or brain is underdeveloped or absent). Yet some brain/neurological conditions are not identified until the first few years of life. This is the case with cerebral palsy (CP), a condition that stems from abnormal brain development. It is the most common type of motor disability among those born in the United States, affecting three in 1,000 children. CP cannot be cured; those with severe CP have a dramatically shorter life expectancy than national averages. In contrast, microcephaly—a condition characterized by abnormally small head and skull size due to underdevelopment of the brain—is often detected prior to birth during a fetal ultrasound. Yet disabilities that stem from brain/neurological disorders may develop at any time. For example, while epilepsy—characterized by seizures that are a consequence of atypical electrical activity in the brain—is most often diagnosed in childhood (from birth to age 20), it is also common among those over age 60. Similarly, both encephalitis (abnormal swelling of the brain) and hydrocephalus (abnormal buildup of fluid in the brain) can occur at any point during the lifespan. Other examples of brain/neurological conditions that impact movement include muscular dystrophy, amyotrophic lateral sclerosis (ALS), cerebral aneurysm, multiple sclerosis, stroke, encephalitis, brain tumors, and meningitis. Additionally, the group of nervous system disorders that are commonly referred to as movement disorders affects physical activity and mobility. Examples include ataxia, dystonia, multiple system atrophy, myoclonus, Parkinson's disease, Huntington's disease, essential tremor, and Tourette syndrome.

A second broad category of disabilities relates to cognition. Such disabilities impede learning, information processing, and the ability to make decisions. They are sometimes referred to as intellectual disabilities and affect at least one-fifth of the US population. Cognitive disabilities may occur because of an injury, congenital anomaly, infection, or degenerative conditions that affect the brain and/or spinal column; examples include TBI, spina bifida, Alzheimer's disease, and meningitis. However, cognitive disabilities often stem from atypical neurological development or atypical function of aspects of the nervous system. For example, schizophrenia—characterized by delusions, hallucinations, and disorganized thinking—is caused by issues with neurotransmitters and dopamine function. Learning disabilities are some of the most common types of cognitive disabilities and impair an individual's ability to perceive, process, and otherwise understand information. While they may manifest during adulthood—particularly after a TBI or infection that affects the brain—most learning disabilities are present during childhood. Rates of diagnosis are disproportionately high among cisgender male and low-income populations as well as and

Black, Indigenous, and People of Color (BIPOC) subgroups. Learning disabilities may be linked to in utero exposure to teratogens, hereditary factors, specific health conditions, malnutrition, and/or environmental factors (e.g., exposure to lead or mercury). Some of the most common types of learning disabilities diagnosed during childhood include dyslexia (difficulty reading printed text), dyscalculia (difficulty understanding numerical information), and dysgraphia (difficulty transmitting thoughts into graphic forms, including via writing or drawing). It is estimated that one-fifth of all Americans have dyslexia, dyscalculia, and/or dysgraphia, although many remain undiagnosed. Other common types of learning disorders involve difficulty interpreting sounds (known as auditory processing disorder) and difficulty interpreting spoken words (language processing disorder). In addition, nonverbal learning disabilities (NVLD) refers to diminished awareness of and ability to interpret nonverbal cues such as facial expressions, tone of voice, body language, and other nonverbal aspects of communication and social cues. Individuals experiencing NLVD often have difficulty with coordination due to issues with motor and spatial-visual skills. Another subcategory of learning-related disabilities, visual perceptual and visual motor disorders (VPVMD), stems from irregular eye movement. Such irregularities lead to challenges in perceiving, organizing, and processing visual information and can contribute to difficulties with attention (especially in class or meetings), understanding written texts, memorization, interpreting maps, and navigating physical spaces (e.g., home, school, and recreational settings).

Other common developmental disabilities that impact cognition include autism spectrum disorder (ASD), sensory processing disorder (SPD), and attention deficit/hyperactivity disorder (ADHD). In individuals with ASD, the areas of the brain responsible for social interaction, perceiving danger, processing sensations, social interaction, and communication—including the amygdala, the cerebral cortex, and the temporal lobe—are functionally different from individuals without ASD. In addition, and due to atypical function of neurons and glial cells, the synapses of the brain in individuals with ASD do not connect and transmit information efficiently or effectively. Thus, it is common for people with ASD to experience difficulties with communication and social interaction; repetitive behaviors such as rocking, hand flapping, and spinning are often present. Such individuals may easily become upset by changes in their environment or routine and may also become fixated on certain people or activities. Nearly 5.5 million adults and 1.5 million children have ASD; cisgender boys and men comprise nearly 80 percent of those with ASD. Although it is common for individuals with ASD to also experience SPD, they are not the same thing. The sensory organs of individuals with SPD function in a typical manner, but their brains process sensory stimuli in a manner that is associated with over- or under-sensitivity to sights, sounds, tastes, smells, and sensations. One, some, or all senses may be affected. Those with SPD often experience issues with coordination. While some may feel overwhelmed by sensory input (e.g., loud noises such as vacuums, airplanes, fireworks; physical stimulation such as being hugged, having their hair brushed, feeling of rough textured clothing), others exhibit a delayed response to stimuli. For example, those with diminished awareness of physical touch/sensation may take longer to respond to stimuli (e.g., extreme heat and sharp objects). Thus, physical injuries such as burns, bruising, and cuts are sometimes more common among those with SPD. It is estimated that 10–20 percent of Americans have some manifestation of SPD. Some also have ADHD—sometimes referred to as ADD—which is typically characterized by short attention span, restlessness, problems with time management, difficulty focusing on tasks, and/or impulsiveness. ADHD most directly affects learning but can also lead to mood irregularities. It is most often diagnosed in children and adolescents, affecting about 10 percent of all minors. Yet some are not diagnosed until adulthood.

Finally, psychological disabilities—sometimes referred to as psychosocial and psychiatric disabilities—are those that significantly impair mental health. Some of the most common among these include anxiety disorders, major depressive disorder (MDD), personality disorders, eating disorders, and behavioral/emotional disorders. Not all manifestations of mental health struggles are disabling. For example, an individual may experience some level of anxiety in certain situations, but it may not alter their mental well-being to the point that major life activities are impacted. For those with significant and pervasive mental health challenges, however, nearly every aspect of their life may be affected. Anxiety disorders involve atypically high levels of fear, worry, and tension; while they may arise in certain situations (e.g., public settings or large groups) or in response to specific stimuli (e.g., spiders and heights), this is not always the case. Common anxiety disorders include social anxiety, panic disorders, phobia disorders, post-traumatic stress disorder (PTSD), obsessive compulsive disorder (OCD), and generalized anxiety disorder (GAD). One-third of Americans will experience an anxiety disorder during their lifetime, yet only one in five with an anxiety disorder will experience it in a severe form. In contrast, MDD includes persistent sadness, hopelessness, and loss of interest in pleasurable activities. MDD is a major contributor to disabilities in the United States, affecting about 20 million people. Affected individuals often experience disruption in sleeping and eating patterns, impaired cognitive function, mood swings, irritability, and the desire to socially withdraw. MDD is also associated with increased risk of non-suicidal self-harming behaviors as well as suicidal ideation and suicide attempts.

A third group of psychological disabilities is personality disorders. These affect between 10 and 15 percent of the US population. Personality disorders can and do overlap to some degree with anxiety disorders and MDD, particularly as symptoms are sometimes similar. However, those with personality disorders experience significant disruptions in patterns of thinking that make it difficult for them to create and maintain healthy social relationships. Such disorders are typically organized into three subgroups. The first subgroup includes disorders that typically lead to erratic or highly unusual behaviors. These include paranoid, schizotypal, and schizoid personality disorders. Individuals with such disorders are often distrustful of others, avoid social interactions, and may express a limited range of emotions. The second subgroup of personality disorders is typified by intense or dramatic responses to relatively benign occurrences, inability to take responsibility for actions, emotional dysregulation, impulsivity, and/or erratic social behaviors. It includes antisocial, histrionic, narcissistic, and borderline personality disorders. The third subgroup is characterized by intense fear and anxiety and includes obsessive compulsive personality disorder (OCPD), avoidant personality disorder, and dependent personality disorder. OCPD should not be confused with OCD. Whereas individuals with OCD engage in repetitive behaviors at times when they feel especially anxious or stressed, individuals with OCPD try to maintain rigid control and strive for perfection in nearly all aspects of their lives, even on seemingly small tasks.

The final two types of psychological disabilities that will be discussed include eating disorders and behavioral disorders. Eating disorders manifest in unhealthy relationships with food and stem from serious psychological issues related to self-esteem, appearance, and body image, including weight, size, and shape. The most common types of eating disorders include anorexia nervosa, bulimia nervosa, binge eating disorder, and avoidant/restrictive food intake disorder. They are most common among cisgender-heterosexual (cishet) girls and women during adolescence and early adulthood, yet rates are also disproportionately high among lesbian, gay, bisexual, transgender, queer, intersex, and asexual (LGBTQIA) populations. Eating disorders also affect cishet boys and men. Such disorders have been documented throughout the lifespan. Eating disorders may lead to dramatic changes in body weight and to impaired function of immune, neurological, musculoskeletal, digestive, and cardiovascular systems. In some cases, they can lead to death. Ten percent of Americans will experience an eating disorder during their lifetime. Behavioral disorders are typified by actions that are extreme and aggressive, lack of empathy for others, and emotional outbursts. Examples of such disorders include oppositional defiant disorder (ODD) and conduct disorder (CD). They are most often diagnosed in school-aged children and can impair learning and socialization. Rates are disproportionately high among cisgender boys and men.

ECONOMIC FACTORS

Income, debt, and other economic factors bear considerably on the lives and well-being of PWD. They are overrepresented among low-income households and typically have higher-than-average medical expenses, even if they have health insurance coverage. Consequently, many struggle to meet basic needs. Furthermore, PWD continue to encounter biases that impede job opportunities; such biases also contribute to lower wages, marginalization, and fewer opportunities for promotion. PWD also tend to be overrepresented in part-time and low-wage jobs yet underrepresented in higher-paying professional positions that include benefits. Such factors have both short-term and long-term consequences.

Income and Employment

There is a two-way connection between poverty and disability. Populations with incomes below 200 percent of the Federal Poverty Level (FPL) have significantly higher rates of disabilities than those with higher incomes. Low-income populations are also more likely to have disabilities, to experience multiple disabilities, and to experience disabilities that are more severe. Conversely, PWD have disproportionately low incomes when compared to those who do not have disabilities; their income also tends to be less consistent and, therefore, they are more likely to experience fluctuation between periods when household income is adequate to meet basic needs and periods when it is not. At present, and even though average incomes among PWD have increased somewhat in recent decades, one-fourth live in households with incomes below the FPL; thus, the poverty rate among PWD is nearly twice as high as among nondisabled Americans. Approximately half of all PWD have a household income of $35,000 or less. On average, earnings are one-third lower than among nondisabled workers. Consequently, those with disabilities are more likely to have difficulty meeting basic needs related to food, shelter, clothing, medical care, and other necessities. They are also more likely to rely on so-called safety net programs designed to support low-income populations; at least two-thirds participate in such programs at some point during their lives. Examples include the Supplemental Nutrition Assistance Program (SNAP), Section 8 rental assistance, Temporary Aid to Needy Families (TANF), unemployment, the Children's Health Insurance Program (CHIP), Medicare, and/or Medicaid. Some also qualify for Social Security Insurance (SSI) or Social Security Disability Insurance (SSDI). Although half of working-age adults with disabilities do derive income from wages or salary, they are more likely than their nondisabled peers to rely on financial support from family members who do not live with them, Social Security retirement benefits, and early withdrawals from employer-sponsored retirement accounts.

PWD are more likely than nondisabled people to be absent from the labor force—that is, to be both unemployed and to not be actively seeking employment. However, many are active participants in the US labor force. The US Bureau of Labor Statistics did not begin tracking rates of labor force participation for PWD until 2008; however, historical data indicates they were largely excluded from the workforce throughout the nineteenth and well into the twentieth century. Although their workforce participation rates have increased gradually in recent years, they remain overrepresented among underemployed (e.g., seeking full-time employment but only able to secure a part-time job and/or unable to find a job that makes full use of the knowledge, training, and skills) and unemployed Americans. Rates of part-time employment are twice as high among PWD; while part-time work can be meaningful and provide access to much-needed income, such employment typically does not provide access to employer-sponsored health insurance or other benefits such as sick leave, flexible spending accounts, flex time, and retirement savings. There are also disparities among subgroups, with PWD who identify as BIPOC, cisgender women, or members of the LGBTQIA community overrepresented among those who are underemployed and unemployed. At present, nearly 40 percent of working-age adults with disabilities participate in the labor force. While this does represent a significant increase over pre-pandemic rates, it remains only about half as high as labor force participation among nondisabled populations. Employment rates are highest among those with sensory disabilities related to hearing and vision but significantly lower for those with disabilities that affect physical movement, cognition, emotions, behavior, and ability to engage in self-care and independent living. PWD are overrepresented in lower-paying industries, including in service (e.g., cashiers, retail sales, call center, and restaurant staff), clerical, production, and transportation industries but remain underrepresented in professional and managerial positions, including those in business, finance, health care, government, entertainment (e.g., film, television, music, and broadcasting), and STEM (science, technology, engineering, and math) fields. They are also overrepresented among sex workers.

Despite the anti-discrimination provisions that govern employment as outlined in the ADA, the reality is that workplace discrimination continues to affect PWD. Such discrimination influences hiring, promotion, and wages. Among job applicants with similar training, education, and professional credentials, PWD are less likely to be hired than nondisabled applicants. They are also less likely to be promoted and receive employer-sponsored opportunities for advanced training. The disability wage gap is also a significant consideration. Among full-time employees, PWD earn only 87 cents for every dollar earned by nondisabled full-time employees; the gap is even greater when both full- and part-time workers are considered as those with disabilities earn 32 percent less than nondisabled populations. Additionally, and despite increasing attention to diversity, equity, and inclusion (DEI) in many workplaces, the reality is that PWD remain marginalized in employment settings. Some of this stems from the lack of accessible workspaces and lack of accommodations. Other times, it is reflected in biased behaviors and statements from supervisors and co-workers. Examples include overlooking the dietary needs of individuals with food allergies or food sensitivities when organizing workplace events or celebrations; making ableist comments or telling jokes related to disabilities; making statements that reinforce negative stereotypes of PWD; or making assumptions about the skills, knowledge, and needs of PWD. Such biases are a major contributor to work-related stress as well as turnover rates among such workers.

Debt and Expenses, Assets and Wealth Accumulation

Burdens associated with economic insecurity are major contributors to stress for PWD. They are twice as likely as nondisabled people to have difficulty paying bills on time and in full. For some, this stems from medical costs. Average out-of-pocket annual expenses for PWD are more than twice as high as such expenses for those without disabilities. When compared to those without disabilities, PWD tend to have more frequent outpatient medical appointments, emergency room visits, surgical procedures, and overnight hospital stays; they also tend to be more reliant on prescription medication, to take multiple types of medication, and may require assistive devices, medical equipment in their homes, specialized transportation services to attend medical appointment, and in-home care. Nearly 40 percent have past due medical bills. However, those with employer-sponsored health insurance are more likely to have past due medical bills than individuals with public health insurance. Additionally, the cost burden of medical care tends to consume a greater portion of income and household budget for PWD and, in some cases, can rival monthly housing and food costs. In fact, disproportionately high medical expenses have been identified as a key contributor to food insecurity and housing insecurity among such individuals. Rates of food insecurity are three times higher in households that include at least one person with a disability. The risk of food insecurity is highest among households that include an individual with two or more disabilities, especially if that individual is an adult who is not employed. Due to a combination of lower-than-average household income and increasing housing prices (including both rent and mortgages), housing insecurity is also a concern for many. Half of adults with disabilities and nearly one-fourth of all children with disabilities are housing insecure; up to 40 percent of all housing insecure adults have at least one disability. Such expenses and related debt are associated with decreased health-seeking behaviors among PWD; they are nearly twice as likely as nondisabled people to refuse medical tests, skip medical appointments, not fill a prescription, and otherwise delay necessary medical care (e.g., treatment, surgical procedures, prosthetics, or other assistive devices) due to costs.

Other measures also provide evidence of the financial vulnerability of PWD. Nearly 80 percent identify personal finances as a source of stress; 40 percent indicate that they do not have adequate financial resources to meet their day-to-day needs. Among adult populations, and regardless of age, gender identity, employment status, and race/ethnicity, they are more likely than nondisabled populations to be late with mortgage or rent payments, to overdraw their checking account, and to have difficulty paying regular household expenses (e.g., phone, water, utilities, maintenance and repair, and consumable goods) and transportation costs. Those with retirement accounts are nearly three times as likely as their nondisabled colleagues to take a hardship withdrawal or hardship loan from such accounts. While this can provide much-needed income in times of crisis, it can also have long-term impacts on financial stability by decreasing funds available for retirement. Interestingly, PWD are as likely than those without disabilities to create a household budget; however, they tend to focus more on short-term economic needs (e.g., for next one to three months) than mid-term or long-term financial goals (e.g., saving for a down payment on a house, child's college education, or retirement; paying off credit cards, student loans, or mortgage). Less than 20 percent have a financial plan that extends from one to five years; less than 10 percent have a financial plan that extends beyond five years. They are also less likely to have debt that is associated with long-term financial stability and increased income—specifically, mortgage debt and educational debt. However, among those with student loan debt, such debt tends to be higher than among nondisabled people. PWD are also more likely to have credit card debt or high-interest payday loans. They are 30 percent less likely as those without disabilities to own a home; among those with a home mortgage, nearly one-third owe more than their home is worth. They are also twice as likely as nondisabled people to rely on reloadable prepaid credit cards to pay bills and to have no savings account or credit cards. While using reloadable prepaid credit cards can help them avoid the high-interest rates that are associated with some credit cards, it also reduces their ability to build a strong credit history. Among those who do have interest-bearing credit cards, over half cannot make payments on time, pay only the minimum amount, use their card to get cash advances, spend beyond their maximum limit, or otherwise engage in behaviors that contribute to high-interest rates, fees, and poor credit history.

When compared to nondisabled populations, PWD tend to have less wealth and fewer assets; they also tend to have a higher debt to income ratio. Such economic considerations not only diminish their ability to engage in health promotion and health-seeking behaviors due to issues of affordability but also contribute to their financial vulnerability. More than half do not have financial resources (e.g., savings, certificates of deposits, and other liquid assets) to cover an emergency. Such vulnerability is especially pronounced among BIPOC populations, cisgender women, and those over age 64 as well as those with incomes below the FPL, who do not have a college degree, and/or are not employed. PWD also tend to have fewer material assets (e.g., high-end jewelry, rare coins, automobiles, and land) or to earn substantial income from rental properties or self-owned businesses. While most PWD have good understanding of simple interest rates and mortgages, they demonstrate less financial literacy in other areas. Less than half have a good understanding of inflation, compound interest, and financial risk. The average net worth of households that include an adult with a disability is about 40 percent lower than among households that include only nondisabled adults. One-third of those over age 64 do not have any financial assets or accumulated wealth. Yet even those who enter retirement with relatively good savings and other wealth may find that such resources are insufficient to meet expenses and stay out of poverty.

EDUCATIONAL ACCESS AND QUALITY

In early America, PWD were not provided with education. Yet in the 1800s, some educators opened schools specifically for children with disabilities. In subsequent decades, efforts toward inclusive education led to legislation that protects the right to education for PWD as well as educational practices that aim to provide appropriate resources to help support their academic achievement. However, such populations remain marginalized in US educational institutions. This is evident not only in the stigmatization, harassment, and biases they encounter from peers as well as educators but also in the disproportionately low rates of academic achievement and degree completion rates of such students.

Historical Considerations

Throughout the sixteenth, seventeenth, and into the eighteenth centuries, disabilities were thought to stem from vice and immorality and were, therefore, deemed a punishment from God. Consequently, PWD were excluded from educational settings. In some cases, they were confined to the home, and although some were provided with cursory educational instruction via tutoring, such options were limited to more affluent families. Most were placed in institutions. In the early 1800s, however, and due to the influences of social reformers, educators, and religious leaders, schools for students with disabilities began to open. Early examples include the American School for the Deaf, founded in 1817 in Hartford, Connecticut; the Perkins School for the Blind which opened in 1829 in Watertown, Massachusetts; and the Massachusetts School for Idiotic and Feeble-Minded Youth, founded in 1848 in Boston. Such schools symbolized a shift to more humane treatment of those with disabilities. These schools tended to be small; students received instruction in social skills, daily self-care tasks, and physical activity to improve health. Most included only basic academic content. However, by the late nineteenth century, and prompted largely by eugenics ideology and xenophobia, there was increasing concern about so-called deviant populations (e.g., those with low IQs, immigrants, alcoholics, prostitutes, criminals, and the poor). PWD were believed to weaken the gene pool and, thus, were deemed a fundamental threat to American society. Consequently, large institutions were created to separate them from those without disabilities.

In the early twentieth century, however, some educators began to experiment with what became known as special education. This included the creation of classes for those with low IQs. Such classes were typically provided in public education settings; however, some teachers traveled to and provided classes to the residents of the types of institutions described above. Initially, special education classes were offered in large urban areas. However, as awareness concerning the horrors of Nazi Germany increased, some social reformers and politicians began to draw parallels between the Third Reich's extermination of PWD and the inhumane treatment of PWD in America. During this period, parents of children with disabilities also formed community groups; although initially created as a means for parents to provide support to one another, many evolved into advocacy groups that promoted social inclusion as well as increased support and services for children with disabilities. By 1953, and with the support of the American Association on Mental Deficiency, advocacy groups combined to create the National Association for Retarded

Children (NARC). While NARC drew attention to mistreatment of those who had been institutionalized, it also promoted inclusion of and expanded support for children with disabilities in all aspects of American society, including educational settings. Failure to do so, they argued, was both dehumanizing and a fundamental violation of constitutional rights. In the 1960s, bolstered by the recommendations of the Panel on Mental Retardation that had been organized by President Kennedy, NARC and other disability rights organizations expanded their influence. In addition to helping shift social attitudes toward PWD, their efforts were instrumental in securing passage of the Education for All Handicapped Children Act in 1975. It affirmed the constitutional right to free, public, and developmentally appropriate education for all children with disabilities. It was reauthorized in 1990 when it became known as the Individuals with Disabilities Education Act (IDEA). At present, IDEA continues to provide the primary foundation for free K-12 public education and related support services for children with disabilities. IDEA also supports early educational interventions for children who are born with disabilities as well as for those who develop disabilities prior to beginning kindergarten.

Elementary and Secondary Education

Educational services designed specifically to meet the needs of and promote educational equity for students with disabilities are generally referred to by the term "special education." Such services may include a wide variety of educational modifications and support related to instruction, academic content, scheduling, setting, and assessment. For example, certain students may require one-on-one or small group instruction as opposed to larger classroom settings, while others may need tutoring services, access to notes or lectures, and extra time or a quiet environment for taking exams. Still others may benefit from counseling, physical therapy, or adaptive devices/technologies (e.g., text-to-speech systems, large print materials, and tactile aids). In most public pre-K through twelfth-grade schools, the parents or guardians of students with disabilities are required to apply for an Individualized Education Program (IEP) for their child; an IEP is sometimes referred to as a 504 plan. Over 7 million children—or roughly 15 percent of all those in K-12 public schools—currently have an IEP. It is more common among cisgender boys than cisgender girls. In addition, Black and American Indian/Alaska Native (AI/AN) students are more likely to receive support via an IEP than students from other racial and ethnic subgroups. Additionally, children from low-income families are more likely to have an IEP. Roughly one-third of those with IEPs receive services and support related to specific learning disabilities. Creation and implementation of an IEP requires documentation from a certified medical professional; such documentation must specify the specific support and services that should be provided. In addition, it is common for a 504 plan to identify appropriate types of discipline for an individual student. Ideally, an IEP provides a tailored plan for meeting the specific needs of a student with disabilities. However, many parents are unfamiliar with the process for obtaining an IEP and/or may not understand their child's right to an IEP. Additionally, it is common for schools to have a standard 504 plan for specific types of disabilities; this is especially true for learning disabilities. While there may be common needs among students who experience the same type of disability, the reality is that different students have different needs. Thus, a standard IEP may not meet the needs of all learners. And even when an IEP is in place, educators do not always follow it.

Within K-12 educational settings, there remains a considerable gap in academic achievement among students with disabilities. Pre-K programs such as Head Start and Early Childhood Special Education provide education to over 1 million children with disabilities aged 3 to 5 each year. However, children with disabilities are less likely than their nondisabled peers to meet academic and social readiness measures by the time they enter kindergarten. On fourth grade standardized reading tests, over 90 percent of students with disabilities perform below grade-level expectations; on fourth grade standardized math tests, 83 percent do not meet grade-level expectations. Similar outcomes have been noted on both eighth grade and twelfth grade standardized tests. Data from school districts across the country indicate that academic performance among students with disabilities is about three years behind that of their nondisabled peers. They are also more likely to repeat a grade level, something that increases their risk of dropping out of school. Rates of successful degree completion continue to lag among high school students with disabilities. Whereas 85 percent of all students in the United States earn their regular high school diploma within four years of starting ninth grade, only 70 percent of students with disabilities do the same. However, there is significant variation by state. While the on-time high school graduation rates of students with disabilities are 75 percent or higher in nine states, it remains 65 percent or lower in thirteen states and is below 60 percent in South Carolina, Ohio, Alaska, the District of Columbia, Idaho, Michigan, and Mississippi. Additionally, the graduation gap between students with disabilities and those without varies considerably among states. Only four states—Arkansas, Florida, Kansas, Montana, and New Mexico—have a gap of less than 10 percent. The gap is lowest in Arkansas where 84.6 percent of students with disabilities and 89.2 percent of students without disabilities graduate on time. However, in twenty-one states, the gap is 20 percent or more; it is highest in Mississippi at 45.6 percent.

Social dynamics within K-12 settings also have a significant influence on the experiences of students with disabilities. When compared to their nondisabled peers, children with disabilities tend to be more socially isolated. They are often stigmatized and marginalized due to their disability and report higher rates of loneliness and social exclusion. They are less frequently invited to join group projects, recreational activities during recess, and school-sponsored sports teams, academic clubs, or other extracurricular groups. They are also frequently excluded from peer-related social events that occur outside of school, including sleepovers, playdates, parties, and dating activities. In addition, and even though bullying of students based on their disability status violates federal and state laws that prohibit discrimination and harassment, such students are three to five times more likely to be bullied by their peers both in and out of the classroom. This sometimes comes in the form of jokes that demean or belittle them due to their disability, name-calling, or use of slurs related to their disability. Other times, it involves acts that highlight the student's disability. Examples include knowingly eating food containing peanuts near a student with a severe peanut allergy; placing furniture or other obstacles in the path of a student with a mobility impairment; and hiding an assistive device or specialized educational materials that a student needs to participate in academic activities. In some cases, it also includes threats, acts of physical violence, sexual harassment, and/or sexual assault. The social stigmatization, marginalization, and bullying experienced by students with disabilities significantly diminish their academic achievement and school completion rates. Such factors have also been linked to diminished sense of belonging among such students and, consequently, to increased risk of anxiety, depression, and suicidal ideation, particularly among those in middle and high school.

Yet the social environment of educational settings is also heavily influenced by the actions and attitudes of teachers, tutors, administrators, parent volunteers, and other staff members. For example, IDEA requires that students with disabilities are placed in the least restrictive environment possible within educational settings. This means, quite simply, that such students may not be placed in special education classrooms and/or separated from their nondisabled peers unless doing so is justified by their specific disability-related needs and is formalized via their IEP. Despite this, and although students with disabilities are spending an increasing amount of time in general education classrooms, one-third spend 80 percent or more of their school day in a special education classroom. Placement in special education classrooms may help to support their specific learning needs; however, even those who are separated from nondisabled students for a portion of the day can experience increased feelings of marginalization and exclusion. Furthermore, while most states require that those who teach special education classes have proper training to do so—and in some districts, such individuals must have a master's degree to be certified in special education—the reality is that many who teach K-12 general education classes lack such specialized training. Consequently, they may lack an adequate understanding of how to fully and equitably integrate students with disabilities into the classroom and support their educational needs. Yet in other cases, educational professionals knowingly discriminate against students with disabilities. Examples include refusing to adapt teaching methods or curriculum as identified on a student's IEP; excluding PWD from academic or extracurricular activities; using demeaning language to colleagues, students, or parents. Such explicit biases violate the rights of students with disabilities and can diminish their sense of belonging and educational achievement.

Postsecondary Education and Training

Students with disabilities who earn a high school diploma or General Education Development (GED) credential are only about half as likely as their nondisabled peers to pursue postsecondary education and training. This is especially true for those with impaired cognition and profound physical impairments. Overall, students with disabilities represent about 20 percent of all undergraduate students and 12 percent of those pursuing graduate degrees. Among those who do enroll in educational programs after high school, they are more likely to participate in technical and vocational programs (e.g., culinary arts, cosmetology, graphic design, auto repair and maintenance, and dental assistant) than their nondisabled peers. While such programs can be less costly and time-consuming than four-year degree programs, the employment opportunities associated with such fields also tend to be lower paying and, thus, diminish lifetime earning potential; they are also more likely to include part-time rather than full-time work and, therefore, may not include benefits such as health insurance. After completing high school, students with disabilities pursue a college degree at only about half the rate as their nondisabled peers. This is sometimes due to financial reasons, but other times it is due to concerns about their ability to adjust to the college academics and social dynamics. Although students with disabilities continue to demonstrate that they can be successful in postsecondary environments, the reality is that the services and support provided to students are different in college than in public K-12 environments. IDEA governs early elementary and secondary public-school settings; however, it does not apply to postsecondary contexts.

All colleges and universities that receive federal funding—including via student financial aid—are required under the ADA to provide appropriate accommodations, including in relation to academic, residential, and dining services as well as nonacademic programs (e.g., athletics, student clubs, and organizations). Such institutions must also protect students with disabilities against identity-based harassment. However, any IEP/504 plan that a student had in high school does not automatically transfer to the postsecondary context. Instead, students must go through a new process of applying for accommodation, typically through the school's disability services office (DSO). This process requires students to register with the DSO; they must then obtain and submit recent medical documentation—typically no more than 18–24 months old—to confirm their need for accommodation. Their application and documentation are then reviewed by the DSO coordinator to determine if they meet legal eligibility guidelines. If they do, their accommodation is specified in a letter provided to the student. If not, their request is denied. Common examples of accommodations for college students include extended time on exams or other assignments, the option to take exams in a low-noise environment, special parking spaces, note-taking services, and use of a recording device during lectures. The student is then responsible for communicating with their professors and providing a copy of their accommodation letter; they must do so separately for each class. Postsecondary institutions are only required to provide reasonable accommodation. For example, if an institution does not provide any on-campus parking located near student housing, then a request for parking within 50 yards of a student's dormitory would not be considered reasonable accommodation. Similarly, while providing a student with extended time to take exams is a common accommodation, it is not reasonable to expect that a student would not be required to take any exams in courses that require them of other students. Because college students are legally adults, their parents are not permitted to provide input regarding the accommodation process unless the student provides written permission. The process can be lengthy, particularly for students who need to secure medical documentation. Obtaining documentation can be expensive and, thus, may pose a barrier to accommodation for low-income students. Additionally, students who are unaware of how to obtain accommodation often do not begin that process before starting college classes. Thus, students may find themselves beginning their studies without the accommodation they need to promote their academic success. Unlike K-12 settings, there is no equivalent of an IEP team at the postsecondary level. Consequently, students typically must navigate the process of securing and communicating with professors about academic accommodation on their own.

At the time they begin college, many students with disabilities lack a formal transition plan to help them adjust to the less-structured yet more demanding academic environment. Those who have strong awareness of their academic strengths and needs, are skilled at navigating new social contexts—including with postsecondary peers, faculty, and staff members—and who have developed strong skills in the realm of self-advocacy are better able to manage the academic, social, and psychological/emotional adjustments that are common among new college students. Students with strong academic support (e.g., tutors, academic coaches, and health-care providers) and social support from family, friends, and academic mentors are more likely to make a smooth transition to college. However, those without such resources, skills, and/or support can quickly become overwhelmed and are at increased risk of poor academic performance and dropping out. At present, only about half of students with disabilities who start college complete their degree. In addition, the type of social isolation and marginalization that occurs in K-12 educational settings is also present on many college campuses. PWD continue to be marginalized in course content and academic research; there are less than twenty institutions in the United States that offer a degree in disability studies. Furthermore, less than 5 percent of postsecondary faculty and staff have a disability.

HEALTH-CARE ACCESS AND QUALITY

Historically, PWD were treated as sinners, criminals, and witches; consequently, there was little medical care provided to such populations. Additionally, they were sometimes subjected to unethical medical experiments and treatments, including lobotomies and forced sterilization. While the disability rights movement has helped to promote more ethical and inclusive health care for those with disabilities, the reality is that such populations continue to experience barriers that limit both their access to care and the quality of health care they receive.

A History of Medical Discrimination

Historically, dominant attitudes toward disability within the medical field were based on the notion of disability as a flaw, defect, or pathology that needs to be cured. In early America, disability was typically regarded as incontrovertible evidence of sin including witchcraft, infidelity, and moral depravity. Thus, if a child was born with a significant physical anomaly, many believed that their parents had done something to cause it; if a teenager or adult had an illness or injury that led to a disability, it was thought that they had committed an egregious sin and, therefore, God was punishing them. Individuals with cognitive or psychosocial disabilities were believed to have been possessed by evil spirits or that the devil was influencing them. Consequently, they were shunned by their families and communities. This sometimes included refusing to provide them with food, shelter, or other necessities; other times, it meant expelling them from their communities; parents sometimes practiced infanticide, particularly to hide their supposed sin from others. Doctors and healers provided little care to PWD during this period. However, they did sometimes attempt to treat such individuals through use of herbal remedies, bloodletting, and/or drilling holes in the skull to allow evil spirits to escape the body. Religious leaders and members of the community would sometimes support such efforts using prayer. In some cases, those with disabilities were thought to be witches or wards of the devil and, consequently, were burned, drowned, or hanged.

During the eighteenth and nineteenth centuries, however, and due to the influence of expanding medical knowledge as well as the social changes that resulted from the industrial revolution, attitudes toward PWD shifted. Disability was no longer equated with evidence of sin or spirit possession. Instead, it was increasingly deemed a problem that was sometimes a consequence of bad genetics. This explanation was most common in relation to cognitive and psychosocial disabilities but was sometimes used for birth defects.

Other times, however, disabilities were believed to stem from bad luck; this was especially common as an explanation for the type of serious workplace injuries that occurred in industrial settings, and minimized the systemic safety issues common in such settings by emphasizing the ideas that such tragedies were unavoidable. Those with disabilities that stemmed from work-related injuries were extended a moderate degree of sympathy and physicians did provide various types of care to such individuals—including measures to try to limit infection and complications as well as the creation of rudimentary prosthetics and other assistive devices. Yet people with cognitive and psychosocial disabilities fared much worse. In most cases, they were put in jails, prisons, almshouses, poorhouses, or asylums and treated like criminals. Inhumane treatment and deplorable living conditions were common. Health-care services were virtually nonexistent. Due to the increasing influence of eugenics ideology, some physicians sterilized residents without their consent.

In the first half of the twentieth century, however, attitudes toward PWD again shifted. Influenced by legislation such as the 1918 Soldier's Rehabilitation Act, the Smith-Fess Act of 1920, and the Social Security Act of 1935, rehabilitation care for individuals with physical disabilities expanded considerably. In addition, and as medical discoveries increased the safety of surgical procedures, physicians were able to promote increased mobility and function for individuals with certain types of physical disabilities. Rehabilitation services also expanded during this period. Yet health-care professionals regarded physical disabilities as problems inherent in the individual rather than a reflection of the way society was structured. Thus, their focus was on curing physical disabilities rather than accepting them. Individuals with cognitive and psychosocial disabilities were treated much differently by health-care professionals. Methods such as electroconvulsive therapy, lobotomies, and heavy doses of sedatives were common and intended to control rather than to provide medical support to such individuals. They were also sometimes subjected to medical experimentation that they had not consented to and/or that was otherwise unethical, including being injected with or exposed to infectious diseases (e.g., influenza, malaria, and hepatitis), exposed to known toxins and carcinogens, and subjected to unnecessary surgeries and forced sterilizations. Yet by the second half of the century, and due largely to the influence of the burgeoning disability rights movement and increasing public awareness about disabilities, health-care providers increasingly questioned the medicalization of disability. They began to understand disabilities as part of the diversity of human experience rather than a problem to be cured. Despite this, many health-care professionals continue to rely on stereotypes of PWD. Examples include the beliefs that they are less sensitive to pain than nondisabled populations, are asexual, and have a poorer quality of life than nondisabled people. In addition, implicit and explicit biases continue to influence health-care providers' attitudes toward PWD as well as the care they provide to them. PWD remain underrepresented in clinical research, something that limits the applicability of the findings of such research.

Access to Care: Economic and Geographic Factors

The cost of health-care remains a significant barrier to health care for many PWD. When compared to those without disabilities, they tend to rely on health services more and to have higher costs associated with necessary health care. In the early twentieth century, new laws helped promote rehabilitation services for veterans who had been injured in combat, thereby reducing direct costs to such individuals. In addition, the Social Security Act of 1935 established a system of economic benefits for certain groups that were deemed socially and financially vulnerable, including certain PWD, thereby making it easier for them to afford health care. Additionally, the Medicare and Medicaid Act of 1965 expanded financial support for and helped provide health insurance to some PWD, including elderly populations, low-income populations, and those no longer able to work due to disability. Yet many continued to experience employment-related discrimination as employers often refused to hire them due to the costs of disability-related health insurance benefits. Passage of the ADA in 1990, however, prohibited such discrimination and, consequently, promoted increased access to health insurance. Passage of the Patient Protection and Affordable Care Act (ACA) of 2010 improved home and community health programs, prohibited employers from restricting access to health insurance for those with preexisting conditions, expanded coverage for essential benefits (e.g., prescription drugs, rehabilitation services, mental health and substance abuse treatment, and management of chronic diseases), and increased availability of accessible equipment in health-care settings. At present, 90 percent of Americans with disabilities have health insurance coverage; this is higher than among nondisabled populations. Despite this, many PWD continue to have difficulty accessing health care due to financial barriers. The bureaucracy associated with insurance processes often results in delayed access to care and can discourage them from seeking care altogether. Additionally, some politicians and economists have indicated that funding for Social Security, Medicare, and other programs that promote health insurance for PWD will run out in the next decade.

Access to care for PWD continues to be impeded by geographic factors. Within the US health-care system, care related to specific disabilities is often considered specialty care that requires a referral to a specialist. For example, an infant born with spina bifida is typically treated by a pediatric neurosurgeon; an individual who lost a leg in a vehicle accident might initially receive care from an orthopedic surgeon but then would also be cared for by a prosthetist if they wish to receive a prosthetic leg. These types of specialty care have the potential to vastly improve the health and quality of life for patients with disabilities. However, access to such care varies significantly by location. Individuals in major metropolitan areas typically have better health-care access due to the higher concentration of health-care professionals in such areas; however, those in rural areas often must travel further to receive specialty care, and for those living in remote rural areas, the distance can be significant. While such travel may be more manageable during times of the year when the weather is good and in areas with well-maintained roads, it becomes more burdensome in areas that receive heavy snowfall or rainfall as well as those with poor-quality roads. Such factors also diminish access to community transportation services provided specifically for disabled populations and to public transportation services. Recent research indicates that access to specialty care can also be challenging for those who live in urban areas, particularly those who live in poor, inner-city neighborhoods where health-care services tend to be scarce and access to transportation services is often lacking.

Access to Care: Physical, Informational, and Cultural Factors

Some of the most common barriers that impede access to health care for PWD include structural features of health-care settings. These are known as physical barriers. While principles of universal design have been around since at least the 1980s, the physical space of many health-care clinics and hospitals continues to be organized in ways that do not adequately accommodate people of varying abilities, sizes, and needs. For example, many facilities lack accessible sidewalk curbs and entry ramps for those who use wheelchairs, canes, walkers, or similar assistive devices. In some locations, elevators are in out-of-the-way locations or require users to access them through side or back doors of the health-care facility. Diagnostic equipment (e.g., X-ray machines used to complete mammograms) are often not height-adjustable and scales used to weigh patients sometimes do not accommodate wheelchairs or walkers. Additionally, doors are sometimes very heavy and/or do not have a delayed closure mechanism to permit individuals to move through them at their own pace. Yet the layout of waiting rooms can also create physical barriers, particularly if furnishings and other items (e.g., informational displays, plants, and lamps) are positioned in ways that create clutter. Exam rooms with narrow doorways that lack lift bars to help patients reposition themselves or that do not have height-adjustable exam tables increase barriers to care.

Informational barriers are also an ongoing concern. Principles regarding informed consent require that patients have the right to be fully informed about their health status as well as treatment options available to them; they also have the right to make decisions about their health voluntarily and without threat, coercion, or manipulation. In addition, they have a right to receive information about their health in the format and language of their preference, and at a level that is appropriate given their educational background and their cognitive abilities. Yet PWD are often denied their right to informed consent. Historical examples include medical experiments performed without their knowledge as well as the forced sterilization of such populations. However, such practices persist. Examples include using medical jargon to explain medical procedures to those with cognitive disabilities, failing to provide certified medical translators to those with limited English proficiency (LEP), and exclusively using written materials rather than providing information in various formats (e.g., audio, braille, and graphic) to accommodate those with hearing, vision, and cognitive disabilities. Failure to provide informed consent is a violation of patients' legal rights. However, it is also associated with diminished health outcomes, decreased patient satisfaction, and reduced likelihood of future health-care-seeking behaviors.

Cultural barriers also continue to impede access to care for many PWD. National standards regarding culturally and linguistically appropriate services (CLAS) were established in 2000 by the US Department of Health and Human Services, Office of Minority Health, and continue to govern health-care services throughout the country. CLAS standards are grounded in the reality that culture has a significant influence on both ideas and practices related to health, wellness, and healing. Additionally, such standards recognize that different patient populations have different linguistic preferences and different levels of health literacy. Thus, they promote a comprehensive approach that incorporates cultural and linguistic factors into the care provided to each patient, particularly as doing so can help promote health equity and reduce health disparities. However, many providers lack understanding of the cultural dimensions of health, including as such dimensions are grounded in disability culture. Even fewer have been trained in promoting cultural competence as a core element of health care to patients with disabilities. Consequently, many providers rely exclusively on the medical model of disability and, in doing so, not only perpetuate stereotypes of PWD but also use language and otherwise interact with such patients in ways that demean, pity, and dehumanize them and, of equal importance, diminish the quality of care provided to such patients. Examples include using outdated and discriminatory terms, focusing on the disability rather than the individual, and assuming patients with similar disabilities have the same needs and experiences.

LIVING ENVIRONMENT AND SOCIAL CONTEXT

In communities across America, the construction of housing, public spaces, and commercial locations such as stores, restaurants, and entertainment venues continues to impede PWD. Social attitudes toward such populations are heavily influenced by media and popular culture representations; such representations continue to rely on well-worn stereotypes that depict them in harmful and inaccurate ways. While such stereotypes impact the way that those without disabilities respond to and interact with PWD, they are also internalized by those with disabilities. Violence and victimization also continue to shape the experiences of PWD.

Housing and Community

The built environment of most homes and communities in the United States continues to pose significant challenges for PWD. One of the most significant concerns is accessible housing. Although the ADA provides the legal foundation for accessible housing, physical barriers remain common, especially for those with mobility-related and other physical disabilities. For example, lack of ramps, elevators, roll-in showers, handles instead of knobs on faucets and doors, accessible light switches and HVAC controls, safety bars in showers and around toilets, and first-floor bathrooms and bedrooms in multistory units are common barriers in home and apartment buildings, particularly those that are older. Additionally, structural elements such as narrow hallways and doors, steps between different rooms, and cabinets and/or countertops that are too high can pose significant challenges. While some homes and apartments can be modified to make them more accessible, such modifications can be expensive. Furthermore, modifications are not always possible—for example, an individual who rents a house or apartment is typically not permitted to make structural changes to their rental unit. Given the disproportionately high rates of poverty among PWD, many who are homeowners cannot afford to make even minor modifications to their homes. Although about one-third of current US housing stock is potentially modifiable to promote increased accessibility for individuals with minor or moderate disabilities that affect mobility, most structures are not. In addition, research suggests that less than 2 percent of the current US housing stock is fully accessible for those who use assistive devices to promote mobility.

Issues related to access and physical barriers are also evident in public spaces. For example, sidewalks and roads that are in poor repair can make it both difficult and dangerous for those with mobility impairments and profound vision impairments to move around their communities. While some may rely on public transportation to help them move from one location to another, the reality is that communities that do not have public spaces that are in good repair discourage PWD from accessing and participating in such spaces. Many parks, recreational trails, restaurants, lodging, shopping, and entertainment venues do not adhere to principles of universal design. Restaurant tables and bar counters are often too high; noise levels in some public settings can be distressing to individuals with certain cognitive or psychosocial disabilities. In addition, the recent trend of self-checkout machines in grocery stores, restaurants, and other venues can make it difficult—and, in some cases, impossible—for PWD to make retail transactions. Such machines are often not at an appropriate height for wheelchair users, and they often do not have features that accommodate the needs of those with visual or hearing-related sensory impairments. Thus, tasks such as shopping for groceries or household supplies, going out to eat, participating in outdoor recreational activities, and attending a sporting event or concert can be challenging.

Social Attitudes, Stereotypes, and Representations

Despite ongoing efforts related to equity and inclusion, negative social attitudes toward PWD persist. Such attitudes can minimize or overlook the challenges that those with disabilities experience, devalue their contributions, and perpetuate the dehumanization and marginalization of such populations. Negative attitudes are often expressed via reliance on stereotypes. Such stereotypes are found in personal conversations, business meetings, political cartoons, and literature. They also continue to permeate American media and popular culture. For example, a dominant stereotype equates certain types of disabilities with violent tendencies. This is especially common with depictions of individuals with schizophrenia, bipolar disorder, autism, major depressive disorder, and ADHD, particularly in thriller movies and crime-drama television programs with plotlines that include violent crimes such as homicide, rape and sexual assault, and aggravated assault. Another common stereotype depicts PWD as asexual and/or aromantic; other times, they are portrayed as sexual deviants and/or sexual predators. Other common tropes portray such populations as pitiable, superheroes, helpless, always angry, asocial, inherently courageous, in constant pain, and/or unable to live a meaningful and independent life. They are often the target of punchlines, with disabilities sometimes used as a plot device meant to evoke laughter from the viewing audience. Those with disabilities comprise less than 3 percent of all characters in American film and television. Critics have pointed out that characters with disabilities are commonly portrayed by nondisabled actors. This is not particularly surprising, however, given that PWD remain underrepresented as writers, directors, producers, and actors. Similar stereotypes are also found in social media, print advertisements, and news coverage.

Stereotypes are not innocuous. Instead, and given the central role of media and popular culture in socialization, they play an important role in shaping attitudes and behaviors. Among nondisabled populations, media and popular culture depictions influence their understanding of not only the skills and abilities of PWD but also socially accepted ways to treat such populations. Thus, they influence personal relationships and can also be found in workplaces, educational institutions, and health-care settings. Research shows that many nondisabled Americans have, to some degree, internalized the stereotypes they encounter in media and popular culture and that such stereotypes do inform their choice of friends and dating partners as well as their interactions with classmates and co-workers with disabilities. Such stereotypes are also found in political discourse and, thus, they influence not only politicians' perceptions of PWD and their respective needs but also legislation. Yet it is also common for PWD to internalize the stereotypes they encounter. Such internalization is associated with decreased self-esteem and increased feelings of shame and self-blaming. Those who internalize such stereotypes are also more likely to self-isolate and, consequently, to experience increased depression, anxiety, and loneliness.

Violence and Victimization

When compared to nondisabled populations, PWD are approximately four times more likely to experience violence during their lifetimes. The US Department of Justice indicates that rates of violent victimization among such populations have increased in the past 15 years. They are victims in one-fourth of all nonfatal violent crimes including robbery, aggravated assault, sexual assault, and rape. In addition, they are more likely than nondisabled people to experience intimate partner violence (IPV)—that is, violence perpetrated by a current or former spouse or partner. IPV may include physical violence, psychological abuse, sexual abuse (including rape), stalking, and cyberstalking (e.g., using social media platforms to intimidate, threaten, or otherwise harass an individual). Rates of such violence are lower among those with physical or sensory disabilities but higher among those with cognitive or psychosocial disabilities. Some violent crimes against PWD are also hate crimes. Such crimes often target the nature of an individual's disability. Examples include destroying assistive devices, attacking emotional support animals or guide dogs, and verbal abuse that relies on ableist slurs. Although there is little data on homicide perpetuated against PWD, evidence suggests that rates of fatal violence against them are also disproportionately high. They are also disproportionately subjected to police violence; it is estimated that up to half of those who are killed by police have cognitive or psychosocial disabilities.

Rates of violent victimization are somewhat higher among LGBTQIA, cisgender women, and BIPOC individuals with disabilities. Among populations aged 65 and older, rates of victimization are similar between those with disabilities and nondisabled populations; however, when compared to nondisabled populations, PWD aged 12–64 are three times more likely to be victimized. Similarly, rates of abuse—including emotional, physical, and sexual—are disproportionately high among children under the age of 12. While perpetrators of such violence are sometimes strangers, the majority are known to the victim and typically include family members, intimate partners, caregivers, neighbors, classmates, and acquaintances. In some cases, health-care providers and support staff (e.g., home health workers and transportation aides) are the perpetrators of such violence. Less than half of such crimes are reported to the police, and only about one-tenth of reported cases end in a conviction.

CHAPTER FOUR

Elderly Populations

Individuals who have entered the later stages of adulthood are commonly referred to as elderly. However, they are also sometimes referred to as elders, aging adults, seniors, senior citizens, golden-agers, or retirees/pensioners (regardless of whether or not they have worked for wages during their lifetimes). Over the past century, the US population has undergone a dramatic demographic shift. Quite simply, and due to a combination of increased public health measures, improved health-care prevention and treatment options, technological advances, and the implementation of various social and economic support programs, individuals in the United States are living longer than they were 100 years ago. Average life expectancy (ALE) in 1920 was 53 years. It steadily increased through the twentieth century and into the twenty-first century; by 2020, ALE had reached 79 years. More people in the United States are living to early-, middle-, and late-old age. At present, seniors represent 16 percent of the total US population; it is estimated that their numbers will double in the next decade and a half, thus reaching over 80 million by 2040.

Relying on the parameters of late adulthood that are commonly used by the US Department of Health and Human Services as well as health-care practitioners and researchers, this chapter focuses on social determinants of health in order to explain some of the most prominent health issues and related inequities among those aged 65 and above. Elderly adults are a diverse population with correspondingly diverse health needs. There are often clear patterns of diseases and disorders among different demographic groups of senior citizens. Such patterns are evident by race, gender identity and expression, sex, ability, sexual orientation, educational status, socioeconomic status, and other socially constructed identities. When compared to younger populations, however, aging adults share common concerns related to physical, mental, and social wellness. They tend to be in worse health than other age groups and, consequently, to require a greater variety and frequency of health services. Their needs related to material and social support are also great yet often go unmet.

CURRENT STATE OF HEALTH

As a natural part of the aging process, cells within the human body begin to slow their division as an individual enters late adulthood; in some cases, cell division ceases altogether or becomes otherwise abnormal. Thus, body tissues (e.g., muscle, skin, bone, nerves, and connective tissues) and organ systems become less efficient and more prone to abnormalities in structure and function. As a result of such changes, it is common for elderly adults to experience a decline in physical health. At least four out of five senior citizens have a chronic physical health condition. Most common among these are heart disease, diabetes, respiratory disease (e.g., chronic pulmonary obstructive disease, or CPOD), cancer, high blood pressure, high cholesterol, osteoporosis, stroke, kidney diseases, and osteoarthritis. Yet due to decreased efficiency and responsiveness of the immune system that typically occurs with aging, older populations are also more susceptible to acute conditions (e.g., influenza, the common cold, and bacterial infections). They are also more likely than younger populations to die from acute conditions; approximately 60 percent of those who die from influenza each year are elderly. Diminished immune functions also render seniors more susceptible to autoimmune disorders (e.g., inflammatory bowel disease, lupus, rheumatoid arthritis, and psoriatic arthritis). In addition, oral health is often compromised. Dental caries, gum disease, and oral cancers are disproportionately high among elderly populations. At least 20 percent of seniors have lost all of their teeth. Poor oral health is highest among those with heart disease, COPD, and diabetes as well as those who use tobacco products.

Aging-related physical changes also impact body composition. In early-old age, risk of being overweight or obese increases. This is often due to decreased physical activity and/or hormonal changes. There is, therefore, a tendency to accumulate body fat while simultaneously experiencing a decrease in muscle mass among those in their 60s and 70s. Yet the risk of being overweight decreases for seniors in their 80s; such individuals are more likely to be normal body weight or even underweight and many require high-calorie, nutrient-dense dietary supplements to help promote health. During late-old age, unintentional weight loss and being underweight are often a result of decreasing efficiency of the digestive system. However, decreasing body weight may also be a consequence of various diseases (e.g., cancer, Parkinson's disease, and HIV), food insecurity, sensory decline (e.g., smell and taste), swallowing disorders, medical treatment (e.g., prescription medication and surgery), and physical disabilities or cognitive impairments that impede ability to obtain, prepare, and consume food.

Other common physical health issues stem from loss of aerobic capacity, muscle mass, joint health, and bone density (a condition known as osteoporosis). Such changes contribute to decreased strength, flexibility, endurance, dexterity, and balance. Thus, older adults are at increased risk of injuries such as sprains, joint dislocation, fractures, bruises, burns, and cuts. Physical changes can make it more difficult for seniors to engage in activities of daily living (ADLs), including bathing, grooming, cooking, eating, getting dressed, using the restroom, taking medication, and walking/mobility. Falls are also common; risk increases during certain activities (e.g., climbing the stairs, walking on a wet or otherwise slippery surface, and standing on a ladder). Yet two-thirds of all falls among elderly populations occur within the home or in surrounding areas (e.g., yard, garden, garage, or driveway). The majority take place on flat surfaces and when an individual is standing up, sitting down, or walking from one room to another. Fall-related injuries among individuals over age 65 result in over $50 billion in health-care costs each year; nearly 1 million elderly individuals are hospitalized annually due to significant fall-related injuries including joint dislocations (e.g., hip, shoulder, and wrist) and fractures of the bones in the pelvis or limbs. Falls can also cause traumatic brain injuries (TBIs)—including concussions, contusions (bruising of brain tissue), cerebral hemorrhages and hematomas, and penetrating brain injuries (e.g., when an object pierces the cranium and enters the brain tissue)—among seniors. The risk of death after suffering a TBI is highest among those over 75 years of age.

Sensory deprivation is also a concern for many older adults. Aging-related hearing loss—known as presbycusis—is linked to deterioration in the structure and function of the ear canal, tympanic membrane, cochlea, auditory nerves, and the joints and bones both within and surrounding the ear structure. One-third of seniors aged 65–75 have diminished hearing; hearing loss is most pronounced in late-old age when it tends to be classified as moderate, severe, or profound. Even mild hearing loss can impede effective communication and diminish quality of life. It is also common for elderly populations to experience vision loss and decreased sense of taste, sense of smell, and sensitivity to touch. This is sometimes due to physiological changes that occur as part of the aging process, including changes to sensory organs. However, it can also be caused or aggravated by illness, injury, medication, or environmental concerns (e.g., loud noises, poor air quality, and temperature extremes). Reduced sensory function can affect nearly all aspects of life. For example, diminished vision and diminished sense of touch are associated with loss of fine motor skills in elderly populations; thus, it may be difficult to write, type, use scissors and utensils, operate electronic devices (e.g., cellular phones, television remotes, and medical equipment), and manipulate buttons, belts, shoelaces, and zippers. Sensory impairment can also contribute to confusion, frustration, and social unease. It increases risk of social isolation, anxiety, depression, and low self-esteem. While age-related sensory impairments cannot be reversed, assistive devices may help enhance function and improve quality of life. For example, hearing aids can enhance communication. However, issues with function (e.g., feedback and distortion of sound), comfort, and affordability of such devices are common.

Brain function also diminishes over time and becomes less efficient at processing information. This is known as cognitive aging; it typically occurs gradually and becomes more prominent over time. Yet cognitive problems among elderly populations can also result from vitamin deficiencies, use of certain types of medication (e.g., antidepressants, antihistamines, statins, corticosteroids, and pain relievers), substances use and abuse disorders (SUAD), TBI, sleep disorders, and infectious diseases. Regardless of the cause, elders who experience cognitive decline often have difficulty with processing and remembering new information; they may also encounter challenges with concentration, reasoning, emotional regulation, and coping with stress. Additionally, those with cognitive decline often experience difficulties with executive functions such as problem-solving, planning, and adapting to unfamiliar situations. Regardless of the cause, cognitive decline contributes to increased risk and severity of anxiety, depression, and agitation in elderly individuals. Interestingly, many seniors develop what is known as a positivity bias in order to cope with cognitive problems; this means they avoid situations that contribute to stress while gravitating to events, people, and other stimuli that foster positive feelings. It is often done unconsciously. While this can help them avoid negative emotions to a certain degree, it can also contribute to social isolation and even prevent them from engaging in necessary tasks (e.g., seeking health care, paying bills, and shopping for groceries).

Some seniors develop severe cognitive impairments due to dementia disorders. Such disorders interfere with their ability to live independently. Over 7 million elderly adults in the United States are currently living with some type of dementia disorder; rates have steadily increased over the past two decades. The most common type of dementia disorder among seniors is Alzheimer's disease; it is characterized by progressive and irreversible shrinking of brain tissues, abnormal accumulation of proteins around brain cells, and death of brain cells. Although Alzheimer's disease can occur in individuals under the age of 65—referred to as early onset—elderly populations represent 96 percent of all Americans living with the disease. In the past 20 years, rates of Alzheimer's disease have increased by nearly 25 percent in the United States. Symptoms become worse over time and are not reversible. At present, there are ongoing studies into medications to treat Alzheimer's disease; some have been shown to reduce severity of symptoms, but there is currently no preventative option. Other types of dementia include those related to other health conditions such as Parkinson's disease, stroke, and abnormal buildup of fluid in the area around the brain (Hydrocephalus). Those with early-stage dementia disorders may wander; repeat questions; misplace things; forget common words or phrases; and have a difficult time recalling names, addresses, or phone numbers. In the later stages of dementia, common symptoms include decreased interest in daily activities, diminished communication, loss of balance, emotional unpredictability (e.g., agitation and aggression), confusion, paranoia, and hallucinations. Those with middle- or late-stage dementia disorders require around-the-clock care. Life expectancy is 8–10 years after a dementia disorder diagnosis.

Physical and cognitive health problems common among elderly populations can also contribute to mental health issues. Quite simply, the changes that are common as part of the aging process can impair the ability of seniors to work, exercise, shop, travel, vote, and participate in social activities and educational opportunities. Such changes can also cause many seniors to become more withdrawn and less socially engaged. Thus, they are less likely to participate in leisure, social, and recreational activities. Importantly, social connectedness and strong relationships with family, friends, and neighbors can actually help promote good physical health, mental health, and cognitive well-being among elderly populations. Seniors with strong social support networks have lower rates of chronic diseases, are more likely to stay physically active, and have stronger immune systems than those who are socially isolated. Additionally, those with strong social connections have lower rates of depression, SUAD, and anxiety; regular, healthy social interactions also help slow the rate of cognitive aging and dementia disorders. In contrast, seniors who are socially isolated and/or lack healthy social networks are at increased risk of illness, injury, cognitive decline, and death. They are also more likely to be victims of physical, psychological, sexual, and financial abuse. Social isolation also increases risk of suicidal ideation and suicide attempts among seniors, especially for those struggling with economic challenges, chronic pain, cognitive impairment, and death of age group peers (e.g., spouse, siblings, and friends). Rates of suicidal ideation are disproportionately high among seniors, especially those over age 75; lesbian, gay, bisexual, transgender, and queer (LGBTQ+) populations; and cisgender men. One-fourth of seniors who attempt suicide will die as a result.

However, the aging process is influenced by a myriad of factors including genetics, income, lifestyle (e.g., habits and practices related to diet, exercise, smoking, alcohol consumption, and use of illicit drugs), environment, and social factors. For example, cisgender female populations tend to live longer than cisgender male populations: 81 years versus 77 years, respectively. This is linked to certain biological influences, including hormonal differences that contribute to greater accumulation of fat around internal organs and higher levels of cholesterol in cisgender males but more subcutaneous fat and lower cholesterol in cisgender women. Additionally, hormonal changes that occur during and after menopause have been linked to increase risk of osteoporosis among cisgender women—while one in four experiences significant loss of bone density during late adulthood, the rate is only one in twenty for cisgender men. Behavioral factors are also significant. Cisgender women of all racial and ethnic groups tend to seek out health services more often than their male counterparts. Cisgender women are also more likely to engage in preventative health behaviors (e.g., vaccines and health screenings) and to follow advice from medical professionals.

Other important differences in health status have also been noted among different elderly populations by racial and ethnic identity, sexual orientation, gender identity, educational attainment, and income. Black, Indigenous, and Hispanic/Latinx/Chicanx (HLC) seniors have disproportionately high rates of sensory deprivation, mobility impairments, and physical disabilities. Rates of premature death are also higher among Black and Indigenous elders. In contrast, HLC and Asian senior citizens tend to have a slightly longer-than-average life expectancy; this is true for both cisgender women and cisgender men. Elderly Asians also have lower rates of cancer, heart disease, and stroke than other racial and ethnic groups; however, rates of diabetes, tuberculosis, hepatitis, and lupus are disproportionately high among Asians. Among LGBTQ+ elderly populations, certain chronic health conditions—including various types of cancer (e.g., prostate, colon, breast, testicular, and cervical)—are more common than among heterosexual and cisgender seniors. LGBTQ+ seniors are also more likely to smoke and abuse alcohol. While about 5 percent of cisgender seniors experience suicidal ideation, the rate is 50 percent for transgender seniors. Rates of sexually transmitted infections (STIs) continue to increase among seniors, including rates of chlamydia, gonorrhea, hepatitis B, human papilloma virus (HPV), and human immunodeficiency virus (HIV). They are disproportionately high among cisgender men who are divorced or widowed, especially those who have sex with other cisgender men. Educational attainment also influences senior health. Dementia disorders are less common among those with enhanced educational attainment. Only about one in twenty seniors who have earned a college degree will develop dementia; the rate is about one in five for those who never attended college. Low-income elderly populations tend to be in worse health and have lower-than-average life expectancy than their more affluent peers. They are also more likely to experience declines in mental health and cognitive abilities following hospitalization.

ECONOMIC FACTORS

The total portion of elderly populations as part of the overall US labor force has increased in recent years and it is anticipated that this trend will continue. For many seniors, wages constitute a significant source of income. They may also receive income from a variety of other sources, including Social Security benefits, retirement benefits, investments, and sale of liquid assets. However, total average debt among those over age 65 continues to increase. Furthermore, poverty and resource scarcity remain pressing concerns for many seniors.

Employment and Income

Many individuals retire in their mid- to late sixties. But others continue to work well past the age when they are entitled to full retirement benefits (typically at 65–67 years of age, depending on year of birth). Since the start of the twenty-first century, it has become increasingly common for seniors to be employed; over the past two decades, the share of seniors in the workforce has increased by one-third. By 2050, seniors are expected to comprise one-fourth of the US labor force. At present, about 12 million senior citizens work for wages. Among those aged 65–74 years old, 25 percent are employed; by contrast, the rate is only about 8 percent for those aged 75 and above. Some seniors work full-time, often maintaining jobs they held prior to reaching late adulthood; this is common among those with careers in management, education, health care, accounting, and law. However, even those who work in other industries often continue to work into their 70s and beyond. Some delay retirement a few years; others officially retire so they may secure Social Security benefits but also continue to earn income via a full-time or part-time job. Adults over the age of 60 are twice as likely to be self-employed as adults aged 25–59.

Social security, pensions, and retirement benefits constitute the most significant sources of income among elderly populations. Some also receive income from investments, rental properties, or the sale of real estate or liquid assets (e.g., stocks, bonds, jewelry, coins, and mutual funds). Yet for those who are employed, earnings represent about one-fourth of annual income. Thus, employment can help promote financial security for aging adults. This may be especially important for those with dependents. Yet working past retirement age is also common among seniors who simply wish to maintain a standard of living they would not be able to support if they only received Social Security and retirement benefits. In some cases, seniors forgo retirement altogether, although reasons for this vary. Some continue to work because doing so provides a sense of purpose and meaning to their lives. Others value the social interactions that are a common part of work life. Yet for many, the decision is based on economic necessity.

Health-Care Expenditures and Medicare

Seniors spend, on average, about 15 percent of their annual income on health care; this is nearly double the average amount of health-care spending among all US households. Expenditures related to prescription medication and medical supplies are nearly 50 percent higher among elderly populations than adults under age 65. Seniors spend one-third more than non-senior adults for health insurance coverage. Consequently, out-of-pocket health costs can consume a considerable portion of income, even for those seniors who are financially stable. Seniors with a substantial employment history and who paid Medicare taxes for 40 fiscal quarters (a period equivalent to 10 years) or more typically qualify for free health insurance through Medicare—it is sometimes referred to as traditional Medicare (TM), also known as Medicare Part A. It covers medically necessary hospitalization, skilled nursing facilities, surgical procedures, and home health care. TM is also available to seniors who did not work for wages or who worked only for a relatively short period of time, but they must pay a monthly premium. Those who paid Medicare taxes for 30–39 fiscal quarters (7.5 to 9.75 years) may obtain TM for $274 per month; for those who paid Medicare taxes for less than 30 fiscal quarters, the monthly cost is $499.

TM covers only a portion of medical costs. Those with Part A are responsible for a $1,556 deductible for each benefit period (e.g., each hospitalization or stay in a skilled nursing facility). Those who require lengthier treatment (more than 60 days) also incur a daily co-insurance fee. For days 61–90, co-insurance fees are just under $400/day; they are nearly $800/day beyond 90 days. In addition, those who wish to add coverage beyond basic TM incur additional costs. For example, the monthly premium for Part B—it covers certain medical tests, equipment, outpatient services, ambulance service, and office visits—is $170. Those who opt for Part B must pay an annual deductible of $233; they are also responsible for 20 percent of costs for approved medical services. Seniors with TM may also opt for Part D coverage for prescription medication. The monthly premium for Part D ranges from $7to $155, depending on coverage level.

Additionally, Medigap is an option; this supplemental insurance is intended to cover some medical costs not covered under TM. An individual can expect to pay a premium of $200–$2,200 per month for coverage via TM plus Part B, Part D, and Medigap. Some seniors opt for another health insurance option called Medicare Advantage (MA), often called Medicare Part C. MA includes all the benefits of TM plus Part B and Part D. When compared to TM, monthly premiums are typically lower for MA; although they do differ by coverage level, plan type (HMO or PPO), and geographic location, they are typically $200–400 per month.

Poverty, Debt, and Resource Scarcity

One-third of seniors live below 200 percent of the Federal Poverty Level (FPL). Yet under the Supplemental Poverty Measure (SPM)—it adjusts poverty thresholds based on geographic location, housing status (e.g., owning versus renting), taxes, and average expenditures for food, health care, and other necessities—at least 42 percent of seniors are living in poverty. Poverty rates are highest among those over age 75. There are, however, economic disparities among different demographic groups. Such disparities are a consequence of the social and economic inequities that persist in the United States and that result in fewer opportunities and resources (e.g., wages, retirement benefits, discretionary income, and assets) for certain groups as a consequence of the intersecting influences of racism, sexism, homophobia, and other structural barriers. While such inequities have been documented among all age groups, there is a cumulative lifetime effect. Those born into poverty and who experience poverty during childhood are more likely to be poor throughout the life span. Although Supplemental Security Income (SSI) is available for seniors who have limited incomes, the average monthly SSI payment is under $500; it is insufficient to cover basic necessities.

At present, poverty rates among the elderly in the United States are disproportionately high among certain racial and ethnic groups. Whereas one in ten of all seniors lives below the FPL, the rate is twice as high among Indigenous, Black, and HLC seniors. In contrast, around 8 percent of elderly whites have incomes below the FPL; additionally, elderly Asians are about one and a half times more likely to be poor than elderly whites. However, there are also differences in income level within broad racial and ethnic demographic groups. For example, among elderly populations who identify as Japanese, Filipino, or Asian Indian, poverty rates are lower than average. Yet poverty rates are disproportionately high—17 percent or more—among seniors who are Cambodian, Bangladeshi, Korean, Vietnamese, and Chinese. There are also differences by sex, gender, and sexual orientation. Elderly LGBTQ+ populations are three times as likely to be poor as non-LGBTQ+ seniors. Regardless of racial or ethnic identity, elderly cisgender women are more likely to be poor than cisgender males. Such disparities have been linked to the gender wage gap and the reality that cisgender women typically have less in retirement accounts and fewer assets than cisgender men. Cisgender women also tend to live longer than their male counterparts and to incur greater total living expenses and medical expenses in late adulthood.

Debt among elderly populations continues to increase. The average debt load for senior citizens has more than quadrupled in the past three decades. Seniors aged 65–74 average nearly $100,000 in debt while the average amount is just over $40,000 for those aged 75 and above. The COVID-19 pandemic has increased the average debt among senior citizens. Their most common sources of debt include mortgages, auto loans, credit cards, and medical debt. However, the percent of seniors with educational debt continues to increase. Some may obtain loan forgiveness through the Public Service Loan Forgiveness (PSLF) Program while those who are totally and permanently disabled may have their loans discharged. Yet seniors with limited incomes are at increased risk of defaulting on student loans; if they do so, a portion of their Social Security benefits may be withheld in order to offset their remaining student loan debt. This increases their risk of living below the FPL and makes it less likely that they can afford basic needs.

Many elders have difficulty paying for housing, food, medical care, and other necessities. Housing insecurity among older adult populations has increased since the late twentieth century. In the early 1990s, around one in ten of homeless adults in the United States was over the age of 50. At present, seniors represent nearly half of all adults who lack safe, adequate, permanent shelter. It is expected that the number of homeless seniors will nearly triple in the coming decade. In addition, food insecurity is an ongoing challenge for many seniors. Although rates of food insecurity are lower on average among seniors than among the overall US populations, at least 3 million individuals over the age of 65 live in a food insecure household. Food insecurity and related caloric deficits and nutritional deficiencies (e.g., protein, iron, calcium, and vitamin C) are most common among those who live alone, reside in rural areas, or have multiple chronic health conditions. Rates are also disproportionately high among cisgender women; Black, Indigenous, and People of Color (BIPOC) populations; and LGBTQ+ populations. Community food banks can help seniors better meet their nutritional needs. Yet issues with access to such facilities, available quantities and types of foods (e.g., dairy alternatives for those with food allergies/sensitivities), and limited supply persist.

Medical expenses and related debt are burdens for many seniors, even for those with health insurance. Among US households headed by a senior citizen, health-care spending averages $7,000 per year. Health care represents one of the most significant categories of spending among seniors, second only to housing. One-third of seniors do not have enough in savings or other liquid assets to cover a medical emergency. Households headed by seniors are somewhat less likely to have unpaid medical debt than households headed by those under age 65. Yet nearly 5 million seniors—roughly one in four—have unpaid medical debt. Such debt is disproportionately high among cisgender women; Black, HLC, and Indigenous populations; those with chronic health conditions; LGBTQ+ populations; and those with incomes below 200 percent of the FPL.

EDUCATIONAL ACCESS AND QUALITY

Senior citizens living in the twenty-first century are more likely to have successfully completed high school and earned a college degree than previous generations. However, they tend to be less educated than adults in their 40s and 50s. Advanced educational attainment is associated with a variety of physical, mental, cognitive, and social benefits for those in late adulthood. Educational programs for senior citizens continue to expand in both number and scope. However, economic, social, and literacy-related challenges pose barriers to education for many senior citizens.

Educational Attainment

At present, elderly populations have higher rates of educational attainment than among previous generations. Ninety percent have earned a high school degree. In addition, it is increasingly common for seniors to have attended college during their lifetime. In the mid-twentieth century, only about one in twenty individuals aged 65 and over held a bachelor's degree; at present, the rate is nearly one in three. However, those who are part of the baby boomer generation (born between 1946 and 1964) are less likely to hold any type of postsecondary degree (e.g., associate's, bachelor's, master's, and doctoral) than adults aged 25–64. It has long been recognized that advanced educational attainment has a protective effect on health and well-being. Senior citizens who have not earned a high school diploma are more likely than their more educated peers to die prematurely (i.e., prior to ALE). In addition, those who have earned an undergraduate degree live about 8 years longer than those who do not. ALE is highest among those who have earned a graduate degree; on average, those who hold such degrees live 14 years longer than their less educated peers. Increased educational attainment is also associated with better health. Senior citizens who have earned a college degree have slower rates of cognitive aging as well as improved overall mental health when compared to their less-educated peers. Those with college degrees are also less likely to develop dementia disorders. It is unclear, however, if this is due to the impact that education has on the neurological system or due to the fact that enhanced educational attainment is associated with better employment opportunities and economic gains that promote a better overall quality of life (e.g., access to health care, housing security, and safe living environment).

In recent years, the number and types of education programs aimed at seniors have increased. These so-called lifelong learning or continued learning programs are often offered through senior citizen centers or senior recreation centers; such centers are funded, in part, by taxes and often provide classes at a reduced cost or even free of charge to elderly populations. Individuals may be charged an annual fee for membership at such centers (typically less than $50). Examples of classes offered via such centers generally include painting, pottery, music appreciation, foreign language, creative writing, dance, literature, botany, and woodworking. Participation in such activities is associated with an increased sense of social connectedness and decreased feelings of loneliness, depression, and isolation among seniors. Participation is also associated with an increased sense of personal achievement and purpose. Exercise classes such as weight-lifting, Pilates, aerobics, rock climbing, spin, yoga, and swimming can also help seniors maintain and even improve balance, flexibility, endurance, respiratory capacity, and strength. At some senior facilities, transportation is provided for those without a vehicle or driver's license or who do not live on a bus line; sponsored transportation is more common in urban and suburban areas than in rural ones. Some senior centers also offer lunch services to help promote participants' nutritional health. Elders who qualify for government-sponsored programs for low-income populations may receive reduced-price or free lunch at some centers.

It has become increasingly common for state governments and institutions of higher education to offer free or reduced tuition for senior citizens who wish to pursue postsecondary education and training. Senior citizens currently represent under one-half of 1 percent of all postsecondary students. Their motivations for pursuing higher education vary. Some enroll in college-level courses to promote memory, concentration, and other cognitive skills. Others are motivated by personal achievement; this is especially common among those who did not have the opportunity to attend college earlier in life due to familial responsibilities or limited income. Yet for seniors who are employed, postsecondary education and training programs can help them obtain knowledge, skills, and credentials that help them remain competitive members of the workforce and make it possible for them to advance in their current career or transfer to a new line of work.

Barriers to Education

Within the context of postsecondary settings, tuition reductions and waivers can help promote improved access to higher education for elderly populations. However, individuals are typically responsible for the costs associated with books, student fees, and supplies. For seniors with limited incomes and significant debt, such expenses may render education unaffordable. Those who can afford such education-related expenses often encounter other barriers to academic success. Many older adults feel marginalized and socially excluded by their traditional college-aged student peers as well as by faculty members and staff. Furthermore, while many senior citizens are adept at various types of educational technology, it is estimated that two-fifths of those aged 65 and over lack the basic digital literacy skills necessary to locate digital resources, identify reputable digital sources, and navigate the unique elements of digital environments (e.g., drop down menus, hyperlinks, search engines, and features such as save, send, and submit). Digital methods of communication and engagement have become central features of contemporary postsecondary education and students are required to use them to register for classes, conduct research, submit assignments, and collaborate with peers on group projects. Consequently, seniors with limited skills and familiarity with digital communication are at increased risk of sub-par academic performance and dropping out. Problems related to navigating digital platforms can also increase feelings of frustration and anxiety and contribute to feelings of low self-worth among elderly students. Some communities have programs that pair young adults with elderly populations in order to help seniors improve their digital literacy skills. However, such programs typically offer only basic help and, therefore, are unlikely to provide the type of advanced digital literacy required for postsecondary success. Furthermore, lack of access to computers and the internet can render participation in college classes impossible for some seniors, especially for those in remote rural areas where broadband connectivity is often lacking.

Challenges related to literacy and numeracy persist among senior populations. Approximately one-fourth of elderly individuals lack the basic literacy skills to effectively communicate (e.g., read, write, and analyze printed texts) and/or the basic numeracy skills needed to understand and manage basic household expenses. Among those aged 80 and above, nearly one in three has low literacy and/or low numeracy. In addition, literacy and numeracy rates are lowest among low-income and BIPOC populations as well as seniors with Limited English Proficiency (LEP), including those for whom English is a second language. Approximately 15 percent of seniors speak a language other than English at home. Seniors with limited English fluency often find it difficult to participate in educational programs, particularly as most programs—even those aimed at seniors—are offered in English. While some community-based recreational and educational facilities have implemented bilingual programs for seniors, the majority have not. Seniors who lack functional literacy and numeracy are also less likely to have good health literacy. Only two-fifths of elders have health literacy skills that are classified as intermediate or proficient. Seniors with basic health literacy or low health literacy are less likely to seek preventative health services (e.g., vaccines and screenings) and less likely to seek treatment for health conditions. They often have difficulty understanding their health status—including diagnoses, treatment options, and medication schedules/dosing—and have higher rates of illnesses and lower ALE than seniors with higher health literacy.

HEALTH-CARE ACCESS AND QUALITY

Many elderly individuals have chronic health conditions. Yet even those in relatively good health tend to use health services more frequently than younger populations. Various types of health insurance programs aim to promote access to health care for seniors, yet rising costs represent a barrier to health care for many. In addition, physical and geographic factors as well as limited access to culturally appropriate, discrimination-free services continue to diminish both access to and quality of care provided to seniors.

Financial Considerations

The vast majority of elderly adults have some type of health insurance coverage. Roughly two-fifths are covered by private insurance; an additional two-fifths have some form of Medicare coverage, including TM or MA. Of the remaining one-fifth, nearly half have Medicare plus private insurance; the other half have some other form of health insurance (e.g., coverage via the TRICARE program for retired military). In fact, health insurance coverage among senior citizens is higher than among any other age group in the United States. Less than 2 percent of seniors lack health insurance. Although health insurance promotes access to health care, it does not guarantee access to all types of care. For example, routine screenings, dental care and eye care are not covered for those with TM. Additionally, prescription medications are only covered for TM recipients who have opted for part D. Coverage for health services also varies with other forms of health insurance. The costs associated with co-pays, deductibles, and health services not covered by insurance can discourage some elderly individuals from seeking care. This is especially true for those on fixed incomes, who do not have significant liquid assets, and/or with incomes below the FPL. When compared to younger populations, seniors are more likely to skip medication, go without filling a prescription, and go without health care due to lack of affordability. Economic barriers to care are most pronounced for seniors with disabilities as well as senior LGBTQ+ populations, BIPOC populations, and cisgender women.

Physical and Geographic Factors

Many seniors also encounter geographic and physical barriers when attempting to secure health care. Some individuals continue to drive a personal vehicle well into middle-old age and, in some cases, into late-old age. However, due to common aging-related health concerns (e.g., sensory impairments and cognitive decline), others discontinue driving; over half a million elderly individuals stop driving each year due to such issues. Still others sell their personal vehicle in order to reduce expenses or liquidate assets so they can secure additional income. Consequently, seniors are more likely than adults under age 65 to identify transportation issues as diminishing their access to health care. Those who reside in urban and suburban areas may be able to rely on public transportation to address health-related needs. However, this is not an option for some. It can take significant time and effort to travel from home to a bus or train stop. Additionally, train platforms and staired entrances of buses may be difficult to navigate, especially if they do not have appropriate ramps, lifts, or handrails. Entrance doors on subways are often on a timer and remain open only for a short period of time; thus, they can be difficult to navigate, especially for those with mobility impairments, muscle weakness, or sensory impairments.

Seniors in rural areas typically have less access to public transportation than those in more urban communities. They often must rely on family members, friends, and even neighbors for travel-related needs. Yet this is not always an option due to scheduling issues, particularly for family members who work or attend school. Other times, elderly individuals do not ask for transportation assistance because they are worried others will regard them as a burden. Some rural communities have implemented transportation programs as part of so-called Aging in Place programs. Through such programs, seniors can obtain transportation to attend medical appointments, go shopping, and tend to other needs. Such options, however, remain limited, especially in rural areas. This may be due, in part, to lack of awareness of grants and other funding (e.g., resources available via the Fixing America's Surface Transportation (FAST) Act of 2015) to help offset costs of such services. Yet even when they do exist, transportation programs for aging populations often operate irregularly due to staffing shortages and/or inclement weather (e.g., heavy snowfall in northern states).

The physical features of health-care facilities can also impede access to care. Under the Americans with Disabilities Act (ADA), health-care facilities (e.g., medical offices, hospitals, clinics, surgical centers, and pharmacies) must make reasonable accommodations so they are more accessible to individuals with physical, mental, sensory, and cognitive impairments. However, this does not necessarily mean that all medical buildings are easy to navigate for elderly populations. Individuals with mobility impairments and/or who use assistive devices such as a cane, walker, or wheelchair often encounter difficulties navigating medical facilities. In some cases, entering and exiting such facilities are challenging due to lack of ramps or poor condition of existing ramps and sidewalks (e.g., snow or ice accumulation, uneven surfaces, steep incline, and lack of handrails). Access can also be impeded due to lack of functioning elevators, or elevators that are difficult to use due to narrow entrance doors, buttons that are located too high for wheelchair users, or simply because the elevator is in an out-of-the way location and/or otherwise difficult to locate due to lack of clear and accessible signage. The interior space of health-care settings can also be a challenge to navigate for elderly individuals with mobility impairments, particularly when such spaces are cluttered and/or lack appropriate furniture such as adjustable chairs, exam tables, and medical equipment (e.g., mammography machines).

Sensory, Informational, Linguistic, and Cultural Considerations

Seniors with sensory deprivation often encounter barriers to health care. The text on signs and monitors and health documents (e.g., intake forms), brochures, posters, and even magazines in waiting areas may be too small for those with vision impairments. Many health facilities continue to lack large-text or braille options for print materials. In recent years, clinics and other facilities have increasingly turned to electronic devices to help reduce paperwork and improve efficiency. These are sometimes used for patient education purposes (e.g., electronic tablets used for educational videos) or for intake forms and consent documents. Yet for elderly patients who have vision or hearing impairments or have issues that diminish their dexterity, such devices may be difficult to operate. In the short term, this can contribute to increased feelings of frustration and dissatisfaction with health-care experiences. Yet it can also have long-term consequences and contribute to seniors' decreased motivation for seeking health care in the future.

Cognitive aging and mental impairments (e.g., dementia disorders) can make it more difficult for some elderly populations to understand health information. Such factors, combined with the fact that health conditions and health status often become increasingly complex with age, typically necessitate a slower pace of communication for elderly patients. Thus, it is beneficial to schedule longer appointment times for elderly populations in order to promote enhanced communication between them and health providers. But within the fast-paced, profit-driven, and chronically understaffed US health-care system, the average length of an office visit with a primary care physician is less than 16 minutes. Many seniors report feeling rushed by medical providers and that they leave their appointments without a clear understanding of their health conditions and treatment options. In addition, linguistic and cultural factors continue to impede access to care for many seniors, including those classified as LEP. Although there has been increasing attention to the importance of providing language access services (LAS) in health-care settings, availability and quality of such services remain insufficient to meet demand. In addition, cultural differences impact attitudes about body language and touch (e.g., handshakes, hugs, and eye contact), diet, treatment options, communication, and who should provide medical care (e.g., gender norms among Muslims). Despite this, many health-care providers are not adequately trained in principles and methods of culturally competent care. Thus, lack of responsiveness to the unique cultural needs of elderly patients continues to impede their access to health care.

One of the most obvious and pervasive demonstrations of lack of culturally appropriate care is ageism. This refers to beliefs about and resulting actions toward elderly populations that are based on stereotypes, assumptions, or even discrimination. Health providers may, for example, disregard complaints of physical pain from elderly patients by attributing such pain to the aging process rather than performing a physical exam. Consequently, underlying health issues (e.g., musculoskeletal disorders, arthritis, and cancer) may remain undiagnosed until the condition has become more advanced. Similarly, many health-care providers do not address issues of sexuality with elderly patients, often because providers are embarrassed, or they assume senior citizens are not sexually active. In other cases, providers have not been adequately trained to understand the specific sexual health needs of elderly populations, especially LGBTQ+ seniors. Approximately half of seniors are sexually active. However, many think they no longer need to engage in safe-sex practices because pregnancy is not possible after menopause or they believe their risk of contracting an STI is low. Additionally, many elders are uncomfortable discussing issues of sexuality, especially safe-sex practices. Since 2014, rates of STIs have more than doubled among elderly populations. The most common STIs among elderly populations include gonorrhea, chlamydia, HIV, genital herpes, syphilis, and human papilloma virus (HPV).

Other common examples of ageism within health-care settings include providers talking down to elderly patients (e.g., using a tone and words that demean or infantilize them); speaking to family members rather than to the patient; characterizing elderly patients as demanding or difficult; and making elderly patients wait longer to receive treatment than younger patients. Failure to provide culturally competent care to seniors can impair their physical and mental health; it can also diminish their trust in providers. Seniors who lack access to non-discriminatory, culturally competent care are less likely to provide accurate information to health-care providers, adhere to prescribed treatment, and seek preventative care.

LIVING ENVIRONMENT AND SOCIAL CONTEXT

Definitions of old age and experiences of late adulthood vary considerably by time period, geographic location, and even in relation to various social identities. Within the United States, one of the most prevalent factors that influences meaning of late adulthood and attitudes about senior citizens is societal attitudes toward elderly populations. Negative stereotypes of older adults can be found in various forms of media and popular culture. Such stereotypes are evidence of ageism and have been linked to the ongoing social marginalization and exclusion of senior populations as well as to types of neglect, violence, and other types of abuse. Although a healthy living environment and supportive community can help promote good health for senior citizens, those who lack such things are at increased risk of poor health, disability, and death.

Meanings and Experiences of Old Age

Social definitions of late adulthood vary considerably. The United Nations has adopted a global definition that deems anyone aged 60 or older to be elderly. Yet definitions vary considerably from one culture to another; in nations with lower-than-average life expectancy, those who have reached their mid-40s are often considered elderly while in countries with longer life expectancy, an individual is not regarded as senior citizens until they have reached their 70s. Within the context of the United States, medical literature, health practitioners, and social institutions often use different guidelines for defining elderly populations. In some cases, adults over 74 years of age are deemed seniors; in other cases, adults aged 65–74 who have significant health issues or functional impairments (including both physical and cognitive) are also included. Other times, elderly is used to refer to anyone who is at least 60 years of age. Furthermore, medical professionals who specialize in aging adult populations—known as gerontologists and geriatricians—often distinguish between different phases of late adulthood based on age: early-old age occurs from ages 65 to 74; middle-old age includes the period from 75 to 84 years of age; finally, late-old age refers to the period of life from 85 years and beyond. Stages of late adulthood are also sometimes defined in accordance with levels of autonomy, physical capacity, and cognitive function and corresponding stages of independence, interdependence, and dependence.

Typically, seniors move from independence to interdependence and then to dependence, thereby requiring additional levels of support and assistance as they age in order to help address health, financial, and social needs. Dependence and related need for substantial support are especially common during the final years of life. Yet not all seniors move through these stages in the same way. Those with disabilities, chronic health issues, and cognitive impairments typically require a greater deal of support and assistance throughout late adulthood and, therefore, are less likely to have periods of independence during this portion of their lives. In contrast, those who are in excellent physical and mental health and have a rewarding social life may reach the end of life without entering a stage of dependency. Yet others may have periods of dependence following a serious illness or accident but then encounter subsequent periods of independence or interdependence after recovery. Aging is not, after all, a linear process or experience.

Ageism in US Society

Attitudes and actions that demean and devalue senior populations are well documented. They reflect youth-focused, anti-aging values that are prominent in US society. Such values are evident in media and popular culture. Senior citizens are underrepresented in mainstream film and television. When they are included, they are most often white, cisgender males. Among all seniors in popular films and television shows, only one-third are cisgender women and one-fourth are Black, HLC, Asian, Indigenous, or of mixed race. Elderly LGBTQ+ characters in any role (leading or supporting) are nearly invisible and appear in less than 2 percent of all films and television shows. In addition, the vast majority of senior characters are part of the supporting cast rather than main characters and they seldom have speaking parts. When seniors are cast in leading roles, the plot tends to focus on end of life issues, struggles with maintaining independence in late adulthood, dementia disorders, and aging-related physical decline. Additionally, film and television tend to rely on well-worn and overwhelmingly negative stereotypes that depict seniors as mentally incompetent, physically frail, asexual, in poor health, lonely, and as a burden to their families and to society. Common caricatures of elderly individuals found in media and popular culture include the perpetually grumpy elderly man; the lovable-but-incoherent grandmother; the elderly villain; the scheming elder who is trying to break the rules (e.g., stay out past curfew at the assisted living facility); the elderly victim; and the ill-but-rebellious senior who throws caution to the wind in an effort to fulfill their dying wish. Such caricatures are also present in children's literature and cartoons.

Senior characters are often infantilized in popular culture; this is often done by having non-senior characters address them using the type of speed, intonation, vocabulary, and sing-song cadence typically used to address young children (this is sometimes referred to as "baby talk"). In addition, elderly characters are often addressed by non-elderly characters via terms of endearment (e.g., honey, dear, sweetie, my love, cutie, handsome, darling, sugar, or sweetheart). Some may regard such terms as innocuous or even charming, but the use of such terms further infantilizes elderly characters and presents them as a "generic old person" rather than a uniquely named individual. Such representations influence both individual and collective attitudes toward elderly populations. They have been shown to impact assumptions about the physical and cognitive abilities of elderly populations. They also contribute to the ongoing stigmatization of aging and the resulting social marginalization of seniors that permeate US culture. Such stigmatization and marginalization can be found in both the attitudes and actions of non-senior populations as well as in various social institutions (e.g., employment, politics, and health care). Yet they are also internalized by elderly populations and can contribute to depression, loneliness, low self-esteem, and decreased quality of life. Ageism has also been linked to increased rates of disability and premature death among elderly populations.

Perhaps one of the most obvious manifestations of ageism in US society is elder abuse. It is rooted in societal attitudes that demean, marginalize, and even disregard individuals who are elderly. Elder abuse takes various forms including physical violence, neglect, sexual abuse, financial exploitation, and emotional abuse (e.g., coercion, name-calling, isolation, and body shaming). The majority of elder abuse is perpetrated by family members such as a spouse, children, or grandchildren. However, elder abuse may also be committed by neighbors, friends, strangers, service providers (e.g., housekeeper, dog walker, and maintenance personnel), other seniors, or even health-care providers. Government reports indicate that 10 percent of senior citizens are victims of some type of elder abuse each year. However, like other forms of interpersonal violence, elder abuse is underreported. Elder abuse occurs among all demographic groups. Yet individuals with disabilities, LEP populations, members of the LGBTQ+ community, and cisgender women are at increased risk of such abuse. Elder abuse is associated with lower quality of life and increased mortality due to various physical health consequences (e.g., bruising, STIs, and traumatic injuries) and mental health consequences (e.g., depression, anxiety, post-traumatic stress disorder, and suicidal ideation) that are common with abuse. In 2010, the Elder Justice Act (EJA) was implemented as part of the Affordable Care Act. It provides funding to help states to promote awareness of and measures to combat elder abuse.

Living Environment and Social Integration

Quality of living environment has a significant impact on the health and well-being of elderly populations. Factors such as noise pollution, water pollution, and air pollution can reduce quality of life for those in late adulthood and contribute to increased morbidity and mortality. For example, poor air quality—both outdoors and indoors—is associated with increased risk of dementia disorders; it also contributes to various respiratory ailments such as COPD, allergies, and asthma. Furthermore, seniors who live in substandard housing with problems related to dampness, mold, and lack of adequate ventilation are at increased risk of poor respiratory health. Such factors can also impair immune function, thereby making seniors more susceptible to communicable diseases (e.g., colds, influenza, and COVID-19). Due to increased incidence of liver and kidney problems among senior populations, water quality is also an important consideration. When compared to non-senior populations, elderly individuals are at increased risk of health problems due to exposure to water contaminants such as viruses, chemicals, metals, and bacteria. Yet there is a scarcity of affordable, high-quality, and accessible housing for older adults.

Community context and social support also figure prominently in the health and well-being of the elderly. The relative age-friendliness of a neighborhood matters a great deal. In areas that provide specialized services to elderly populations (e.g., senior community centers, recreational classes, living communities, educational programs, transportation services, holiday celebrations, and meal delivery services), such populations have an overall better quality of life and higher levels of social connectedness. In contrast, seniors living in areas that lack such services have higher rates of social isolation and loneliness; they are also more likely to report feeling that they are not valued members of their communities. Inclusion programs may be especially important for LGBTQ+ seniors, particularly as they are more likely than non-LGBTQ+ seniors to be socially isolated and lack the type of social support networks crucial to maintaining some measure of independence in late adulthood (e.g., remaining in their homes). Due to the combination of limited social support and the ongoing influences of homophobia, biphobia, transphobia, and gender-normativity in US society, the risks associated with certain chronic physical health conditions, disability, and premature death are disproportionately high among LGBTQ+ seniors, particularly for those who are low-income, immigrants, and/or identify as Black, Indigenous, or HLC. When compared to non-LGBTQ+ seniors, they also have higher rates of anxiety, depression, suicidal ideation, and suicide attempts.

CHAPTER FIVE

Hispanic, Latinx, and Chicanx (HLC) Populations

Those individuals who were born in or have ancestral ties to Mexico, Spain, or countries in Central America, South America, and the Caribbean and/or whose first language is Spanish are often collectively referred to by the pan-ethnic term "Hispanic." This is the terminology most often used by researchers as well as governmental entities to gather, organize, and report data related to birth and death rates, education, employment, income, household composition, and health of such populations. However, in recent years, it has become increasingly common to opt for the gender-neutral terms Latinx (those born in or with ancestral ties to countries in Latin America) and Chicanx (those born in or with ancestral ties to Mexico). This is especially common among those who aim to be more inclusive of the unique perspectives of sexual minorities, transgender, and gender nonconforming populations. Consequently, throughout this chapter, the acronym HLC—Hispanic, Latinx, and Chicanx—will be used to both acknowledge mainstream use of terminology and to promote inclusivity.

There are over 60 million residents of the United States who identify as HLC; they represent nearly one-fifth of the total US population and collectively are the largest racial and ethnic minority group in the nation. The concentration of HLC populations is highest in areas that were part of Mexico prior to the Treaty of Guadalupe Hidalgo (1848), especially in California, Texas, Arizona, and New Mexico. However, Illinois, Georgia, Florida, New York, and New Jersey also have large HLC populations. Overall, the largest subgroups are those with ties to Mexico (60 percent), Central America (10 percent), and Puerto Rico (10 percent). At present, HLC populations are the fastest growing of all racial/ethnic groups in the United States; estimates indicate they will represent one-third of the total US population by 2050. HLC populations are diverse. Nearly two-thirds are born in the United States while others immigrate to the country. Just over 70 percent primarily speak a language other than English at home, most commonly Spanish. Yet some rely primarily on one of the various indigenous languages of Mexico, Central America, or South America (e.g., Quechua; Miskito; Embera; and various Mayan dialects such as

Maleku Jaika, Yucatec, and Tzeltal). Approximately 60 percent are bilingual in Spanish and English. Yet HLC populations share some common concerns related to health and well-being. These are fundamentally linked to the ongoing social, political, educational, and economic marginalization of HLC populations in the United States.

CURRENT STATE OF HEALTH

For decades, researchers and health professionals have been fascinated by the so-called Hispanic Paradox or Hispanic Morality Advantage (henceforth referred to as "the HLC paradox"). First coined in the mid-twentieth century, it references the gap between the social and economic realities of HLC populations and their actual health status, mortality rates, and life expectancy. The HLC paradox is most pronounced in first- and second-generation populations but decreases thereafter. As a group, HLC populations tend to have lower-than-average socioeconomic status and rates of educational attainment. Additionally, they tend to live in areas with less healthy environmental conditions and experience significant barriers to health care. Despite such disadvantages, average life expectancy (ALE) among HLC populations is consistently higher than the national average. In 2017, ALE for all populations in the United States was 78.6 years. For HLC populations, however, it was 81.8 years. In addition, HLC cisgender women had the second highest ALE: on average, they lived 84.8 years (only non-HLC Asian cisgender women had a higher ALE, at 85.8 years). Such longevity among HLC populations has been linked to epigenetics as well as health-related behaviors such as lower-than-average rates of smoking and higher-than-average consumption of fruits, vegetables, and legumes. In addition, close-knit familial and community networks have been noted as significant factors in promoting physical and mental health of HLC populations. However, during the COVID-19 pandemic, ALE among HLC populations declined by approximately three years. Various factors have been associated with this decline, including multigenerational households, large family size, disproportionate concentration in jobs that require regular social interaction, and limited availability of culturally and linguistically appropriate health services related to COVID-19 prevention and treatment.

Some of the most prominent health concerns among HLC populations include chronic diseases. HLC adults are more likely to be diagnosed with and die from type 2 diabetes than non-HLC whites. Rates of high blood pressure, chronic liver diseases, and obesity are also higher. They are also more likely to be diagnosed with chronic kidney disease, experience kidney failure, need a kidney transplant, and die from kidney disease than non-HLC populations. Alzheimer's disease and other memory loss disorders are also a significant concern; HLC populations have the highest rate of such disorders among all racial and ethnic groups. For those who engage in physically demanding jobs (e.g., custodial, construction, or agricultural labor), musculoskeletal injuries are common and can contribute to disability. Rates of HIV are also disproportionately high; most new cases are transmitted via male-to-male sexual contact. Leading causes of death among HLC populations include heart disease, cancer, accidental injuries, stroke, and diabetes. Yet they are less likely to die from heart disease and cancer than the general US population. Rates of infection and hospitalization due to COVID-19 have been unduly high among HLC populations. In 2020, COVID-19 was the leading cause of death for HLC adults in some states.

There are also significant differences in frequency and severity of chronic conditions among HLC subgroups. Rates of heart disease, high cholesterol, and cancer are twice as high among HLC populations born in the United States than among those who immigrate. Nearly half of HLC adults are obese and rates are highest among second- and third-generation populations born in the United States. Rising rates of obesity are expected to diminish life expectancy among HLC populations in coming decades. In contrast, those born abroad have higher rates of cancers related to infections of the liver and stomach as well as cancers that stem from certain sexually transmitted infections (STIs), especially cervical cancer. Additionally, and while rates of chronic obstructive pulmonary disease (COPD) are two-thirds lower among HLC populations than among Black and white groups, there is variation in rates of the disease among different HLC subgroups. COPD occurs in about 5 percent of Mexican, 10 percent of Cuban, and 14 percent of Puerto Rican populations on the US mainland. Such disparities have been linked to differing attitudes toward smoking and variations in incidence and detection of early-onset asthma.

Fertility rates among HLC populations are the highest among all racial and ethnic groups in the United States. In recent years, and although rates of prenatal care during the first trimester of pregnancy have increased overall in the United States, such rates have declined among HLC populations. Rates of preterm birth—birth that occurs prior to the thirty-seventh week of pregnancy—have simultaneously increased among HLC groups but remain below the national average for all racial and ethnic groups. Rates of stillbirth and miscarriage among HLC cisgender women are also lower than the national average and are similar to such rates among non-HLC white populations. Similarly, rates of maternal mortality for HLC cisgender women are below the national average; however, rates of complications during pregnancy, labor, and delivery are nearly twice as high among HLC populations when compared to non-HLC whites, especially among foreign-born Puerto Rican, Mexican, and Dominican populations; those who are undocumented; and those with Limited English Proficiency (LEP). Rates of teen pregnancy and childbearing in HLC communities are among the highest in the nation. Congenital malformations—especially related to the brain and spine—and mortality rates are disproportionately high among HLC newborns, although there are some variations by subgroup (e.g., lowest among Cuban populations and highest among Mexican populations).

Among HLC youth, one of the most prominent physical health concerns is obesity. Rates of obesity are nearly twice as high among HLC children as their non-HLC white peers. Such disparities have been observed as early as kindergarten and can contribute to high blood pressure, high triglyceride levels, dysglycemia (unstable blood sugar levels), and fatty liver disease. Obesity in HLC children is also associated with increased risk of metabolic syndrome, a disorder characterized by a combination of high blood sugar, high blood pressure, excess fat around the abdomen, and high cholesterol. Metabolic syndrome during childhood is associated with increased lifetime risk of diabetes and heart disease. It also increases risk of being overweight or obese in adulthood. Asthma is common among HLC youth, especially Puerto Ricans.

Rates of mental illness among HLC populations have increased by 50 percent over the past decade. Factors linked to such increases include poverty, language barriers, limited access to mental health screening and treatment services, cultural marginalization, and ongoing stigma related to mental health disorders. For foreign-born HLC populations, the stress associated with immigration and acculturation can contribute to poor mental health. However, rates of mental illness are higher among those born in the United States and are especially pronounced among HLC adolescents and young adults. However, given that HLC cisgender women tend to live longer, they are at increased risk of poor mental health due to social isolation and loneliness during old age; such risks are especially pronounced for foreign-born LEP populations. Individuals who identify as lesbian, gay, bisexual, transgender, queer, intersex, or asexual (LGBTQIA) are also at increased risk of poor mental health due to stigma and ostracism. Some of the most common mental health disorders among HLC populations include anxiety, major depressive disorders, and stress-related disorders, including post-traumatic stress disorder (PTSD). Those with poor mental health are more likely to engage in high-risk behaviors (e.g., smoking, excessive alcohol consumption, abuse of illicit drugs, and unprotected sex). Intimate partner violence (IPV) and reproductive coercion remain ongoing concerns among HLC populations and have been linked to normative gender ideologies, especially *machismo* and *marianismo*.

ECONOMIC FACTORS

When compared to the US population overall, HLC populations tend to have lower net worth and household income. They earn lower wages and more likely to live below the Federal Poverty Level (FPL). Such disparities persist despite educational attainment and are especially pronounced for HLC cisgender women and LGTBQIA individuals. HLC populations are overrepresented in entry-level jobs yet underrepresented in professions that provide higher wages, benefits, and opportunities for career advancement. The ongoing economic marginalization of HLC populations has both short- and long-term consequences for their financial security and continues to impair their health and well-being.

Economic Status of HLC Populations

There is a good degree of economic diversity among HLC populations. Whereas foreign-born Cubans and South Americans tend to fare better economically and are more likely to be middle class, Mexican and Puerto Rican populations born in the United States are among those most likely to be low-income. However, there has been relatively little change in the overall socioeconomic status of HLC populations as a group over the past four decades. The HLC middle class has expanded slightly yet the percent who are among America's upper middle class is approximately the same now as it was in 1980. In 2020, the median household income among HLC populations was approximately 20 percent lower than the national average for all racial and ethnic group and 24 percent lower than among non-HLC white households. Additionally, the average net worth of HLC households is less than one-fourth of that for non-HLC white populations. The rate of poverty among HLC populations has fluctuated somewhat in recent decades. While it remained fairly consistent at just over 20 percent from 1970 through 1980, it hovered around 30 percent for a 15-year period from 1980 until the mid-1990s. After decreasing in the early years of the twenty-first century, it increased during the Great Recession. It then declined steadily from 2010 onward; by 2019, the poverty rate among HLC populations reached a historic low of just under 16 percent. However, it remains nearly 1.5 times higher than national averages and more than twice as high as the poverty rate among non-HLC whites and non-HLC Asians. Furthermore, HLC individuals are more likely than non-HLC whites and non-HLC Asians to experience deep poverty (when household income is less than half of the FPL).

Consequently, HLC populations remain overrepresented among the poor. While they comprise only around 18 percent of the total US population, they represent nearly 30 percent of those living in poverty. They are also overrepresented among those who are homeless or housing insecure, food insecure, and uninsured. Rates of poverty, homelessness, and food insecurity are highest among HLC individuals who are members of the LGBTQIA community. Such populations are also more likely to live below the FPL and to rely on government-sponsored health insurance for low-income populations, needs-based food programs, and similar social service programs. The COVID-19 pandemic increased the percent of HLC households living below the FPL. It is anticipated that rates of poverty among HLC populations will remain higher than pre-pandemic levels for at least 5 years. Such economic insecurity has been identified as a key source of chronic stress, anxiety, and depression among HLC populations.

In addition, HLC populations are nearly twice as likely as non-HLC white populations to experience what is commonly referred to as liquid assets poverty (LAP). This occurs when a household lacks the economic resources necessary to cover basic living expenses for a three month period if the primary wage-earner loses their job or are otherwise unable to work due to injury, illness, natural disaster, or other catastrophic circumstances (e.g., the COVID-19 pandemic). Examples of such economic resources include savings, investments, real estate, retirement accounts, and items that can be sold (e.g., automobiles, jewelry, rare coins, art, and antiques). In addition, and despite the fact that HLC populations are only about half as likely to own homes as non-HLC whites, home equity comprises a greater portion of their total wealth. Thus, when they encounter circumstances that require them to liquidate assets, HLC populations are more likely to sell their primary residence. While doing so may help them meet immediate economic obligations, it can have long-term consequences and diminish their ability to plan ahead for expenses related to college education and retirement. It is estimated that only 20 percent of HLC working adults have $10,000 or more in a retirement account. Furthermore, those with limited liquid assets are especially vulnerable if unexpected expenses arise, even those that are relatively low-cost. HLC working adults are twice as likely as their non-HLC white counterparts to be unable to afford a $400 emergency expense.

Wages and Employment Patterns

At present, there are approximately 29 million HLC adults in the paid labor force. It is anticipated that HLC employees will represent 78 percent of net new workers by 2030. When compared to all employees in the United States, HLC populations earn less, are more likely to be unemployed, and are less likely to work in skilled industries. Whereas average weekly earnings for all employees aged 16 and over in the United States are just over $1,000, the average is only around $800 for HLC populations. This earnings gap increases with age. When compared to national averages, weekly earnings for HLC populations are approximately 5 percent lower among those aged 16–24; they are 21 percent lower among those aged 25–54; and 24 percent lower among those aged 55 and older. Furthermore, there are significant disparities by sex. On average, HLC cisgender men earn nearly $850 per week, approximately $250 less than the national average for all cisgender men. Yet HLC cisgender women earn around $100 per week less than HLC cisgender men. Additionally, HLC cisgender women earn about 16 percent less than the average for cisgender women of all racial and ethnic groups; they earn 22 percent less than non-HLC white cisgender women.

At present, and despite ongoing attention to the racial/ethnic and sex disparities in wages, HLC cisgender women who work full-time earn less than 56 cents for every dollar earned by non-HLC white cisgender men. This translates to approximately $30,000 less in earnings per year. For those with minor children, average earnings are only 46 cents for every dollar earned by non-HLC white cisgender men. Consequently, over the course of their lifetimes, HLC cisgender women will earn about half a million dollars less than non-HLC white cisgender women and over 1 million dollars less than non-HLC white cisgender men. The wage gap can and does have immediate impacts on mental health, particularly as it contributes to anxiety and depression and reduces job satisfaction. It is also associated with stress-related physical symptoms such as headaches, stomachaches, and musculoskeletal problems. Furthermore, it increases risk of displacement and food insecurity and makes it more difficult to afford health care. However, the cumulative impact is also significant as it diminishes resources for retirement. Although education is often promoted as a strategy for increasing lifetime earnings, in reality the wage gap between non-HLC white cisgender men and HLC cisgender women increases with advanced educational attainment: it is higher among those with a college degree than those with a high school diploma. There has been a minimal narrowing of the wage gap for HLC populations in recent decades. However, at the current rate, it will take over 300 years for HLC cisgender women to earn fair and equal wages. The gap is even more pronounced for HLC populations who are members of the LGBTQIA community.

HLC populations are more likely to participate in paid employment during their lifetimes than non-HLC Blacks and non-HLC whites, yet they have some of the highest unemployment rates of all racial and ethnic groups. Such rates have decreased since the Great Recession (2007–9); however, they remain higher than national averages. The COVID-19 pandemic has exacerbated such disparities. Immediately prior to 2020, HLC populations constituted about one-fifth of the paid labor force; however, they represented 23 percent of workers who lost their jobs during the first year of the pandemic. In fact, from March 2020 through the end of February 2022, rates of unemployment among HLC populations were one-third higher than national averages. In December 2020, 100 percent of job losses in the United States occurred among cisgender women; nearly half of those losses occurred among HLC women. Overall, rates of unemployment during the pandemic have been nearly 60 percent higher among HLC cisgender women than their non-HLC white counterparts. However, members of the LGBTQIA community are among those HLC populations most likely to be unemployed and encounter discrimination in the workplace; over 80 percent also report feeling unsafe in their workplace. While a variety of job training programs aim to help unemployed populations gains skills necessary to secure higher-paying jobs, few of these programs specifically target HLC populations or have been adapted to meet their specific cultural and linguistic needs. Furthermore, systemic discrimination remains a significant factor in hiring, pay, and promotion. HLC populations are nearly twice as likely as non-HLC whites to encounter discrimination in the workplace. Yet they often do not report such discrimination, often because they believe their complaints will not be taken seriously or fear retaliation from employers or co-workers. Yet in other cases, it is because they lack the economic resources needed to pursue legal action or are worried that they and their family will be targeted for investigation by Immigration and Naturalization Services (INS), regardless of their immigration status. Other times, they endure such discrimination because they fear they will lose their job.

As a group, HLC populations are underrepresented in a variety of employment fields, particularly those associated with higher wages, more generous employment benefits, and opportunities for advancement. Examples include media, television, film, and publishing; STEM fields (Science, Technology, Engineering, and Mathematics); research; the legal field (including among lawyers and judges); business administration and management; public administration; teachers and principals; higher education faculty and administrators; elected officials; and among health-care professionals including surgeons, physicians, dentists, registered nurses, and health-care administrators. In addition, HLC populations tend to be concentrated in industries that rely primarily on low-wage, unskilled labor. They constitute one-third of employees in construction; crop production and harvesting; food manufacturing (e.g., slaughterhouses, canneries, and mass production bakeries); dry cleaning and laundry services; and food service industries. In addition, HLC populations represent roughly one-fourth of employees in furniture manufacturing; textile and apparel manufacturing (including nearly 40 percent of those who cut and sew garments, purses, and accessories); truck drivers; auto repair and maintenance; and the leisure and hospitality industry. They also make up nearly 40 percent of employees who clean, repair, and otherwise maintain buildings and grounds of schools, hospitals, stores, offices, and government buildings. HLC populations represent 85 percent of day laborers, the majority of whom are cisgender men. Such individuals work on a day-to-day basis and without a contract, employment benefits, or promise of future work.

Many of the jobs where HLC populations are overrepresented are associated with significant health risks, including musculoskeletal injuries, traumatic injuries, and exposure to toxic substances (e.g., glue, paint, pesticides, herbicides, cleaning products, and chemicals). Many also involve exposure to temperature extremes; this is common in agricultural labor, landscaping and ground maintenance, and day labor. In addition, such jobs are among those most likely to lack employment benefits including paid vacation, paid sick leave, parental leave, retirement benefits, and health insurance. Employment patterns, wages, and benefits are key factors in health-seeking behaviors of HLC populations. Due to financial concerns related to low wages and lack of health-related benefits, they are more likely than non-HLC populations to delay health care, worry about medical bills, and go without medication. They are also more likely to either have problems paying or be unable to pay medical bills.

EDUCATIONAL ACCESS AND QUALITY

Access to education and educational completion rates are lower among HLC populations than national averages. This is true not only from pre-K through grade 12 but also throughout postsecondary programs. There are some differences in educational attainment when comparing foreign-born versus native-born HLC populations; furthermore, there are differences in educational attainment when comparing first generation to second- and third-generation HLC populations. However, and while HLC enrollment rates have increased in recent years, such populations remain underrepresented among those who complete vocational training or who earn professional licensures, bachelor's, master's, and professional degrees.

Pre-K through Grade 12

Enrollment among HLC students attending public education programs from pre-K through twelfth grade has increased in the past decade. They constituted approximately 22 percent of all students in 2009 but 27 percent of all students in 2019. However, they are least likely of all racial and ethnic groups to be enrolled in private K-12 schools. HLC families with preschool-aged children often report significant difficulties accessing high-quality educational programs, primarily due to cost, quality, and location of available programs. HLC students are overrepresented among single-parent-headed households. Furthermore, rates of poverty among students under the age of 18 are nearly one and a half times as high among HLC populations when compared to national averages; such rates are especially high among children living in households headed by unmarried cisgender women. Children in HLC families are more likely to participate in extracurricular sports teams than children from other racial and ethnic groups. Yet they are less likely than their non-HLC white peers to engage in extracurricular activities or learning opportunities such as visiting a library, art gallery, or museum or attending a live performing arts event. However, their parents are as likely as those from other racial and ethnic groups to read stories to their children, do arts and crafts, and play games with their children. HLC parents are also more likely than parents from other racial and ethnic groups to regularly discuss family history and heritage with their children. Rates of pre-K enrollment are lower among HLC populations than the overall US population; however, their enrollment throughout elementary and middle school is on par with national averages. Throughout their pre-K through grade 12 educational experiences, HLC students are more likely to attend schools that lack sufficient funding, have less experienced teachers, and have limited options for both remedial and advanced courses (e.g., gifted/talented, advanced placement, and International Baccalaureate).

Among all students who are English language learners (ELL) in pre-K through grade 12, nearly 75 percent are HLC students. Thus, there are nearly 4 million HLC students with limited English proficiency in the US public educational system; approximately three-fourths of them were born in the United States. Under the provisions of the Equal Educational Opportunities Act (EEOA) of 1974, ELL populations are entitled to free educational support so they may fully participate in public education programs and have the same opportunities for educational success and achievement as native English speakers. For beginning learners, such support most often takes the form of ESL (English as a second language) instruction; for those with greater English proficiency, transitional bilingual or dual-language instruction is typically used. Classroom instruction is often combined with subject-specific tutoring either during school hours or via after-school programs. Yet when measured by grade-level academic performance, it is clear that the effectiveness of ELL programs varies considerably by state and even by school district. HLC students who are ELL lag behind their native English-speaking peers with regard to academic performance.

Furthermore, ELL students often experience significant psychological distress; they often find it difficult to communicate in educational settings; develop social relationships with English-speaking peers; and understand basic information about school policies, procedures, homework, and behavioral expectations. Thus, they are at increased risk for chronic stress, anxiety, depression, and negative feelings toward school. During the COVID-19 pandemic, support for ELL students diminished considerably, particularly as many districts lacked adequate funding and staff to provide remote instruction or tutoring. Students whose families could not afford a computer or internet were especially impacted. Consequently, academic performance among HLC students who are ELL declined during the pandemic.

Academic performance in math and reading among HLC students in grades K-8 tends to be lower than national averages. By the time they reach eighth grade, only around 20 percent of HLC students meet grade-level expectations in these subjects. At the secondary level, the academic achievement gap is even more pronounced. Furthermore, while the rate of successful high school completion among all students in the United States is approximately 85 percent, it is 81 percent for HLC students. In at least fourteen states, the rate of high school completion for HLC students is less than 75 percent; such rates are lowest in the District of Columbia (60 percent), Louisiana (67 percent), and Minnesota (70 percent). Dropout rates have declined dramatically among HLC students in recent years; whereas approximately one-third dropped out of high school in the mid-1990s, rates were only around 10 percent in 2020. Yet dropout rates among HLC high school students are still twice as high as among non-HLC white students and more than three times higher than non-HLC Asian students. HLC cisgender males are especially likely to drop out early (at the end of middle school or in the first two years of high school). Those whose parents did not complete high school, do not place significant value on education, are not involved in their child's education, or have low expectations for their children's academic performance are most at risk of dropping out. Those who attend schools where the student population is not racially and ethnically diverse and/or where there is a paucity of HLC teachers and staff are less likely to earn their diploma. The same is true for students who have limited English proficiency (LEP), attend poorly funded schools, must work for wages, and/or must attend to family responsibilities (e.g., caring for younger siblings, aging relatives, or their own children).

Within educational settings, HLC students are more likely to be punished and to receive harsher penalties for dress-code violations, behavioral infractions, tardiness, and skipping school than their non-HLC white and non-HLC Asian peers. Thus, punitive actions by teachers and administrators have been identified as key factors in drop-out rates among HLC students. Such polices, in essence, push students out of educational settings by decreasing their motivation to continue to attend school and stigmatizing them in ways that negatively affect their self-concept as well as their relationships with peers and teachers. In addition, rates of teen pregnancy and teen childbearing among HLC populations are higher than among most other racial and ethnic groups. Title IX of the Educational Amendments Act of 1972 requires that public schools allow pregnant and parenting students to continue their education and prevents schools from forcing such students to attend so-called alternative schools. However, many HLC pregnant teens report feeling stigmatized, marginalized, and unsupported in traditional high school settings. Furthermore, parents and extended family members often pressure pregnant HLC students to leave school, get married, and find a job so they can support their child. Only about 10 percent of HLC students who drop out of high school will eventually earn their GED. Those who drop out or are pushed out of school are more likely to lack functional literacy skills and to have limited health literacy. They also face increased lifetime risk of chronic diseases including diabetes, high blood pressure, obesity, heart disease, and asthma. They are more likely to work in low-wage jobs that do not provide benefits and to live below the FPL.

Adult Education

By the time they reach adulthood, HLC populations represent one-third of Americans who are functionally illiterate. Among foreign-born HLC adults who have been in the United States for 15 years or more, approximately two-thirds do not meet basic literacy standards and do not have the skills necessary to read, write, and communicate effectively. This impairs their ability to navigate various social institutions including the health-care system, government agencies, and educational facilities (including both as students and as parents of students). It also impairs their ability to secure and maintain gainful employment. Over 75 percent of HLC populations who are functionally illiterate are over age 40; nearly 80 percent are cisgender women. Rates of illiteracy and LEP are higher among HLC populations who immigrated to the United States due to war or civil conflict in their country of birth. Among all subpopulations, illiteracy rates are highest among those from Mexico, especially indigenous groups. Illiteracy and LEP among HLC adults are associated with significant shame, embarrassment, and low self-esteem, especially in employment and educational contexts. Increasingly, community and nongovernmental organizations have facilitated programs to help promote literacy for HLC populations. Such programs can be effective. However, HLC individuals who live in poverty, lack free time due to family and employment responsibilities, do not have a computer or internet access, and/or lack basic literacy in their native language often have difficulty accessing and progressing in such programs.

HLC students are more likely to enroll in college than they were two decades ago. Whereas only around one-third of HLC high school students went on to pursue postsecondary education in the late 1990s, nearly half did in 2019. However, due to social and financial factors, college enrollment among HLC students decreased by at least 5 percent during the first year of the pandemic. Those who pursue college are more likely to attend a 2-year institution than a 4-year institution. For many, such decisions are based on family finances, particularly as tuition at 2-year institutions is significantly less than at 4-year public institutions. At the undergraduate level, four out of five HLC students who are enrolled full-time receive need-based financial aid. While there have been an increasing number of HLC-specific scholarships over the past two decades, the funds offered may not be enough to render college affordable for low-income families, particularly in light of escalating tuition. Some HLC parents may discourage their children from going away to college because they fear for their safety and well-being, need them to help care for younger siblings, need them to work so they can contribute to the household income, or because they believe it is important for the family to stay together. Such pressures are especially pronounced for daughters. Yet for other HLC students, lack of adequate academic preparation and mentoring relationships during high school leaves them feeling underprepared for postsecondary education.

At both 2-year and 4-year institutions, HLC students are overrepresented in liberal arts, humanities, and general studies. Yet they constitute only around 15 percent of students who pursue degrees in biology, chemistry, business, management, and health-care studies (including pre-health professional programs), and less than 2 percent of those in engineering and computer sciences. Consequently, they are drastically underrepresented in degree programs that are associated with higher-paying careers. Just over half of HLC students who begin their postsecondary education at 4-year institutions complete their degrees within six years. This is markedly lower than the national average of 63 percent for students of all racial and ethnic groups. Rates of degree completion are higher among HLC cisgender women than HLC cisgender men (58 percent versus 50 percent, respectively). Yet the rate of successful completion among HLC students who start at 2-year institutions is around 33 percent, over 6 percent lower than the national average. And among those who complete their associate's degree before transferring to a 4-year institution, only around 10 percent successfully complete their bachelor's degree. HLC individuals who are part of the LGBTQIA community, however, have higher-than-average educational attainment than heterosexual and cisgender HLC populations.

Rates of successful completion of associate's and bachelor's degree programs are higher among HLC students aged 25 and older when compared to traditional-aged HLC students (those aged 18–24). However, such rates are still lower than national averages. At the undergraduate level, HLC students earn only around one-fifth of all associate's degrees and 15 percent of bachelor's degrees. At the graduate level, they earn only one-tenth of master's or professional degrees and 8 percent of doctoral degrees. Rates of both undergraduate and graduate degree completion are, however, higher among HLC students who attend Hispanic-Serving Institutions (HSI). The student population at such colleges and universities is comprised of at least 25 percent HLC students; furthermore, such institutions have historically aimed to promote educational opportunities and success of HLC students. The number of HSI has expanded dramatically in recent years; in 2020, there were nearly 600 HSI in the United States and Puerto Rico. However, critics contend that many postsecondary institutions are eager to recruit enough HLC students so they can claim the HSI title yet do not adequately understand or respond to the unique needs of HLC students.

HEALTH-CARE ACCESS AND QUALITY

HLC populations face significant barriers to health care. Quite simply, and in light of the high rates of poverty and unemployment plus relatively low rates of health insurance within HLC communities, they often find health care unaffordable. They often face geographic barriers that impede access to primary care providers, pharmacies, and advanced health services. Limited access to linguistically and culturally appropriate care also remains an issue. Furthermore, HLC populations are underrepresented among health-care professionals, something that impedes access to high-quality, culturally competent care for HLC patients and diminishes ongoing efforts to promote diversity within the US health-care system.

Economic and Geographic Considerations

HLC populations have the highest uninsured rates among all racial and ethnic groups in the United States. Rates of private insurance are approximately one-third lower among HLC population than among non-HLC whites yet there is a good deal of variation of such coverage among HLC subgroups. For example, rates of private insurance coverage range from 48 to 58 percent among Mexicans, Puerto Ricans, and Cubans but are less than 35 percent for Central Americans. Only around 50 percent of HLC populations have private insurance. Prior to passage of the Patient Protection and Affordable Care Act of 2010 (ACA), one-third of all HLC populations were uninsured. While uninsured rates among HLC populations dropped significantly after ACA, they remain disproportionately high compared to national averages. At present, nonelderly HLC individuals are nearly three times as likely to be uninsured as non-HLC Asian and non-HLC white populations and nearly twice as likely to be uninsured as non-HLC Blacks. Given that many chronic health conditions are more common among HLC populations and that average incomes among HLC populations are lower than national averages, health-care costs can consume a significant portion of their household budgets. Even those with health insurance often have difficulty affording co-pays and prescription medications. Thus, they tend to seek health care less often and spend less on health services than other racial and ethnic groups. Yet HLC populations also encounter significant lifetime health expenses. This is particularly true for those with chronic health conditions and for cisgender women due to higher-than-average life expectancy. Thus, when measured by both short- and long-term impacts, the cost of health care represents an undue burden for HLC populations.

Approximately 20 percent of HLC populations lack health insurance. Another 30 percent rely on government-sponsored health insurance for low-income populations; such insurance has been shown to promote improved access to health care as well as improved health. However, many low-income HLC populations do not qualify for such insurance. Immigrants are not eligible for Medicaid or CHIP (Children's Health Insurance Program) coverage until 5 years after they are legally recognized as qualified noncitizens (e.g., because they are a lawful permanent resident (LPR), hold a green card, or are residents of certain US territories such as the Marshall Islands or Micronesia). States may waive the 5-year waiting period for refugees and asylees as well as pregnant individuals and minors. However, as of the end of 2021, only 29 states and the District of Columbia had implemented such waivers. Similarly, those over age 65 are not eligible for Medicare until they have worked in the United States for at least 10 years, and they (or a spouse) have paid Medicare taxes. Those who are over age 65 but do not have a work history in the United States do have the option of paying for Medicare Part A coverage (it covers hospitalization, skilled nursing facilities, and hospice). Yet they may only do so after they have legally resided in the United States for at least 5 years. Lack of familiarity with US social service programs can discourage many who are eligible from applying for such coverage. For LEP populations, communication barriers often prohibit them from pursuing government health insurance coverage. Furthermore, anti-immigrant sentiment and the perceived threat of deportation—even for those who have entered the United States through legal channels—continue to discourage eligible individuals from applying.

Geographic information system (GIS) mapping demonstrates that there are relatively few health-care providers located in communities that are predominantly inhabited by HLC populations, particularly when compared to communities predominantly inhabited by non-HLC white populations. Consequently, HLC populations are less likely to have a primary care provider (PCP). Such providers can help facilitate what is referred to as continuity of care wherein the patient and provider establish a long-term, cooperative relationship and work together to establish health goals within the unique social and economic context of the patient's life. However, and given limited access to PCPs, HLC populations are less likely to receive preventative care, treatment when ill or injured, and referrals for secondary or tertiary level care. In cases when HLC populations must be hospitalized, they are less likely to receive care after they are discharged. GIS mapping also indicates that there are fewer pharmacies located in HLC neighborhoods. This inhibits access to medication and has been cited as a key factor in diminished likelihood of adherence to prescribed dosing and frequency for medication, including among HLC youth diagnosed with depression and those with attention deficit/hyperactivity disorder. There are also fewer ambulatory care services, mental health services, and substance abuse treatment services in predominantly HLC communities.

Linguistically and Culturally Appropriate Care

Within the US health-care system, and despite the linguistic diversity of the American population, most care is provided in English. Title VI of the Civil Rights Act of 1964 prohibits discrimination in health-care programs that receive federal funding. It also serves as the legal foundation for requiring linguistically and culturally appropriate health care. However, there remains limited availability of trained medical interpreters to help better meet the needs of those with LEP, including HLC populations. And even when language access services (LAS) are available, patients who require such services often have to wait longer to receive care. Consequently, HLC populations with limited English proficiency and fluency encounter significant challenges understanding insurance, co-pays, scheduling processes, exam and surgical procedures, and their rights within the US health-care system. Furthermore, they frequently have difficulty making sense of hospital discharge instructions, including medication and follow-up appointments; thus, they are at increased risk for poor health outcomes and readmittance. For those with limited literacy in their native language, such challenges are even more pronounced. HLC individuals with LEP typically must travel greater distances to access linguistically appropriate health services. This is especially burdensome for those with mobility impairments, young children, who lack personal transportation, or who do not have good access to public transportation (e.g., in rural areas). For those who are employed, travel to obtain linguistically appropriate health care increases the time spent away from work and, thus, reduces income; for students, it diminishes time in the classroom.

Many HLC populations continue to rely on traditional health practices, sometimes exclusively yet other times in combination with more mainstream treatments. While this is most common among first generation HLC populations, such practices are routinely practiced by second and third generations as well. For example, Mexican, Dominican, and Puerto Rican populations often consult a traditional healer known as a *curandero* or *sobador* or *espiritista* (an individual who is believed to have healing powers) when they are ill. It is also common for them to use herbal remedies to treat various ailments such as headaches, digestive disorders, insomnia, body aches, and even reproductive problems. Haitian populations, who often practice Vodoun, may rely on traditional healers known as shamans, *docte fey*, or *docté xo*, particularly as it is believed that such healers can call upon spirits to aid in health and recovery. Within the biomedical model that dominates the US health-care system, such traditional practices may be misunderstood, belittled, or otherwise dismissed as scientifically invalid. This can leave HLC patients feeling disrespected and contribute to patient dissatisfaction, decreased compliance with prescribed treatment, and reduced incidence of future health-care-seeking behavior. Many have called for increasing attention to the importance of traditional health practices in order to improve care provided to HLC communities. Yet few health-care professionals are aware of such practices; even fewer are adequately trained to incorporate or accommodate such practices in the care they provide to HLC patients.

The values and practices found in the mainstream US health-care system often conflict with HLC cultural norms and beliefs. Many HLC populations have more lenient standards regarding punctuality; thus it is not uncommon for them to be late for medical appointments. Within the US health-care system, such tardiness is often frowned upon by providers and interpreted as a sign is disrespect, laziness, or even disregard for health. Furthermore, cultural norms influence communication and interactions between HLC patients and health-care providers. Among many HLC populations, it is considered rude to question or express doubt about the opinion of authority figures, including medical providers. Thus, HLC patients may agree with or indicate understanding of medical instructions out of respect, even if they do not understand or intend to follow such instructions. Among Brazilian and Puerto Rican populations, it is common to expect that health-care providers will form close, personal relationships with their patients. Within the context of the efficiency-driven model that dominates the US health-care system and that leaves precious little time for providers to develop rapport with patients, such populations can easily feel slighted and as though providers don't really care about them or their well-being. Health-care providers may also be unfamiliar with HLC intragroup dynamics, including as they relate to gender. Many HLC populations regard cisgender adult males as head of the family and responsible for making decisions. Thus, despite the fact that cisgender women are typically responsible for providing care to ill or injured children, spouses, or aging family members, they are expected to defer to men's authority in matters of health. Such deference may not be fully understood by non-HLC health professionals and may even be critiqued or resisted, particularly under the guise of promoting gender equality. When health-care professionals respond in such a manner, HLC patients are likely to feel denigrated and may be discouraged from seeking health care in the future.

In light of the significant HLC population in the United States, ongoing training that aims to promote enhanced linguistic and cultural competence among the health-care workforce has been presented as a strategy for promoting improved health among this population. Such training would foster increased understanding of HLC beliefs, values, and norms overall as well as differences among HLC sub-populations. It would also promote increased awareness of the importance of linguistic competency, thereby helping to promote expansion of LAS and increase the number of providers who are fully trained to provide linguistically appropriate care. Yet perhaps the most efficient and cost-effective strategy to enhance linguistic and cultural competence is to increase the number of HLC individuals employed within the US health-care system. At present, HLC populations comprise just over 13 percent (just over 2 million individuals) of the total health-care workforce in the United States. They are overrepresented in lower-paying positions such as emergency medical technicians (EMTs), paramedics, and nurse's aides. However, they comprise less than 8 percent of all nurses and less than 6 percent of physicians and surgeons. HLC populations represent only around 5 percent of all psychologists and 6 percent of therapists. Furthermore, they occupy only around 3 percent of all health-care leadership positions, including as upper-level administrators (e.g., chief executive officer, chief fiscal officer, chief information officer, chief medical officer, and chief nursing officer); program, clinic, laboratory, or shift managers; directors of human resources; and hospital board members. By increasing the representation of diverse HLC populations throughout varying levels of the health-care system, the unique perspectives and needs of such populations would become more central to that system. This would provide a necessary foundation for improved health outcomes for HLC populations. Certain community health programs have adopted this approach by implementing the *promotores y promotoras de salud* model. It relies on trained HLC peers to provide support and education on various health-related issues within HLC communities. In addition, various community and professional organizations such as the League of United Latin American Citizens (LULAC), Hispanic Federation, National Latino Behavioral Health Association, and National Alliance for Hispanic Health continue to draw attention to and work to combat health disparities for HLC populations.

LIVING ENVIRONMENT AND SOCIAL CONTEXT

Despite their increasing numbers, HLC populations continue to be socially marginalized. They encounter various forms of bias and discrimination in their communities and to live in low-income areas that lack services and amenities and also increase their exposure to environmental risks. Anti-HLC sentiments are reflected in dominant stereotypes that permeate popular culture as well as political discourse. Gender norms also shape the experiences and health of HLC populations. Although such norms they have changed somewhat in recent years, they continue to reinforce heterosexual and cisgender norms and contribute to various types of gender-based violence.

Social Marginalization of HLC Populations

Throughout the United States, HLC populations generally constitute a minority of the population in their communities, including in metropolitan, suburban, and rural areas. Unlike many other minority groups in the United States, most HLC populations—including both native-born and foreign-born—do not cluster in ethnic enclaves. Instead, they are more dispersed throughout neighborhoods and typically represent less than 15 percent of the total population in the areas in which they live. In fact, less than one-third of HLC populations reside in communities where they constitute more than 50 percent of the total population; the majority of those who live in such areas are native Spanish speakers. Those HLC populations who live in predominantly non-HLC white communities are more likely to encounter bias and discrimination than those who live in predominantly HLC communities. Commonly cited examples of such bias and discrimination include underrepresentation in religious, social, and political organizations; lack of community services specifically for HLC populations (e.g., translation services for LEP populations); public demonstrations that espouse anti-immigrant and pro-assimilation agendas; racial profiling by law enforcement officers; and hate crimes targeting HLC populations (e.g., assault, vandalism, arson, destruction of property, rape, and murder). Such crimes have increased in recent years throughout the United States.

Furthermore, bias and discrimination against HLC populations are evident in the geographic marginalization of HLC populations within racially and ethnically diverse communities. Although housing segregation was rendered illegal under the 1968 Fair Housing Act, the reality is that patterns of segregation persist. HLC populations who reside in neighborhoods where the majority of residents are non-HLC whites tend to live in the most racially and ethnically diverse areas of such neighborhoods, typically in the older or lower-income areas. Such areas tend to have fewer government service offices, community amenities (e.g., libraries, parks, and recreational facilities), retail and grocery stores, and health-care facilities. They are also more likely to be food deserts—areas where residents have limited access to fresh, nutritious food options—and to have an abundance of fast-food restaurants. Furthermore, such areas typically have higher concentrations of air pollution and hazardous waste, something that has been linked to increased rates and severity of respiratory illness and other health conditions among HLC populations.

The impact of stereotypes is also significant in shaping the experiences of HLC populations. Such stereotypes are well documented in movies, television, electronic media, and literature. HLC populations remain underrepresented in film; they constitute only about 5 percent of all characters and less than 4 percent of leads or co-leads in mainstream motion pictures. Approximately half of films do not have any HLC characters. Rates of representation are even lower for HLC populations with disabilities and those who are part of the LGBTQIA community. Similar patterns of representations are found in mainstream television programming. Furthermore, such representation relies heavily on stereotypes that portray HLC populations in a negative manner. Most commonly, they are depicted as unintelligent, lazy, relying primarily on Spanish while also having limited ability to speak and understand English, scheming to displace non-HLC white populations in the job market, and immigrants who are attempting to manipulate the system in order to stay in the United States (e.g., having babies in the United States, evading police and immigration officers, and fabricating immigration documents). There are some differences in representation by gender. HLC cisgender males are most often portrayed as villains who are involved in drug smuggling, organized crime, and prone to violence. Yet the most common roles for HLC cisgender females include maid/housekeeper or the hypersexualized and feisty Siren who uses sex to manipulate men. The consequences of such representations are significant, particularly as they reinforce ethnocentrism and anti-HLC sentiments. They are also inherently heteronormative and cisnormative; LGBTQIA individuals are nearly absent among representations of HLC populations. Such stereotypes serve as part of the ideological foundation for Latinophobic and Hispanophobic agendas that continue to permeate both US political discourse and social institutions (e.g., schools, workplace, government, and the legal and judicial system) and contribute to the ongoing denial of equal rights and opportunities to HLC populations. Such stereotypes and related ideologies have been linked to increased rates and severity of chronic stress, depression, low self-esteem, and suicidal ideation among HLC populations.

Gender Norms

Gender norms are an important component of HLC communities and identity. While there are variations in among different subgroups based on ancestry, age, and place of birth (e.g., those born in the United States versus those who immigrate to the United States), the norms of *marianismo* and *machismo* remain prevalent. Rooted in HLC heteronormative, cisgender ideologies and reflecting Christian-based beliefs and values, they have been shown to influence attitudes toward health as well as social, sexual, and health-seeking behaviors. Furthermore, such constructs fundamentally impact cultural attitudes related to gender identity and expression, sexuality, dating, and marital relationships. Simply defined, *marianismo* defines the traditional ideal role of women. Based on the examples of the Virgin Mary and the Virgen de Guadalupe, key features of *marianismo* include subservience to male authority, selflessness, a pleasant disposition, piety, passivity, chastity before marriage, and loyalty to a heterosexual male partner. *Marianismo* encourages cisgender women to prioritize the needs of spouses, children, aging parents, and other family members over their own needs. Consequently, they often minimize attention to self-care, including health care related to both prevention and treatment. *Marianismo* has been shown to discourage physical activity, participation in sports, academic achievement, career advancement, and social connections outside the HLC community. It is also linked to increased stress, anxiety, and depression.

Women and girls who do not live up to the *marianismo* standard may be scorned or otherwise punished by their families and become the subject of gossip and ridicule in their communities. This often occurs, for example, for those who are assertive, do not marry, have sex outside of marriage, have many sexual partners, or give birth while unmarried. Such individuals are often characterized in accordance with the construct of *La Malinche*. It is based on the example of an enslaved young Aztec woman known as Doña Marina who served as guide and translator for the conquistador, Hernan Cortés; she was later his mistress. Given her role in helping Cortés defeat the Aztecs as well as her sexual relationship with him, *La Malinche* is widely regarded as a traitor. Similarly, contemporary cisgender women and girls who do not conform to the *marianismo* ideal are often deemed unfeminine, selfish, and as rejecting cultural values. In recent decades, however, attitudes toward women's empowerment among HLC populations have become increasingly positive, a change that suggests adherence to traditional norms is becoming somewhat less rigid. Further evidence of such change is the fact that HLC communities tend to be more accepting of members of LGBTQIA populations than the general US population.

In contrast, *machismo* is a normative construct of masculinity. It is often associated with aggression, self-reliance, sexual prowess and promiscuity, emotionally distant affect, and dominance in familial and other social relationships (often through the use of intimidation). *Machismo* has been linked to men's engagement in high-risk behaviors such as smoking, excessive alcohol consumption, certain types of violence, and unprotected sex with many partners in order to demonstrate manliness. It also discourages emotional vulnerability and, therefore, is associated with diminished mental health. Yet *caballerismo* is becoming more prominent among younger HLC populations born in the United States. It is a construct of masculinity that promotes connectedness, emotional expressiveness, and a responsibility to nurture and protect both family and community. *Caballerismo* is associated with positive mental health and engagement in health-promoting behaviors among cisgender, heterosexual males as well as transgender, nonconforming, and sexual minority populations.

Despite such changes, gender norms remain key factors in various types of gender-based violence. Although rates of intimate partner violence (IPV) within HLC communities have been similar to national averages over the past two decades, such rates have increased during the COVID-19 pandemic. Rates of physical, emotional, and sexual violence targeting HLC individuals who are members of the LGBTQIA community are disproportionately high.

Furthermore, HLC cisgender women who are victims of such violence experience higher rates of impaired physical and mental health than women from other racial and ethnic groups. Those most likely to be victimized include those with history of childhood sexual abuse, family violence, or drug and alcohol abuse. Unintended pregnancy also increases risk of victimization. In addition, IPV is the leading cause of homicide for HLC cisgender women. Yet HLC victims are less likely to report IPV than those from other racial and ethnic groups, often because they fear retaliation from their abuser, worry they will not be taken seriously by predominantly non-HLC white police forces, or lack access to linguistically appropriate support services. In light of anti-immigrant and anti-HLC sentiment that increased during the Trump administration, others do not report IPV because they fear deportation for themselves or their family members, regardless of their immigration status.

Reproductive coercion is a common form of IPV among HLC populations. It includes the threat or use of force, manipulation, and/or deception in an attempt to control someone's reproduction. Examples include pressuring someone to become pregnant or have many children; undermining effectiveness of birth control (e.g., hiding birth control pills and removing condoms without consent); controlling outcomes of pregnancy (restricting access to abortion or coercing someone to get an abortion); or threatening to out someone who is LGBTQIA—that is, to disclose their gender or sexual identity without their consent—if they do not comply with reproductive wishes of the abuser. When compared to other racial and ethnic groups, HLC cisgender women experience disproportionately high rates of reproductive coercion, including from partners as well as extended family members. Those who identify as LGBTQIA, are unmarried, are immigrants (regardless of status), are victims of physical IPV, and/or do not earn their own income are the most vulnerable to such coercion.

CHAPTER SIX

Homeless and Housing Insecure Populations

Individuals who lack permanent, safe, and adequate shelter are commonly referred to as homeless, unhoused, unsheltered, displaced, or housing insecure populations. Official reports regarding the prevalence of homelessness in America rely heavily on data gathered during the point-in-time study. It occurs one night each January and aims to count the number of people engaged what is commonly referred to as rough living or rough sleeping. Such individuals are living and sleeping on the street, under bridges and highway overpasses, in parks, at construction sites, in abandoned buildings, or in vehicles. Information gleaned from homeless shelters, transitional housing facilities, social service agencies, and community groups that provide support to unhoused populations are also incorporated into governmental estimates of the number of unhoused Americans. According to these combined sources, just over 600,000 individuals were homeless in 2021. However, it is widely recognized that such estimates are inaccurate due to the limits of data collection methods as well as difficulties locating and accurately identifying certain housing insecure populations. Consequently, academic researchers and nongovernmental organizations suggest that 2–4 million individuals are unhoused for at least a period of time each year in America.

Individuals who are unsheltered are often blamed for their situation. This is clear in both historical and contemporary descriptions that depict homelessness as a consequence of poor life decisions. Similar blaming is evident in narratives that contend that certain populations elect to be homeless or that they could secure stable and safe housing if they just tried hard enough. Yet over the past 50 years, there has been increasing recognition that homelessness is a consequence of structural inequities. Economically, it has been linked to increasing inflation, rising housing costs, globalization, expanding urbanization, low-wages, and the shrinking US social safety net. Furthermore, both risk and rates of housing insecurity are disproportionately high among particular demographic groups, particularly those that are politically, economically, and socially marginalized due to structural inequalities including low-income communities; Black, Indigenous, and People of Color (BIPOC) populations; sexual minorities; immigrants; and gender-nonconforming populations. Homelessness is also fundamentally linked to well-being. In some cases, being unhoused causes poor health, yet in other cases, homelessness is a consequence of poor health. It is clear that unsheltered populations face often insurmountable barriers that limit opportunities, diminish quality of life, and increase risk of certain illnesses, injuries, and diseases as well as premature death.

CURRENT STATE OF HEALTH

Unhoused populations face increased risk of certain types of illnesses, injuries, disabilities, social isolation and marginalization, and violence. Such issues are associated with decreased quality of life, abnormally high burden of disease, and reduced life expectancy. Homeless populations tend to be in significantly worse overall health than the general US population. On average, those who are chronically homeless live 15–20 years less than the overall US population. However, due to the various mental and physical health risks they encounter, life expectancy is also reduced for individuals who experience transitional or episodic homelessness. While housing insecurity contributes to poor health, poor health is a leading cause of homelessness. Those with certain chronic physical conditions, disabilities, cognitive and behavioral disorders, substance abuse disorders, and mental illnesses face increased risk of unemployment and poverty. Thus, they are more likely to be displaced during their lifetimes.

Rates of mental illness are two to three times higher among unhoused populations than among the general US population. Nearly half of all homeless individuals have a psychological disorder that impairs their ability to work, learn, care for themselves (e.g., sustain healthy eating, sleeping, and hygiene activities), maintain healthy relationships, and/or communicate effectively. Some of the most common mental illnesses among unhoused populations include depression, anxiety, bipolar disorder, post-traumatic stress disorder (PTSD), and schizophrenia. However, substance use and abuse disorders (SUAD) related to alcohol, prescription drugs (e.g., opioids), and illegal substances are also widespread. Comorbidities of mental health disorders are also common and those with chronic health conditions and/or disabilities are at increased risk of certain mental illnesses. Furthermore, at least one-fourth of homeless Americans suffer from a health condition that impairs cognitive function, behavior, or emotional regulation.

Many individuals have a diagnosed mental health disorder prior to becoming homeless. Such illnesses increase risk of poverty; they are also commonly associated with reduced resiliency and coping skills as well as increased social isolation. For example, nearly two-thirds of homeless veterans suffer from PTSD prior to becoming homeless. Similarly, those diagnosed with schizophrenia or bipolar disorder are among those most likely to become chronically homeless. Risk of housing insecurity increases when mental health disorders are not effectively managed via appropriate medications and psycho-therapies. It is estimated that over 25 percent of all unhoused populations have an undiagnosed mental illness. When compared to those without a history of mental illness, homeless individuals with mental health disorders have a more difficult time securing adequate food, water, health services, and temporary shelter. They are also more likely to engage in high-risk behaviors such as unprotected sex, physical violence, and substance abuse and to be victims of violent crimes such as assault with a deadly weapon, sexual assault, hate crimes, rape, aggravated robbery, and homicide.

Yet the stress associated with being unhoused—even for a short period of time—can and does exacerbate existing mental health issues. Homelessness can even cause poor mental health as it diminishes quality of life and is linked to diminished self-worth and self-esteem. In addition, being without secure and stable housing is recognized by mental health professionals as a traumatic event; it has also been identified as an adverse childhood experience (ACE) that contributes to trauma and, thus, increases risk of PTSD throughout the lifespan. Due to prevailing social and political attitudes toward homeless populations as well as the daily realities they encounter as they attempt to meet basic needs, it is also common for housing insecure populations to feel vulnerable, ashamed, unloved, lonely, hopeless, overwhelmed, unimportant, and invisible. Such feelings are associated with increased risk of depression, SUAD, non-suicidal self-injury, and suicidal ideation as well as suicide attempts, including both during and after periods of displacement. Rates of suicide are five to ten times higher among homeless and recently homeless populations than among the general US population, especially among displaced veterans, males, minors, and individuals who identify as lesbian, gay, bisexual, transgender, queer, intersex, or asexual (LGBTQIA). Moreover, housing insecure populations are at increased risk of long-term consequences associated with undiagnosed and untreated mental health disorders.

Physical health issues are also common among unhoused populations. In some cases, such issues cause homelessness, especially for individuals with illnesses, injuries, or disabilities that make it difficult to work, result in the loss of a job, or lead to costly medical bills that make it difficult for them to afford housing. Individuals with chronic illnesses and disabilities are among the populations most at risk of experiencing homelessness at some point in their lifetimes; it is estimated that over 80 percent of unhoused populations have some type of chronic illness or disability. However, even acute conditions can lead to housing insecurity and displacement, particularly for low-income populations and those without health insurance. Some of the most common physical ailments among homeless populations include respiratory ailments (e.g., tuberculosis (TB), asthma, bronchitis, chronic obstructive pulmonary disease (COPD), and pneumonia), diabetes, hypertension, cardiovascular diseases, stroke, malnutrition (e.g., anemia, low bone mineral density, and vitamin deficiency), and unhealthy body weight (including both underweight and obesity). Limited access to clean water, sanitation, and hygiene (WASH) facilities also impairs the health and well-being of unhoused populations and contributes to poor oral health (e.g., cavities, mouth sores, and gum diseases), skin conditions, and urinary tract infections.

For those with health conditions that existed prior to becoming displaced, the daily realities of being unhoused can exacerbate and aggravate such conditions. Yet such realities can also cause health problems for those that are in good general health. For example, exposure to heat, cold, rain, snow, humidity, heavy winds, and other weather-related conditions can both cause and worsen certain types of respiratory illnesses, immune system disorders, and heart conditions. Climate and weather can also lead to hypothermia, heat stroke, and dehydration. Homelessness also increases risk and severity of musculoskeletal problems, skin diseases and disorders (e.g., rashes, psoriasis, eczema, cancer, and fungal infections), and diseases transmitted by insects (e.g., Lyme disease, West Nile virus, typhus, and trench fever), companion pets, or wild animals (e.g., giardia, toxoplasmosis, roundworm, tapeworm, and hookworm).

Sexual and reproductive health are ongoing concerns. Nearly 75 percent of pregnancies among homeless individuals are unintended. Rates of miscarriage, stillbirth, and pregnancy-related complications are nearly twice as high among unhoused populations as among the general US population. For unhoused individuals who menstruate, lack of affordability of hygiene products—also known as "period poverty"—is a significant concern. Although tampons and menstrual pads are sometimes available at homeless shelters, supplies are limited. Therefore, they will often resort to using rags, newspaper, toilet paper, or other unsanitary items to catch their menstrual flow or to simply allow it to leak through their clothes. Such practices diminish psychological well-being and increase risk of infection in the urinary tract and reproductive tract. However, for transgender and gender nonconforming individuals, they can increase feelings of gender dysphoria; for those who have not openly shared their gender identity, visible menstrual stains increase their risk of violent victimization, including rape and sexual assault. In addition, sexually transmitted diseases (STDs) are common among unhoused populations. Some of the most common include gonorrhea, syphilis, chlamydia, HIV, and hepatitis. STD rates are especially high among those who engage in a practice known as survival sex (e.g., wherein an individual engages in sexual acts in exchange for materials goods, temporary shelter, or protection). In some cases, they are coerced into such activities through threats, violence, or other forms of intimidation.

Homeless populations are often victims of harassment and violence. Over half are victims of physical attacks; two-thirds witness an act of physical violence against another unhoused person. Rates of victimization are similar among cisgender males and females; however, they are highest among LGBTQIA populations, those with cognitive disabilities, and minors. Such violence is associated with increased risk and severity of anxiety, PTSD, and other mental health issues. Physical injuries commonly associated with such victimization include bruises, cuts, broken bones, stab and bullet wounds, and concussion. Although such attacks are sometimes carried out by other homeless individuals, non-homeless strangers and police are often the perpetrators. Harassment of unhoused individuals in public places is common. Yet they are also victimized in jails, shelters, food distribution sites, and health-care settings. Furthermore, some communities have implemented anti-homeless architecture to discourage unhoused populations from inhabiting certain public spaces. Examples include slanted, curved, or segmented benches; metal spikes placed on windowsills and grate covers; uneven sidewalks; and barriers that prohibit access to parks and to areas under bridges and overpasses.

ECONOMIC FACTORS

Homelessness is, in many respects, an economic issue that stems from a combination of lack of safe, high-quality, and affordable housing; limited access to employment that pays a living wage; and pervasive poverty. However, there are other economic considerations as well including the costs of real estate and rental properties. There is a cyclical relationship between poverty and homelessness as each is both affected by and increases risk of the other. Various governmental and community programs do offer economic support to unhoused populations. Yet funding for and success of such programs vary.

Employment, Wages, and Housing Affordability

Systemic economic inequalities are key contributors to homelessness in America. The US gross domestic product (GDP) has continued to increase since the Great Recession (2007–9). Even during the COVID-19 pandemic, corporate profits rose and hit record highs in 2021. Yet the American middle class continues to shrink, rates of poverty continue to expand, and wealth becomes increasingly concentrated among a small portion of the population. Nearly half of unhoused individuals cite unemployment, underemployment, low wages, or lack of economic resources as the direct cause of their lack of housing. It is estimated that at least half of all unhoused adults are unemployed; in some cities, the rate is over 65 percent. In some cases, homeless individuals do not have the types of marketable skills necessary to secure employment. This is especially common for those who did not complete high school, college, or a postsecondary certification program. Yet even individuals with a bachelor's degree can and do struggle in the contemporary job market, particularly given that such credentials only provide access to entry-level positions in many fields. Thus, underemployment also contributes to homelessness. An individual is underemployed if they are actively seeking full-time employment but can only secure part-time work. It also occurs when an individual is unable to find a job that matches their skill set and, therefore, must accept a low-wage position for which they are overqualified. Underemployment is especially common in fields where the supply of qualified job candidates is greater than the number of available jobs (e.g., auto mechanics, electricians, construction workers, telemarketers, administrative assistants, and sales). Approximately one-fourth of unhoused adults are underemployed.

Nationally, over 20 percent of unhoused adults are employed but do not earn enough to pay for housing. Although average wages have increased steadily over the past 40 years, they have not kept pace with inflation. As a result, the real value of wages—what one is able to actually purchase with their earnings—has decreased. Even basic needs have become less affordable. Furthermore, the federal minimum wage has remained unchanged since 2009. By the start of 2022, thirty states and the District of Columbia (DC) had implemented minimum wage laws that exceeded federal standards. In 2022, in California, Oregon, Washington, New Jersey, Connecticut, New York, and Massachusetts as well as the DC, the minimum wage was $13.00 or more per hour. However, fifteen states had laws that were on par with the federal minimum wage of $7.25 per hour, while five others did not have a state minimum wage law. The current federal minimum wage is not a living wage and does not enable most employees to attain a decent standard of living that includes sufficient food, water, clothing, fuel, and transportation as well as access to good-quality education and health care for themselves and their families.

It also diminishes the possibility of home ownership for many. Housing prices have nearly doubled in the past decade, from an average of $211,000 in 2011 to just over $411,000 in 2021. Rent for an apartment is typically less expensive than a mortgage yet may still be unaffordable, especially in communities with a high cost of living. For example, the national average for a one-bedroom apartment in early 2022 was approximately $1,700 per month. However, in cities such as San Diego, Oakland, Los Angeles, Miami, and San Jose, average monthly rent was $2,000–$2,400. And in New York, Boston, and Washington, DC, it was around $3,000. In cities where average rent is substantially higher than the national average, rates of homelessness are among the highest in the nation. In states where the minimum wage is $7.25, even those who are employed full-time often find themselves unable to afford a basic apartment. For example, the fair market rent (FMR) for a one-bedroom apartment in Texas is approximately $950. Thus, an individual who earns minimum wage would need to work approximately 100 hours each week in order to afford rent on such an apartment and still have enough of their take home pay (after taxes and other payroll deductions) available to meet other basic needs. In other states where the minimum wage is also $7.25 per hour, an individual earning such wages would need to work between 70 and 106 hours per week to afford a one-bedroom apartment. Furthermore, in states with the highest FMR, even a minimum wage that far exceeds the national average is often inadequate. In California, an employee who earns the state minimum wage of $14.00 per hour would have to work nearly 90 hours per week—the equivalent of more than two full-time jobs—to afford the average rent on a one-bedroom apartment; they would need to work more than 110 hours each week to afford a two-bedroom apartment. At $15.20 per hour, DC has the highest minimum wage in the nation. Yet an individual earning such a wage would need to work 78 hours per week to afford a one-bedroom apartment and 89 hours per week for a two-bedroom apartment. Individuals who face such a severe cost burden of housing are among those most likely to become homeless.

Barriers to Employment

There are significant barriers to employment for unhoused populations. For example, job applications typically require that an individual list their home address. Many do not have an address. For others, the address of the shelter, transitional housing center, or domestic violence facility where they are staying is the only one available to them. Due to stereotypes commonly associated with homeless populations (e.g., that they are lazy, unmotivated, and dangerous) some employers will not consider hiring individuals who are staying in a shelter. While some have called for banning address requirements until after a formal employment offer has been made, most employers still require this information. Similarly, most application forms include questions about criminal history; some also mandate a credit check before an offer of employment is made. Proponents of such practices argue that they can help assess the character of applicants. However, critics contend that they violate fair hiring practices, particularly due to disproportionately high rates of conviction and incarceration of BIPOC individuals as well as disproportionately high rates of poverty and poor credit history among women and BIPOC populations. In the past decade, there has been an increase in ban the box legislation—also known as fair chance legislation. It prohibits questions about criminal history and associated background checks until a job offer has been made or, for some jobs, eliminates such measures altogether. By 2022, thirty-seven states had adopted such legislation, yet there was no federal law banning such practices.

Telephone communication also remains a barrier to employment for many unhoused individuals. While some do have cell phones, they often have difficulty paying for their service plan and maintaining connectivity and, thus, phone access is sporadic. Other times, their phones are old and not fully functional or lack smart technology and cannot access the internet. Some nonprofit and governmental agencies provide free cell phones to unhoused populations, yet such programs are limited. Pay phones once provided access to low-cost communication. Yet due to increasing reliance on cell phones, the number of pay phones in the United States has declined by more than 90 percent in the past two decades. Some shelters have a so-called house phone. However, it must be shared among all residents and there are generally strict limits on length of calls and time of day when the phone may be used; they typically may not be used for incoming or long-distance calls. Without consistent phone access, homeless populations cannot be contacted by prospective employers and, thus, are less likely to secure employment. For those who are employed, limited phone access can make it more difficult for them to communicate with employers about scheduling, illness, or other issues, thereby increasing their risk of termination.

Workplace dress codes and grooming standards can be burdensome for housing insecure populations. In some cases, codes and standards are required by the Occupational Safety and Health Administration (OSHA), particularly to enhance safety via the use of personal protective equipment (PPE) that can help guard against potential injuries, falls, burns, or sensory deprivation. In other cases, they are required by the Food and Drug Administration to promote safe handling of food, laboratory equipment, or certain controlled substances. Under the Fair Labor Standards Act (FLSA), employers may require employees to wear a uniform or enforce a dress code that requires a uniform or prohibits certain types of clothing. Similarly, employers are legally permitted to implement policies regarding acceptable personal hygiene, grooming, and appearance standards. These are generally implemented as a means of demonstrating professionalism, increasing brand recognition, and boosting morale and productivity of employees. Such standards typically require that employees bathe or shower daily; use deodorant; keep clothing clean, pressed, and free of holes or tears; wear clothing that fits properly; do not have any visible tattoos or piercings; keep nails trimmed; refrain from certain hairstyles or hair colors; be clean-shaven; and wear (or refrain from wearing) makeup. Some employers do provide free uniforms. Others, however, require employees to pay for them; this is legal as long as employees earn minimum wage. In some cases, employees must pay for uniforms up front; other times, employers will deduct the cost of uniforms from the employees' paycheck. If PPE is required by OSHA, employers are required to cover the costs of such equipment. But employers who require use of goggles, safety gloves, footwear, back support devices, or other items not mandated by OSHA may require employees to purchase them.

Limited availability of WASH facilities for displaced populations has been identified as a major public health and human rights concern but also can negatively impact employment. It not only impairs the ability of displaced individuals to obtain safe water for drinking and cooking but also restricts their access to toilets and shower facilities. Diminished access to such facilities impairs physical health, especially due to increased incidence of skin problems as well as various infectious diseases. It also undermines mental health and contributes to embarrassment, low self-esteem, and loss of dignity. Of equal importance, it can make it nearly impossible for homeless populations to adhere to workplace appearance and grooming standards. Even those who are able to access handwashing stations, public toilets, or mobile showers provided by nonprofit organizations are often unable to afford things such as soap, toothbrushes, towels, toothpaste, razors, deodorant, shampoo, menstrual products, and similar items. Furthermore, limited access to laundry facilities can make it nearly impossible for homeless individuals to keep their clothes clean and in good order. Some organizations have recognized this challenge and sought to address it by providing free laundry facilities or clothing items for individuals to wear for job interviews or to work. However, there is a chronic shortage of such services and supplies.

Childcare and transportation are other common barriers to employment for those who are displaced. The average cost of childcare in the United States is over $8,000 per child; it is significantly higher in major urban areas and some suburban communities. There are some programs to help offset costs of childcare for low-income populations. These include vouchers, subsidies, and scholarships as well as head start and early head start programs. However, parents typically must work at least 25 hours per week consistently over a one-month period or more before they become eligible for such assistance. The child and dependent care tax credit can also help ease the burden of childcare for working families. However, it is only available for those who were employed in the previous tax year and who paid for childcare expenses out of pocket. Some childcare assistance programs require participants to provide a permanent address. And while some shelters will permit residents to use the shelter address for such purposes, others do not. Similarly, transportation costs can be burdensome. Many rural areas do not have public transportation. In areas where such options exist, schedules are not always convenient and both bus and subway routes may require multiple connections, thus making them less time-efficient than individual transportation. Yet the costs of purchasing, maintaining, and repairing a vehicle, purchasing fuel, and paying for parking can render vehicle ownership out of reach. Some who are homeless often rely on vehicles for shelter, yet such vehicles are often in poor repair and may not be a reliable source of transportation to and from work.

Strategies for Addressing Economic Barriers

Some have promoted job training programs to help promote employment and increased earnings for unhoused populations. However, in light of inflation, rising housing costs, stagnant wages, and various other economic factors that give rise to poverty and homelessness, such programs alone are insufficient to address the problem. Many unhoused populations may be eligible for Social Security Disability Insurance (SSDI), Supplemental Security Income (SSI), veterans' benefits, or food assistance via the Supplemental Nutrition Assistance Program (SNAP) or Special Supplemental Nutrition Program for Women, Infants, and Children (WIC). However, passage of the Personal Responsibility and Work Opportunities Reconciliation Act of 1996 (PRWORA) has led to decreased funding for and availability of programs that are part of the social safety net for low-income populations. Furthermore, limited transportation and childcare options can make it difficult for individuals to apply for such assistance.

Others have promoted tiny homes—residences that are generally under 300 square feet and often portable—as a cost-effective solution to homelessness. Several major cities throughout the country have created tiny home villages specifically for unhoused populations. But zoning restrictions and building codes—which are often rooted in concerns about property values—often prohibit the presence of homes under 1,000 square feet. In addition, while tiny homes may be appropriate for a single person or couple, they may be less suitable for those with children due to space constraints and safety concerns (particularly as bedrooms in tiny houses are often lofted and accessible only by ladder). Wheelchair users and others with mobility impairments are among those most likely to find tiny houses unsuitable.

Sometimes, in an attempt to reduce their housing expenses, individuals and couples will engage in a practice known as doubling up. This involves moving in together and sharing living expenses. It is typically easier for single adults or couples to engage in this practice but more difficult for those with children, particularly due to limits on the number of residents permitted in a single rental unit. Even those without children may find that living with others is not suitable; they may prefer to have their own space due to personality traits or may find that living with others exacerbates certain mental health conditions. Additionally, those unable to afford housing sometimes move into the homes of family members. Yet some do not have this option because family members lack adequate living space. In other cases, family conflict can render such arrangements stressful or even dangerous. Such conflict is often a cause or contributing factor to homelessness, especially for those who are victims of IPV such as cisgender women and their children as well as LGBTQIA youth and young adults.

EDUCATIONAL ACCESS AND QUALITY

It has long been recognized that access to education promotes housing stability throughout the lifespan. Yet access to various types of educational and training programs remains elusive for those who are housing insecure. Furthermore, the mainstream American educational system is not designed to meet the specific needs of unhoused populations. Various strategies that aim to improve educational access, academic support, and meet the unique social and materials needs of unhoused learners have been implemented over the past 50 years. But adequately identifying students who are homeless and responding to their needs remain barriers to their continued enrollment and academic achievement.

Pre-K through Twelfth Grade

Education is widely regarded as a strategy for reducing homelessness. Children and teens who are not enrolled in formal educational programs are more than four times as likely as those enrolled in school to be housing insecure. It is difficult to obtain an accurate number of homeless students, particularly as they and/or their families may move around frequently. However, it is estimated that the number of housing insecure school-aged minors has nearly doubled since 2007 and some have argued that there is an epidemic of homelessness among students from pre-K through twelfth grade in the United States. Current data indicates that at least 1.2 million students under the age of 18 are unhoused at some point each academic year. Federal law mandates access to free public education for students from pre-K through grade 12 who are experiencing homelessness. Yet there are challenges in enrolling unhoused students, particularly as most public school districts require a permanent address at time of enrollment. This may deter some displaced families from attempting to enroll their children. Among those who are enrolled, the realities of being housing insecure undermine their academic success and completion rates. Disparities in access to education and educational attainment are especially pronounced among housing insecure students with limited English proficiency (LEP), who are not in the care of a parent or other adult family members (typically referred to as unaccompanied minors), and/or with incomes below the Federal Poverty Level (FPL) as well as immigrants, BIPOC, and LGBTQIA students.

Students who lack stable and secure housing are more likely than their housed peers to be chronically absent, experience developmental delays, diagnosed with learning disabilities, underperform academically, lack the academic skills required to advance to the next grade level, and suspended or expelled for behavioral problems. In addition, displaced students are over 75 percent more likely to drop out of school than their housed peers. Individuals who do not earn a high school diploma or successfully complete the general educational development (GED) tests are at least four times more likely to experience homelessness during their lifetimes as students who complete high school. Housing insecure students who earn a high school diploma or GED are less likely to graduate on time. Those who do complete their diploma often have gaps in their educational history; these gaps can range from weeks to months or even years in some cases. Housing insecure students are significantly less likely than housed students to pursue postsecondary education or training. They are also more likely to live in poverty as adults and to encounter periods of homelessness during their adult years.

Homelessness has also been shown to diminish social relationships for children and adolescents from pre-K through twelfth grade. Unhoused students are less likely to develop supportive, mentoring relationships with their teachers, school counselors, and administrators. Due to the uncertainty and instability of their living situation, they generally do not get adequate, restful sleep and this can negatively impact their ability to complete homework, remain attentive in school, and fully participate in class activities. They often do not tell school professionals about their housing circumstances out of embarrassment or because they fear stigmatization. Other times, they do not share such information because they fear they will be placed in foster care; this is especially common for unaccompanied youth. Homeless children and teens often do not have adequate coping skills to share their experiences with others or otherwise form healthy relationships. Unhoused children and adolescents often have difficulty connecting with their peers. They are at increased risk for social marginalization and bullying from classmates. Self-isolation is also common, and they may act out in immature, aggressive, or otherwise inappropriate ways due to the persistent and varied forms of stress they experience. In addition, there are substantial economic and logistical barriers that can make it nearly impossible for them to participate in optional academic enrichment programs (e.g., visual arts, band, choir, and theater), sports, and extracurricular activities.

Various policies and programs aim to promote education for and respond to the specific needs of unhoused students. For example, Title I, Part A of the Elementary and Secondary Education Act of 1965 provides federal funding to help meet the needs of low-income students, including those who are homeless. Some of the most common forms of support provided via Title I programs include reduced fee and free lunches, extra training for teachers, and tutoring programs. Improved access to free lunch was promoted by the Community Eligibility Provision of the 2010 Hunger-Free Kids Act. In 1987, the McKinney-Vento Act (MVA) was approved and then reauthorized under the parameters of the Every Student Succeeds Act (ESSA) of 2015 (specifically Title IX, Part A). MVA requires local educational agencies to have a liaison dedicated to homeless youth. The liaison is responsible for ensuring students get enrolled and remain enrolled, receive appropriate academic support, and receive free transportation to and from school. Furthermore, some volunteer groups provide academic support to students in shelters. Such measures are important. But they fail to reach all unhoused students—especially those who are not staying in shelters or transitional housing and/or who are not already enrolled in school—and do not fully address the scope or severity of the myriad challenges faced by such students.

Adult Populations

Educational attainment and literacy rates among adult homeless populations are lower than among the general US adult population. Although some individuals with advanced education can and do experience homelessness, rates are disproportionately high among those who lack a high school diploma or GED. It is estimated that between 20 and 40 percent of housing insecure adult populations are illiterate or lack basic functional literacy; rates are highest among those with mental illness and/or who experienced housing insecurity during childhood. Individuals are said to be illiterate if they lack even basic skills related to reading, writing, and numerical expression. In contrast, an individual is functionally illiterate if they have some level of ability in these areas but have not developed beyond basic reading, writing, and calculation skills. Thus, they often find it difficult to conduct tasks related to locating and applying for jobs, navigating public transportation, managing personal finances, completing employment tasks, shopping, understanding governmental or community support programs available to them, and other activities that require functional literacy. They are also less likely to have adequate health literacy and, therefore, to find it more difficult to understand prevention and treatment protocols related to diet, exercise, hygiene, and diseases. Many shelters and community programs provide free literacy classes for homeless populations. Such classes are most effective when taught by those well versed in the dynamic and interconnected academic, personal, financial, and health needs of such populations.

Yet not all homeless adults struggle with literacy. In fact, a growing portion of America's homeless population are young adults who are attending college. Nearly 15 percent of those attending two-year and four-year public institutions are homeless. It is common for them to sleep in their cars, tents, homeless shelters, parks, or structures not intended for habitation (including parking structures, storage units, or even academic buildings). However, as a result of the broader economic challenges wrought by the COVID-19 pandemic as well as increasing rates of tuition and other academic-related costs across the country, an increasing number of college students are experiencing basic needs insecurity, including food, shelter, clothing, and medical care. In 2021, over 40 percent of all enrolled undergraduate students in the United States were unable to afford rent, utilities, or other costs associated with housing. Rates are highest among LGBTQIA and BIPOC students; cisgender college women are also somewhat more likely to experience housing insecurity than their cisgender male peers. Such housing insecurity is associated with a variety of health problems for college students and contributes to increased rates of stress, anxiety, depression, sleep disorders, and malnutrition. They are also somewhat more likely to engage in high-risk behaviors related to sexual activity as well as use and abuse of alcohol, tobacco, prescription medication, and illicit drugs. However, it also impairs their social relationships and diminishes academic performance. Thus, it increases their risk of academic probation and suspension. In recent years, postsecondary institutions have made a concerted effort to better understand and respond to the needs of students experiencing basic needs insecurity. Among the most common are campus food pantries, scholarships, and waivers for exam fees or campus housing deposits. Some campuses have also adopted "safe parking programs" that permit unhoused students to park on campus and sleep in their cars overnight; students who do so also have access to campus restrooms, libraries, computing facilities, and Wi-Fi.

There are a variety of educational and vocational training programs for homeless and housing insecure adults. Some focus on a specific subgroup (e.g., veterans, LEP populations, or those who lack functional literacy) while others are open to all populations. Typically, such programs focus on literacy, numeracy, GED preparation, basic computer skills, independent living skills (e.g., creating and managing a household budget, organizing a schedule, and making appointments), and social skills (e.g., self-confidence, communication skills, and interpersonal relationships). Yet many offer job training and work readiness skills to help individuals increase their employability. Internships, transitional employment, and job-specific training (e.g., effective communication skills for those who will work in customer service positions) are also common. Such programs can help individuals secure employment. Yet the training they receive typically only qualifies them for entry-level jobs that do not pay a living wage.

HEALTH-CARE ACCESS AND QUALITY

There is a significant need for health-care services among housing insecure population. Rates of serious chronic health conditions including cardiovascular diseases, diabetes, HIV/AIDS, and respiratory disorders as well as various types of acute illnesses are approximately three times as high among homeless populations as among the general US population. Similarly, rates of disabilities, SUAD, and mental illness are markedly higher among displaced populations. Yet the health care available to homeless individuals is often substandard due to a variety of economic, geographic, informational, and physical barriers. Additionally, such populations are often stigmatized and unwelcomed in health-care settings. Such factors not only diminish the quality of care they receive but also discourage them from seeking care in the future and, therefore, can further diminish their health.

Issues of Access

One of the key barriers that homeless populations face in relation to health care is diminished access. In some cases, this stems from geographic issues. In light of their economic realities, free health services are the most common source of health care for homeless populations. Yet such services are often not evenly distributed over geographic areas, and many operate on a limited schedule due to lack of adequate staffing, funding, and space. While free clinics are more common in major urban areas, they are less common in suburban and rural communities. Consequently, homeless populations in suburban and rural communities who lack private transportation or who must rely on public transportation often have a more difficult time accessing such services. Yet even in urban areas, access is a problem. Free clinics are often not centrally located; thus, it may require considerable time for someone to travel from the area of the city where they are staying to a free health clinic. Many simply cannot afford to pay for a cab or bus fare. Those with companion pets may not have a safe location to leave their pet while they travel to health clinics. Furthermore, the demand for free health services can be high in urban areas and, consequently, it is common for such clinics to have lengthy waiting lists. The time associated with traveling to clinics and waiting for health services can be incredibly burdensome and leaves little time for homeless individuals to engage in the efforts necessary to try to meet their basic needs. Geographic barriers are especially burdensome for those with mobility impairments as well as those who are caring for young children or elderly family members. Consequently, many unhoused populations simply go without health care until there is a health crisis and they must seek emergency care.

A number of strategies have been utilized in an effort to expand access to health care for homeless populations. Some homeless shelters and transitional housing facilities have added small, on-site health clinics; these offer basic care for minor injuries and common illnesses (e.g., colds, the flu, respiratory infections, diarrheal diseases, and STDs). Others partner with Health Care for the Homeless (HCH) facilities in an effort to promote better access to health services. Some communities have partnered with medical schools and various social service and health agencies to create mobile clinics or hold community health fair events that provide vaccines, dental check-ups, eye checks, and other types of basic care to unhoused individuals. Such options can help diminish geographic barriers to care. Yet given that homeless populations may be difficult to identify and that their health needs extend far beyond what can be addressed by basic services, such strategies yield only limited results.

Affordability and Health Insurance Coverage

Like other low-income populations, those who are homeless and housing insecure have a difficult time paying for health care. They are more likely than housed populations to require ongoing care for both acute and chronic conditions as well as to require emergency care and inpatient care. Consequently, the costs associated with health care for housing insecure and unhoused populations are significantly higher than national averages when measured on a per-visit average. However, such averages are also skewed by the fact that unhoused populations rely heavily on emergency care services. Nationally, just over one-third of patients seen in emergency rooms are displaced. Annually, those experiencing homelessness accumulate emergency health-care expenses that are nearly three times higher than among housed patients receiving Medicaid.

Prior to the passage of the Patient Protection and Affordable Care Act of 2010 (ACA), most homeless adults did not qualify for government-sponsored health insurance. Under the provisions of the ACA, however, states could opt to expand Medicaid coverage to adults with incomes up to 138 percent of the FPL, regardless of age, pregnancy status, or disability status. Medicaid expansion programs were implemented in thirty-one states as well as DC. In the ensuing years, the number of homeless adults receiving Medicaid gradually increased. By 2018, less than one-fourth of adults in expansion states were uninsured; in contrast, the rate was approximately two-thirds in non-expansion states. In addition, in states with expanded coverage, the costs associated with providing health care to homeless adults decreased while associated revenues increased. Expanded Medicaid coverage has been noted as especially important in supporting services available via HCH clinics. Other gains include improved quality of care; access to preventative, surgical, dental, and ophthalmological services; and improved training to help providers better meet the unique and complex needs of homeless populations.

Despite such gains, and as part of ongoing efforts to dismantle the ACA, the Trump administration introduced a provision that allowed states to incorporate work requirements for those receiving Medicaid. The provision, initiated in 2018 via the US Department of Health and Human Services, applied to all adults who were not disabled, elderly, or pregnant and mandated that they are employed or engage in preapproved volunteer assignments (sometimes referred to as community engagement assignments) or job training for a minimum number of hours per month (typically 80 or more). The provision did allow states to provide exceptions for those deemed too medically frail to work. However, this exception was widely recognized as far too narrow, particularly as it excluded many with mental health disorders as well as certain physical conditions. Furthermore, some states did not include such exceptions. In Arkansas, nearly 20,000 people lost Medicaid coverage in the first year after the mandatory work requirement was implemented. In addition, and despite evidence that reducing Medicaid coverage would diminish public health and increase rates of homelessness, the Trump administration proposed a federal work requirement for all states who wished to continue to access Medicaid funding. Such mandates were legally blocked by district courts in some states, yet they were approved in others and the issue was slated to go to the US Supreme Court. Ultimately, the Biden administration took action to reverse the work requirement; thus, the court never heard arguments in the case. Yet the issue of Medicaid coverage for homeless populations is far from over, particularly as future administrations could simply reinstate mandatory work provisions or other requirements that limit eligibility.

Stigma, Biases, and Quality of Care

It is common for homeless individuals to report feeling stigmatized within health-care settings. In fact, they identify biases as one of their most prominent barriers to care. Such biases are evident in the organization of the health-care system, including in the lack of facilities and services dedicated to the health of displaced populations. They are also evident in the values of the health-care system, particularly as the emphasis on time and profit generally means that providers typically spend minimal time in direct contact with patients. Under such circumstances, it is difficult for providers to devote appropriate time to getting to know patients and fully understanding the range of factors that influence their health. Given that many homeless individuals are distrustful of authority figures—including health-care providers—it often requires additional time and attention in order to develop the type of rapport with them that is an essential component of effective patient-provider communication.

Furthermore, most health-care professionals have not been adequately trained to understand and meet the needs of displaced populations. For example, many health professionals do not recognize common signs of homelessness or understand the unique challenges that homeless populations face with regard to following treatment plans. Thus, they often lack awareness of how seemingly small things such as prescribing medication that needs to be refrigerated or requiring patients to make appointments via telephone or requiring them to return to the clinic to receive test results can be unduly burdensome for those who are homeless. Rooted in implicit bias, lack of awareness is not intentionally malicious. Yet it can and does diminish the quality of care provided to those who are housing insecure. Other examples include lack of awareness about the full range of community services available to displaced populations; misinterpreting difficulty keeping appointments as a sign of disrespect; or being unaware of the extent of housing insecurity in the community in which they practice.

Yet other times, health professionals are aware of their bias and actively discriminate against patients who are displaced. For example, some may refuse to treat homeless patients because they believe that providing care to them is a waste of resources or because they regard them as inherently difficult to work with (e.g., they believe they exaggerate pain symptoms and otherwise scheme in an attempt to obtain prescription medications that they do not really need). Others may judge the choices that homeless patients make, blame them for their poor health, or ask homeless patients to leave the care facility because of the way they look or because they have noticeable body odor. Such behaviors are especially common among health-care providers when treating displaced patients who use illicit drugs, trade sex for temporary shelter or food, or otherwise engage in activities that are illegal or that the provider regards as immoral. Other commonly cited examples of explicit bias include disregard for patient modesty; failure to honor principles of informed consent and medical ethics (e.g., not explaining exam procedures, diagnosis, or the full range of treatment options); making them wait longer to receive care than housed patients; and speaking to or otherwise treating patients who are homeless in a disrespectful or demeaning manner. In addition, a practice known as "patient dumping" reflects explicit bias. It involves discharging a patient because they cannot afford care yet failing to provide them with an appropriate treatment plan or resources to help promote their recovery. Consequently, such patients are left without adequate shelter, food, water, clothing, and necessary medication as well as support from appropriate social services organizations. Patients discharged in such a manner are more likely to be readmitted, less likely to recover, and more likely to die. Patient dumping is both unethical and illegal; it violates the Emergency Medical Treatment and Active Labor Act (EMTALA) of 1986. However, the practice persists.

LIVING ENVIRONMENT AND SOCIAL CONTEXT

Homelessness and housing insecurity are often organized into different categories based on the amount of time someone is homeless or other specific aspects of their circumstances. Some demographic groups are disproportionately affected by homelessness and housing insecurity. It is clear that the daily realities that homeless populations must contend with are detrimental to their health and well-being. Yet equally important are dominant social attitudes that maintain the structural inequities that give rise to housing insecurity and disparage those who are homeless. Such attitudes are evident in both historical as well as contemporary American social welfare policies.

Categories and Demographics of Contemporary Homelessness

Housing insecurity is generally organized into four subcategories. Transitional homelessness involves a single episode of homelessness that lasts less than one year. It is caused by a major life event or catastrophic incident (e.g., loss of employment, divorce, serious illness or injury, death of a family member, tornado, hurricane, or house fire). The second category is episodic homelessness; it occurs when an individual or family unit has three or more distinct episodes of displacement within a 12-month period. In contrast, an individual who has been unhoused for more than one year or unsheltered four or more times within a three year period is said to experience chronic homelessness. The fourth category is known as hidden homelessness (also known in research literature as provisional homelessness but typically referred to as couch-surfing or crashing in common usage). It is the most common type of housing insecurity and characterized by a pattern of short-term stays at different locations (e.g., motels; vehicles; tents; homes of friends, peers, or co-workers) by individuals who lack permanent shelter. Those who are part of the hidden homeless are typically ineligible for services provided to other homeless populations and, thus, are often excluded from official data. In addition to the above categories, there are special designations for those who are at high risk of becoming homeless (known as imminent homelessness) and those who are unhoused due to intimate partner violence (IPV).

Housing insecurity can and does affect individuals from all demographic groups. Even those who are wealthy are not immune from the possibility of homelessness during their lifetimes (although the likelihood of them becoming homeless is significantly less than for low-income and middle-class populations). On an average night, there are over half a million homeless individuals in the United States who stay in shelters or transitional housing. Yet estimates indicate that there are over 2 million more who are engaged in rough sleeping or couch-surfing. Approximately 70 percent of those who are displaced are single individuals (including both adults and unaccompanied minors) while the remainder are families with minor children or couples. Unaccompanied minors, families with children, and homeless veterans are more likely to stay in shelters or transitional housing than single adults. Those who are chronically homeless are the least likely to stay in shelters.

Certain populations are disproportionately represented among the homeless in the United States. Cisgender men and boys are nearly twice as likely to be homeless as cisgender women and girls. Furthermore, the majority of displaced veterans and formerly incarcerated populations are cisgender men. Such disparities point to the lack of appropriate support services to help such populations successfully transition to post-military and post-incarceration life. In addition, those who are born into poverty are more likely to experience homelessness at some point during their lifetimes. Whites outnumber other racial and ethnic groups among America's homeless, yet historically oppressed racial and ethnic groups are overrepresented among displaced populations. Rates are especially high among Indigenous, Black, and Hispanic/Chicanx/Latinx (HLC) populations. And while the majority of America's homeless are cisgender heterosexuals, LGBTQIA populations are overrepresented, especially among displaced adolescents and young adults. In addition, there are disparities by age. Minors represent less than 20 percent of displaced populations, but nearly three-fourth are over the age of 25. In recent years, the average age of America's homeless population has increased; at present, those over age 50 make up nearly one-third of those who lack safe, permanent, and affordable housing.

Historical and Contemporary Attitudes toward Homelessness

Housing insecurity was first documented in the colonial era. At the time, individuals who were unhoused and often wandered from community to community seeking food and shelter were referred to as vagrants. They were deemed a threat to safety and social order, particularly as they did not conform to social standards that emphasized close-knit families and communities. Additionally, such individuals were regarded as idle; under Puritan norms that dominated social, religious, and political life in the colonies, idleness was deemed a sin and laws were created to punish those deemed idle. Consequently, homeless individuals were either run out of town or were often auctioned off and forced to work as indentured servants. Exceptions were granted for homeless widows and children as they were regarded as inherently blameless and, therefore, deserving of community support. Widows were either supported by community churches or taken in by members of the community. Homeless minors, on the other hand, were placed in homes as apprentices or indentured servants and required to work to cover their room and board. Homelessness increased during and after the American Revolution. However, expanding railroads and industrialization meant that jobs were more plentiful and, consequently, those who could not afford housing were increasingly regarded as lazy and blamed for their situation. Subsequently, county poorhouses (sometimes referred to as almshouses) were created in order to house, feed, and monitor the homeless. Poorhouses were less expensive for the community and required individuals housed there to work (typically at an on-site farm). However, and given that homelessness was believed to be a consequence of individual failings rather than structural inequities, the widespread support for poorhouses was also based on the notion that by institutionalizing homeless individuals would reform them and help them adhere to middle-class morals and values. Importantly, Black and Indigenous populations were generally excluded from poorhouses as it was thought they could not be reformed.

Following the Civil War, attitudes toward homeless populations shifted once again. Widows, orphans, and disabled war veterans were considered deserving of assistance; thus, they were provided with various forms of support—including through civil and religious charity organizations—rather than being put in poorhouses. Yet due largely to the influence of burgeoning eugenics movement in the period, certain poor and homeless populations were deemed undeserving. These included BIPOC populations as well as those born into families that had experienced intergenerational poverty. Such ideas persisted into the twentieth century. Poor and BIPOC populations were blamed for being homeless, while a social safety net was created for those regarded as worthy of public support. Examples of such programs include unemployment benefits, social security, worker's compensation programs, widow's pensions, and Aid to Dependent Children (ADC). Collectively, such programs reduced risk of homelessness for white, heteronormative, and middle-class populations. After the Second World War, and in light of the booming postwar economy, the notion that certain homeless populations were to blame for their situation was reinforced. Again, race and ethnicity were significant: BIPOC populations were regarded as unworthy; in contrast, white, disabled veterans and their families were deemed entitled to support, including housing.

By the late twentieth century, notions of deserving and undeserving poor populations were coupled with conservative "family values" rhetoric and formed the basis for welfare reform. Such reform dramatically altered America's social safety net and reinforced racialized stereotypes of those in need as lazy, unintelligent, dangerous, and manipulating the public welfare system at the expense of taxpayers. Such stereotypes continue to influence public support for programs that aim to help those who are displaced or housing insecure. In recent years, many cities have ordered police and city workers to disperse homeless populations and destroy their encampments, often using bulldozers, tear gas, high-powered water hoses, or simply by setting fire to tents and belongings. City officials often justify such actions as necessary for public safety, arguing that homeless encampments increase crime and promote the spread of disease. Certain types of illegal activities (e.g., drugs, prostitution, theft, property violations, and violence) do occur in such encampments. Yet in most cases, criminal activity precedes the creation of encampments. Put another way, homeless encampments are typically created in areas that are already prone to crime. Thus, the presence of homeless encampments does not necessarily increase incidence of such activities. Furthermore, during the COVID-19 pandemic, the Centers for Disease Control and Prevention (CDC) advised against the practice of clearing homeless encampments, particularly as doing so can make it more difficult for public health agencies to provide support to displaced individuals who contract the disease. It can also undermine contact-tracing efforts and contribute to increased rates of serious illness, disability, and death among unsheltered populations.

Despite the prominence of such attitudes, the social movement to support homeless populations and protect their civil and human rights has gained momentum in recent years. The voices and perspectives of homeless populations remain central to that movement. By sharing their experiences, they have helped to delineate the unique and intersecting challenges they face in relation to not only housing but also health, safety, income, education, employment, and social belonging. Yet the ongoing efforts of allies have also been important. Perhaps the most influential among these have been nonprofit organizations such as the National Alliance to End Homelessness, Coalition for the Homeless, Invisible People, National Health Care for the Homeless Council, and the National Homelessness Law Center as well as various organizations that work at the state and local level to support displaced populations. Such allies have also included academic researchers, politicians, attorneys, religious leaders, and health professionals.

CHAPTER SEVEN

Incarcerated Populations

Individuals involuntarily held in the various local, state, and federal facilities that comprise the American prison industrial complex—including in jails, prisons, and detention centers—are commonly known as incarcerated populations. They are also sometimes referred to as inmates, detainees, convicts, criminals, offenders, and felons, depending on the context and the status of their case within the criminal justice system. Under state and federal laws, an individual may be incarcerated only under certain conditions: if there is an active warrant for their arrest; they have been convicted of a crime; they have been arraigned and formally charged with a crime but are awaiting trial (known as pre-trial detainment); or law enforcement officers have witnessed the individual committing a felony or certain types of misdemeanors. A person may also be detained for up to 24 hours if there is reasonable suspicion that they have committed a crime or possess information about a crime. Debates about incarcerated populations in the United States are highly politicized. Some argue that incarceration is intended to punish those who commit crimes, yet others promote rehabilitation and successful reintegration of inmates into society upon their release.

The health of incarcerated populations has been treated as irrelevant throughout much of American history. Yet it has garnered increasing attention in recent decades. Much of this attention has been prompted by ethical concerns about the treatment of prisoners and increasing evidence of poor living conditions and various types of human rights violations in jails and prisons. It is also fueled by evidence that the social and economic inequities in broader American society—particularly those that result in differential treatment of individuals based on race, sexual orientation, gender identity and expression, socioeconomic status, ability, etc.—are endemic in the US criminal justice and correctional systems. Consequently, the health and well-being of incarcerated populations has emerged as an important yet understudied area of public health. Indeed, mass incarceration has been identified as one of the most significant barriers to health equity in the United States. And while there are some health concerns that affect incarcerated populations overall, certain subpopulations have unique health needs.

CURRENT STATE OF HEALTH

Inmates are often in poor physical health even prior to their incarceration. Low-income populations are overrepresented among inmates. Consequently, so-called diseases of poverty are common among those entering the correctional system. Examples include tuberculosis (TB); sexually transmitted diseases (STDs) such as HIV, hepatitis B, hepatitis C, gonorrhea, syphilis, and chlamydia; certain types of bacterial infections; and various diseases transmitted by animals and insects (e.g., West Nile virus and Lyme disease). However, some chronic diseases are also more common among low-income populations in the United States and, thus, among those entering jails and prisons. Examples include heart disease, high blood pressure, diabetes, cancer (especially lung, liver, skin, and cervical), and various respiratory and pulmonary illnesses (e.g., asthma, chronic obstructive pulmonary disease, and tuberculosis). Incoming inmates are also more likely to be overweight, underweight, or obese and malnourished than the general US population. Physical disabilities are also common.

Many individuals also experience poor mental health prior to incarceration, and critics argue that the correctional system has become the primary method of dealing with mental illness in America. Nearly 40 percent of Americans with a severe mental illness will be incarcerated at some point in their lives. Odds of arrest and imprisonment are especially high in the year after a severe mental illness episode, particularly for those with impulse control disorders, conduct disorders (e.g., uncontrolled anger), post-traumatic stress disorder (PTSD), addiction disorders, bipolar disorders, schizophrenia, delusional disorder, and major depressive disorders. Furthermore, suicidal ideation and suicide attempts are common in the months prior to arrest; many individuals who contemplate or attempt suicide are arrested rather than provided with appropriate mental health care. Additionally, those with developmental disorders (e.g., Autism spectrum disorders and attention-deficit hyperactivity disorder), cognitive disorders, traumatic brain injury (TBI), intellectual disabilities, and memory loss disorders (e.g., dementia and Alzheimer's disease) are overrepresented among detainees. Approximately half a million inmates have some type of cognitive or developmental health issue prior to incarceration. Such issues have been documented among all demographic groups in correctional facilities but are highest among lesbian, gay, bisexual, transgender, queer, intersex, and asexual (LGBTQIA) populations; Black, Indigenous, and People of Color (BIPOC) populations; and individuals convicted of violent crimes.

Yet regardless of their health status at the time of incarceration, the unique physical environment and social dynamics of correctional facilities increase the risk of poor health. When compared to the US population overall, those incarcerated at some point during their lives are in worse health. Even individuals detained for short period of time can and do encounter physical and mental health problems as a result of their incarceration. Yet risk and severity of poor health increase as length of detainment increases. Incarceration is also associated with diminished life expectancy; each year of detainment reduces life expectancy by approximately 2 years. Common causes of death among inmates include cancer, liver disease, heart disease, drug overdose, and respiratory disease; in the past decade, however, suicide has emerged as the leading cause of death. Approximately half of those who die in jails and prisons are awaiting trial because they cannot afford bail.

Chronic physical health conditions are also an ongoing concern. The most common include respiratory diseases (e.g., chronic obstructive pulmonary disease (COPD), asthma, bronchitis, and emphysema), cancer, cardiovascular diseases (e.g., hypertension, coronary artery disease, arrhythmia, heart attack, and stroke), kidney disease, and diabetes. Infectious diseases are also widespread and are easily transmitted among high-density populations. Rates of colds and influenza are higher among incarcerated populations than among the general US public; TB and STDs are among the most common infectious diseases contracted during incarceration. Staphylococcus infections—including Methicillin-Resistant Staphylococcus Aureus (MRSA), a highly contagious and potentially life-threatening condition—have increased in recent years. During the first two years of the COVID-19 pandemic, infection rates were five times higher among inmates than national averages. Among elderly inmates, the physical and cognitive decline that are common parts of the natural aging process are aggravated by the environmental and social conditions common in jails and prisons. Such conditions have also been identified as key factors in diminished health for juveniles, LGBTQIA populations, and inmates with disabilities.

Health problems related to food and nutrition are widespread. Inmates are nearly seven times more likely to suffer from foodborne illnesses than the general US population. Some illnesses occur when prisoners consume foods or beverages that are rotten or that contain parasites, bacteria, viruses, or toxins. Yet others occur when certain undercooked foods (e.g., eggs, meat, poultry, and fish) or contaminated grain products, fruits, or vegetables are eaten. Furthermore, the food provided to inmates is typically not nutritionally balanced. It generally consists of processed foods that are high in sugar, fat, sodium, and refined carbohydrates yet lacking in protein, vitamins, minerals, whole grains, and fresh produce. Consequently, malnutrition is common among incarcerated populations and increases their short- and long-term health risks. Some of these risks include obesity, impaired immune function, diabetes, stroke, cardiovascular diseases, certain cancers, cognitive impairment, anemia, and low bone density.

Physical injuries are also common. Some are the result of accidents such as falls and slips—these are particularly common among elderly populations and those with mobility-related disabilities—or incidents involving machinery, correctional vehicles, or other equipment. Yet the majority of injuries are the result of altercations between inmates or with correctional officers. Some of the most common injuries include bruises, muscle strains, sprains, and fractures. However, lacerations, concussions, and damage to internal organs are not uncommon. Injuries are typically more extensive and potentially life-threatening when multiple attackers are involved; when inmates use knives, razor blades, rocks, clubs, or shanks (homemade daggers), wires, or other objects during attacks; or when officers use handcuffs, clubs, tasers, guns, or similar devices during an altercation with or to punish inmates. Data from governmental agencies indicates that homicide rates in jails and prisons have tripled in the past decade. Official reports indicate that rates of sexual violence—including sexual harassment, coercion, sexual assault, and rape—have also increased dramatically in recent years. Yet some nongovernmental organizations contend that underreporting of inmate victimization related to both homicide and sexual violence is widespread.

Nearly half of inmates develop a serious mental health disorder while serving time. These most often include PTSD, depression, anxiety, mania, antisocial personality disorder, and emotional dysregulation. Yet most go undiagnosed, and comorbidity is common, particularly among those who experience long-term incarceration and/or extended periods of solitary confinement. Poor mental health is also common among inmates who are victims of physical violence, sexual violence, bullying, and inhumane treatment by correctional staff (e.g., designed to cause physical pain and/or mental anguish). Those who witness such violence also face increased risk of impaired mental health due to vicarious traumatization. Over 1 million inmates suffer from substance use and abuse disorders (SUAD) including addiction; many develop SUAD during their incarceration. Rates of death due to drug overdose among inmates have increased six-fold in the past two decades and are highest among those with SUAD. The suicide rate among inmates is at least 4 times higher than among the general US population; rates are highest among Indigenous, juvenile, and LGBTQIA inmates.

ECONOMIC FACTORS

Socioeconomic status and incarceration are inherently intertwined. Low-income populations are overrepresented among inmates. Furthermore, many incur significant debt while serving time, and a criminal record has been shown to increase risk of long-term financial insecurity. The costs associated with providing health care and other necessities to inmates are considerable. And while some of these costs are borne by governments or nonprofit entities, others are incurred by inmates and their families.

Socioeconomic Status before, during, and after Incarceration

Low-income populations are more likely to be incarcerated than those who are more affluent. Prior to their incarceration, nearly 60 percent of inmates have incomes that are near or below the Federal Poverty Level (FPL). Estimates suggest that nearly half of inmates are not employed and often lack stable housing in the years immediately prior to their detainment. Individuals who are unable to afford housing at any time during their life—even for a few months—are more than 10 times as likely to be incarcerated when compared to populations with stable housing. They also have a higher debt burden and are nearly 10 times as likely as never-incarcerated populations to be homeless. Race is a significant consideration in examinations of the socioeconomic dimensions of incarceration, particularly as Black, Indigenous, and Hispanic/Latinx/Chicanx (HLC) populations are overrepresented among America's homeless, poor, and incarcerated populations. Similar patterns are noted among LGBTQIA populations.

Economic barriers permeate the US judicial and correctional systems. Nearly one-fourth of all inmates are arrested but cannot pay bail; many also lack the resources to pay for an attorney. The US Constitution guarantees the right to legal representation for anyone charged with a crime and provides special consideration for indigent individuals. They are typically represented by a public defender. However, such representation is not necessarily free as courts may require defendants to assume a portion of the fees associated with such services. It is widely recognized that public defenders have a heavy caseload and inadequate staffing. In addition, they do not choose the cases they take on and, therefore, may lack the expertise and resources needed to prepare a strong defense.

When compared to those who hire private counsel, individuals represented by public defenders are less likely to have their case dismissed or to receive probation if convicted; they are also more likely to plead guilty, be convicted, and receive longer sentences. Assistance is sometimes available to low-income individuals through legal aid centers or private law firms that offer pro bono services, yet the supply is inadequate to meet the demand. Furthermore, although the Civil Rights Act of 1964 prohibits discrimination on the basis of national origin (including primary language), the availability of linguistically appropriate and affordable legal services to low-income populations is insufficient. Consequently, those with limited English proficiency are often unable to understand the charges against them, their rights, and the legal process; they also face increased risk of conviction and incarceration.

During incarceration, financial concerns generally intensify. Although some inmates can secure employment, the pay is generally low and averages less than $1 per hour. Yet most jails and prisons do not provide wages to inmates. Instead, work assignments may be assigned as a means of helping inmates gain skills that will increase their employability after they are released. This is common, for example, in facilities that offer technical or vocational training programs. More frequently, however, inmates perform forced labor as a condition of their incarceration. Although the 13th Amendment abolished slavery, it permits involuntary servitude as punishment for those convicted of crimes. Thus, inmates are often forced to work. Sometimes, such work occurs within jails or prisons (e.g., groundskeeping, laundry, custodial, food service, and maintenance). Yet it has become increasingly common for correctional facilities to contract with for-profit companies and require inmates to perform labor for such companies, especially those engaged in the manufacture of clothing, shoes, home goods, and even weapons. Critics argue that such practices are a contemporary form of slavery. But judicial decisions have consistently affirmed that inmates are not legally considered employees and, therefore, are not entitled to the same legal protections that apply to the general labor force, including in relation to wages, working hours, and safety.

Incarceration is associated with over $100 billion annually in so-called hidden expenses. These are the various costs borne by inmates or by their family members, including for health care. For those with chronic health conditions, medical costs can accumulate quickly. Yet even relatively healthy individuals often have incarceration-related medical debt after they are released from jail or prison. Some inmates receive assistance from family members to help pay medical bills. However, this use of resources can also increase financial strain for the family unit, especially in low-income communities, and leave them less able to afford food, housing, and other basic needs. Yet there are other hidden expenses as well. Some states rely on a pay-to-stay model wherein inmates must pay for room, board, and even basic necessities. In some cases, inmates are charged a daily flat-rate; these can be as low as $25 but in some cases are over $150. Yet most facilities use the fee-per-item model that includes a separate charge for each food item, beverage, phone call, clothing item, tampon or menstrual pad, tube of toothpaste, roll of toilet paper, etc. Some inmates may have commissary funds (typically transferred to them by family members or friends) to pay for such items, but those from low-income families or who lack supportive social networks often do not. Given their limited access to paid employment, many find even basic hygiene items unaffordable.

There are also other hidden costs of incarceration. Family members and friends of inmates often incur expenses related to phone calls, transportation to and from correctional facilities, legal matters, and time away from work or school to visit inmates. In addition, there are significant costs associated with the job training, education, health care, and legal support provided to inmates by various nonprofit organizations, even when such support is provided by volunteers. Incarcerated parents often incur fees and fines associated with unpaid child support or with the care of their children placed in the foster care system. Predictably, most individuals leave correctional facilities with considerable debt. Such debt can easily represent more than half of their total annual income. It is reported to credit monitoring agencies and, hence, impairs their credit rating. This can increase barriers to employment as well as housing.

Health-Care Expenditures

Government spending related to the operation of correctional facilities exceeds $80 billion per year. Yet less than 12 percent of total spending related to the US correctional system—including local, state, and federal institutions—is dedicated to health-care services. This includes primary care, supplies, prescriptions, mental health services, salaries for health professionals, administration, diagnostic and laboratory services, dental care, and ophthalmological care. Nationally, the average per-inmate health-care expenditure is around $6,000. But health-care spending varies considerably. Whereas Arkansas and Louisiana spend only around one-third of the national average, California spends over three times as much. Such variations are influenced by a number of factors including fiscal management strategies, differences in inmate populations, and rates of certain health conditions that require significant and ongoing care (e.g., HIV, diabetes, cardiovascular diseases, and cancer). However, the structure of health systems, quality of care provided to inmates, and staffing levels are also significant.

General medical care represents nearly 40 percent of all correctional health-care spending. In contrast, hospitalization is around 20 percent; prescriptions and mental health services each represent around 14 percent; and substance abuse treatment, dental health, and administration each comprise less than 5 percent. In some instances, grants can help offset health-care costs and promote improved access to specialized care for certain groups of inmates based on age, geographic location, or particular health conditions. Examples include the Delta Health Care Services Grant Initiative, Tribal Opioid Response Grants, Residential Substance Abuse Treatment for State Prisoners (RSAT) program, Opioid Affective Youth Initiative, Ryan White HIV/AIDS Program, and Justice and Mental Health Collaboration Program.

Some states cover the majority of health-care costs for detainees. However, in federal and most state facilities, inmates are charged a co-pay for each health service they receive. Proponents argue that this practice helps control health-care budgets, reduces requests for frivolous visits to the infirmary, and follows the co-pay model that requires non-incarcerated populations to assume some financial responsibility for the care they receive. However, such co-pays have been identified as an excessive burden for most inmates. In some correctional facilities, co-pays average $2–5; yet in others, they are $10–25. For certain specialized health services (e.g., mental health care), some states have co-pays as high as $100. Both prior to and following incarceration, individuals may be eligible for Medicare and Medicaid. However, access is suspended while serving time. The Affordable Care Act of 2010 (ACA) gave states the option of expanding Medicaid coverage to incarcerated populations; most have not done so.

EDUCATIONAL ACCESS AND QUALITY

There is a two-way connection between education and incarceration. On the one hand, low educational attainment is associated with increased risk of incarceration; conversely, incarceration increases risk of diminished educational attainment and poor academic performance. Thus, access to education has increasingly been recognized as an essential component of broader efforts to rehabilitate inmates and prepare them to successfully transition to life after incarceration. Despite this, prison education programs are generally low quality and plagued by lack of funding and limited academic options.

Educational Attainment among Incarcerated Populations

Inmates are one of the least educated populations in America. Roughly 60 percent of federal inmates and 70 percent of those in local and state facilities do not have a high school diploma or GED. Individuals without such credentials are nearly 4 times more likely to be incarcerated than those who complete high school. In addition, nearly one-fourth of inmates have a disability that impairs learning and cognition. Yet there are significant variations in educational attainment among different demographic groups. White, cisgender, heterosexual inmates are more likely to have a high school diploma, GED (General Educational Development) certificate, or college degree than other incarcerated populations. Among incarcerated LGBTQIA individuals, approximately 70 percent do not have a high school diploma or GED. Approximately 75 percent of incarcerated Indigenous, 30 percent of incarcerated Blacks, and 35 percent of incarcerated HLC populations did not complete high school. Educational disparities persist even after release: among former inmates, over 40 percent of HLC cisgender women and one-third of Black cisgender women do not have a high school diploma or GED; in contrast, the rate is less than 20 percent for white cisgender women. Thus, BIPOC and LGBTQIA populations are among those most likely to lack basic education and literacy skills, including both before and after incarceration.

Within juvenile facilities, eight out of ten detainees meet the criteria for low literacy. Juveniles who do not meet grade-level expectations are more likely to be incarcerated. Similar patterns have been noted among minors who lack strong, supportive connections with teachers and their academic peers; who feel marginalized or stigmatized in school settings; or who lack opportunities or are otherwise unable to participate in extracurricular and social activities available through schools or community organizations. Rates of literacy and educational attainment are similarly low among adult inmates. Over 65 percent of incarcerated adults lack functional literacy skills. Thus, they cannot read, understand, and use information from printed texts such as books, magazines, brochures, letters, or newspapers. Rates of digital literacy (e.g., media, computer, and internet sources) among adult inmates are even lower.

Benefits of Educating Incarcerated Populations: Health and Beyond

Inmates who participate in education programs tend to have better overall physical and mental health than those who do not. They also have higher rates of health literacy, more often engage in preventative health measures, and are more likely to follow treatment protocols related to both acute and chronic health issues. Rates of physical and sexual violence among inmates are lower in facilities with postsecondary vocational, technical, or degree programs; thus, risks to physical and mental health are diminished. Inmates who participate in educational programs typically report increased confidence and enhanced sense of purpose. Such changes have been shown to be especially significant for those with a history of familial or intimate partner abuse, particularly as individuals with a healthy self-concept are less likely to tolerate or perpetrate physical, psychological, or sexual abuse. Furthermore, access to education increases likelihood of post-incarceration economic stability; this has obvious implications in regard to the ability to afford basic needs such as food, shelter, clothing, and health care. Former inmates with postsecondary education and training are more likely to earn a living wage and, therefore, are less likely to experience the type of chronic stress associated with poverty as well as the various acute and chronic diseases more common among low-income populations. Increased access to education is also linked to reduced rates of drug use, abuse, and addiction both during and after incarceration.

Educating inmates also promotes benefits for their families and society. Inmates who have completed educational programs are better equipped to understand and engage in parenting practices that promote healthy child development; more likely to be involved in their children's education; and more likely to promote educational achievement in their families. Thus, their children are less likely to be chronically absent from school, more likely to do well in school, and more likely to complete high school and pursue higher education. Former inmates with advanced credentials are also more likely to secure a job that provides health insurance and other benefits. This reduces their reliance on government-sponsored health insurance and other services for low-income populations. Moreover, recidivism and reincarceration rates are substantially lower among those who have access to education. Although such decreases are most pronounced for inmates who earn a postsecondary degree, they have also been noted among those who participate in literacy enhancement, GED, technical, and vocational programs. It is estimated that each dollar invested in prisoner education saves over four taxpayer dollars in judicial and correctional spending.

Education within Correctional Facilities: Options and Barriers

Nearly nine out of ten state and federal facilities offer educational programs. Within local and county facilities, programs are generally limited to basic adult education, GED preparation, ESL, and life skills. Such programs can help meet the educational needs of some incarcerated populations but offer only limited benefits in relation to long-term self-sufficiency and financial security. In addition, many are taught by volunteers or those who lack teaching credentials; thus, quality and frequency can be inconsistent. Some facilities also offer vocational training in landscaping, culinary arts, agriculture, welding, carpentry, auto maintenance and repair, and HVAC (heating, ventilation, and air conditioning) and other trades to help promote post-incarceration job opportunities. Facilities that offer training in trades that require a government-issued license (e.g., electricians, plumbers, and cosmetologists) may offer certification exams but often do not cover exam-related fees.

Some state and federal facilities do offer postsecondary options. In some states, however, certain prisoners are prohibited from participating in such programs due to the length of their sentence or the crime associated with their conviction. Yet even where such restrictions do not exist, an inmate must first obtain permission from the warden in order to enroll in college-level courses. There is growing evidence that biases related to race, gender, sexuality, socioeconomic status, and other identities influence the granting or denial of such permission. Inmates must pay for college applications as well as pay for and pass the American College Test (ACT), Scholastic Assessment Test (SAT), or similar admissions texts. Applications and exams can be challenging as many inmates are unfamiliar with these types of documents and there is limited support available to them. In addition, bureaucratic barriers can make it difficult to obtain high school academic records or other documents that must be submitted with college applications. Individuals who encounter such barriers are less likely to persist with postsecondary opportunities.

Affordability is another obstacle to education. The low-income status of many inmates leaves them unable to pay for tuition, books, and supplies. Some are able to secure grants or scholarships through foundations or corporations while others rely on veterans benefits or tuition subsidies. But many must rely on family financial support. Limited access to computers and the internet can make it difficult for inmates to complete the Federal Application for Student Aid (FAFSA) which is required for most grants and scholarships. Due to the Omnibus Crime Bill of 1995, incarcerated populations were excluded from receiving federal student loans as well as Pell Grants for nearly 20 years. In 2015, the Second Chance Pell (SCP) experiment reinstated Pell Grants for inmates on a limited basis. The program was expanded in December 2020; in April 2021, the ban on Pell Grants for incarcerated students was repealed. From 2015 through the end of 2021, however, less than 40,000 inmates were approved for such grants.

When college degree programs are available, they are often sporadic, offer only a limited range of courses, and frequently rely on instructors who have limited teaching experience or lack understanding of the unique needs of incarcerated students. Many prisons have libraries; however, they are generally underfunded and lack the types of resources needed for college-level courses. Although online academic options do exist in some correctional settings, the digital divide—including lack of regular computer and internet access as well as knowledge of how to successfully navigate online learning platforms—continues to hamper inmates' access to and success in online programs. This divide has been linked to higher rates of academic-related anxiety, diminished self-esteem, and poor academic performance among inmates. Inmates are especially at risk of academic failure or withdrawal from academic programs if they are transferred to a different facility, do not receive sufficient support from instructors, or are disciplined in ways that limit their ability to complete assignments (e.g., if they are put in solitary confinement or lose computer privileges). Only a small percentage of inmates complete a postsecondary degree.

HEALTH-CARE ACCESS AND QUALITY

Although they are legally entitled to health care, inmates encounter numerous barriers to such care. Available services are often low quality, may offer only basic services, and are generally insufficient to meet diverse health needs. Specialized services for those with unique or advanced health conditions and access to culturally appropriate services for diverse patient populations are similarly lacking. Consequently, the health care available to inmates can aggravate and even cause health problems.

Legal and Ethical Considerations

Under the US Constitution, incarcerated populations are entitled to adequate health care and, to some degree, to be protected from conditions known to cause undue and significant health risks. In the decision in *Estelle v. Gamble (1976)*, the Supreme Court of the United States (SCOTUS) declared that correctional employees must respond in a timely and medically appropriate manner to health issues that cause or have the potential to cause significant pain, disability, or death for inmates. In *Wilson v. Seiter (1991)*, the court established that while intentional denial of medical care was the most obvious violation of prisoners' right to health care, indifference to their health-care needs or willfully delaying access to care for obvious health problems constitutes cruel and unjust treatment. Other judicial decisions—such as *Ingraham v. Wright (1977)*, *Hudson v. McMillian (1992)*, and *Hope v. Pelzer (2002)*—established limits on use of physical punishment by correctional staff against inmates, particularly as such punishment carries inherent health risks. Still other decisions—including *Helling v. McKinney (1993)* and *Brown v. Plata (2001)*—addressed living conditions in jails and prisons, asserting that exposure to harmful substances (e.g., second-hand smoke) and overcrowded conditions constitute cruel and unusual punishment.

Yet other judicial decisions have placed limits on prisoners' rights regarding health care. In most cases, inmates may refuse treatment and retain their rights to both informed consent and due process in matters related to health. However, in *Washington v. Harper (1990)*, SCOTUS established that if a health issue poses a significant threat to the safety or health of others (e.g., other inmates, guards, and health-care providers), an inmate may be required to undergo treatment (e.g., forced to take anti-psychotic medication) without their consent. Those with tuberculosis and HIV may also be forced to undergo treatment aimed at controlling and preventing the spread of such diseases. In some states, certain diagnostic tests and vaccines may also be required. Inmates who believe their right to health care has been violated are entitled to pursue legal action. However, under the Prison Litigation Reform Act of 1996 (PLRA), they must first follow and exhaust formal grievance procedures within the correctional system. In addition, PLRA requires inmates to demonstrate that they suffered physical harm. It does not, however, provide recourse for impaired mental health due to lack of medical care, harsh treatment (e.g., extended solitary confinement and denial of food or water), or abuse by staff or other inmates.

Health-Care Structure and Services

There are four primary structural models that govern the provision of health care to incarcerated populations. In the direct provision model, care is provided by health-care professionals employed by the department of corrections. Roughly one-third of states use this model. Although direct provision can help control health-care costs, chronic staffing shortages and limited availability of certain health services have been identified as significant barriers to care in direct provision. In contrast, the contracted provision model involves outsourcing care to private corporations. Such corporations generally have agreements to provide care in multiple correctional facilities in a specific state or region, yet there are some that work throughout the country. In addition to providing health services, contracted corporations may also assume health-related administrative responsibilities. Private facilities typically outsource health care, although approximately 40 percent of state prisons also use the contracted provision model. It is often associated with cost savings. However, understaffing and high staff turnover rates have been shown to diminish the quality and consistency of care provided via this model.

The third model combines the direct and contracted provision model; thus, some health services are provided by correctional system employees while others are offered by contracted providers. While this can help balance the various strengths and weaknesses of the two models, it can also lead to bureaucratic complications when responsibilities for expenditures, quality, and administration are not clearly defined. Finally, a handful of states rely on students in medical, nursing, or other advanced health-training programs to provide the majority of health care to inmates. Advocates argue that doing so reduces operating costs while also providing students with practical experience. Yet critics contend it offers inferior care, particularly as students may not be adequately trained to diagnosis anything beyond common ailments.

Typically, an inmate receives a general physical examination when they enter a correctional facility. In general, mental health is not assessed during such examinations except when an individual is known to have a preexisting mental illness or if the circumstances of their arrest and incarceration suggest that such an illness is likely. For individuals incarcerated for less than a year, the intake exam is likely the only physical they will receive. Long-term inmates, however, are generally given a physical once per year. Beyond basic intake and annual physical examinations, inmates only receive medical care when ill, injured, or if they have a chronic condition. Preventative care is not common. For example, although the Federal Bureau of Prisons has endorsed vaccines for inmate populations as a basic public health measure, correctional facilities are not required to offer vaccines. Even when inmates have injuries or illness that is obvious, accessing care is not easy. In most cases, they must receive permission to visit the infirmary; this can take several days. If they are prescribed medications, they must stand in line each day to receive them; this can be especially burdensome for those who are elderly, have mobility impairments, or have health conditions that render them weak or fatigued (e.g., diabetes, nutritional deficiencies, cancer, and fibromyalgia) or make walking or standing difficult (e.g., leg, back, or head injuries).

Most correctional infirmaries are not equipped to provide advanced care. Therefore, inmates with serious health conditions are typically transported to hospitals. If the condition is deemed immediately life-threatening (e.g., a heart attack or stroke), transport occurs via ambulance. Yet if it is not, correctional buses or vans are used; such transport occurs only after additional guards can be located to supervise the inmate for the duration of transport, examination, and hospitalization. Such delays can increase risk of complications for certain medical conditions. In addition, transportation in correctional vehicles can aggravate pain and discomfort, particularly for those with musculoskeletal injuries. Inmates are often handcuffed or shackled to their beds while in the hospital setting, a practice that increases risk of physical injuries and mental suffering. Although both the American Medical Association (AMA) and American College of Obstetricians and Gynecologists (ACOG) have denounced the practice as humiliating and cruel, more than half of all states still permit the shackling and handcuffing of inmates during childbirth.

Biases in Health Care

One of the most prominent factors that influences access to and quality of care for incarcerated populations is bias. Pervasive stereotypes of inmates dominate American culture including mainstream movies, television, music, cartoons, and other forms of popular culture and depict inmates as inherently violent, untrustworthy, simple-minded, unmotivated, selfish, antisocial, and uncaring. In addition, both crime suspects and convicted criminals are most often portrayed as Black, HLC, Indigenous, or of Middle-Eastern descent; immigrants; poor; unmarried; sexual minorities; gender queer; cisgender males; and those involved in gang activities (especially related to drugs, weapons trafficking, prostitution, and violence). In contrast, law enforcement officers, judges, and correctional staff are generally depicted as white, American-born, middle-class, heterosexual, and cisgender. Such stereotypes are at the core of systemic inequalities that disproportionately target and punish certain populations. In policing practices, for example, such biases are evident in racial profiling as related to the surveillance of particular communities, treatment of suspects, and arrest rates. Such biases also influence both political and public attitudes, something that has been documented in crime legislation, jurors' perceptions of defendants, conviction rates, and sentencing patterns.

Implicit and explicit biases also influence access to and quality of health care available to incarcerated populations. The health-care system in most facilities reflects a one-size-fits-all approach that denies the very real and important differences among inmates. Such differences bear considerably on the health status of inmates. For example, those with a history of intimate partner violence and/or sexual abuse often have PTSD, anxiety, depression, and may experience panic attacks. Yet the health care available to inmates generally does not include regular screening for mental health issues and offers few options for treatment. Cultural background and social identity of inmates also influence their understanding of and acceptance of specific types of treatment as well as their need for certain types of health care. Yet culturally competent care—that is, care that acknowledges, respects, and incorporates the diverse cultural values, beliefs, and practices of patient populations—is a rarity of correctional settings. Obvious examples include the lack of dietary accommodations for different religious groups (such as those that adhere to a vegan diet or who do not consume pork products), failure to provide trained medical interpreters for inmates with limited English proficiency, and lack of health services that respond to the unique physical and mental health needs of transgender and gender nonconforming populations. Limited access to reproductive/sexual health care as well as geriatric care is also indicative of the systemic biases inherent in correctional health care. And while the Americans with Disabilities Act of 1990 require accommodations for inmates with disabilities, their unique health needs are routinely overlooked.

Biases are also evident in the attitudes and actions of health-care providers and correctional staff. They are more likely to interpret behaviors associated with certain types of mental illness (e.g., confusion, verbal outburst, restlessness, and involuntary movements) as aggressive when exhibited by Black, HLC, and Indigenous inmates as compared to similar behavior in white populations and, thus, to endorse punishment of BIPOC inmates as well as the use of handcuffs and shackles when providing medical care to these populations. In addition, stereotypes related to sex, gender expression, and sexuality have been shown to influence staff responses to inmate requests to visit the infirmary, particularly as the stereotype that cisgender women and LGBTQIA populations are overly emotional is often used to diminish their symptoms (including their levels of pain). Furthermore, while sexual victimization occurs among all demographic groups of inmates, LBGTQIA individuals and cisgender women are often blamed by staff for their victimization; thus, their reports of sexual victimization by inmates or staff are often not taken seriously. Blaming is also a common thread in staff treatment of inmates with drug abuse or addiction issues. Those who suffer from mental health issues, cognitive decline, or developmental disabilities are often infantilized or treated as incompetent. In addition, staff members sometimes willfully ignore medical and scientific guidelines when providing care to inmates. For example, several inmates sued an Arkansas jail after they were given high doses of Ivermectin to treat COVID-19. Ivermectin is an anti-parasitic commonly used to treat horses and livestock. Although it is also sometimes used to treat head lice and certain skin conditions in humans, both the US Federal Drug Administration and the Centers for Disease Control and Prevention continue to warn against its use to prevent or treat COVID-19.

LIVING ENVIRONMENT AND SOCIAL CONTEXT

Both historical and contemporary data indicate that the United States is a pro-incarceration nation. It is widely recognized that the unique physical environment of jails, prisons, and detention centers diminishes the health and well-being of inmates. However, disproportionate rates of incarceration among certain demographic groups, combined with the social dynamics and power hierarchy within correctional facilities, mean that certain subpopulations bear the brunt of incarceration-related physical and mental health risks that can be detrimental to both short- and long-term well-being.

Pro-incarceration Nation

The United States incarcerates a greater portion of its population than any other nation. Rates of incarceration in America have increased four-fold in the last 50 years and the current rate is approximately 700 prisoners per 100,000 population. In contrast, rates are below 150 in the UK, Canada, France, Italy, and Denmark. Yet there is a good degree of variation in rates of incarceration throughout the United States. More than twenty states have rates that exceed the national average; such rates are highest in southern states including Louisiana, Mississippi, Oklahoma, Georgia, Arkansas, Alabama, and Kentucky. Yet other states have rates well below the national average, especially in the northeast: Massachusetts, Rhode Island, Vermont, Maine, and New Hampshire all have incarceration rates below 200 per 100,000 population. However, Minnesota's rate is also below 200.

Since the start of the twenty-first century, there has been a notable decrease in public support for mass incarceration. Despite this shift, the United States maintains an extensive system of mass incarceration. It includes over 7,000 jails, prisons, and detention centers. While some are public institutions operated by local, state, or federal governments, others are private facilities managed by for-profit corporations. Nearly 90 percent of inmates are held in public facilities. There are currently over 2.1 million individuals imprisoned in the United States. This represents a decrease from peak levels in 2008 when the population exceeded 2.3 million. This decrease is linked, in part, to declining rates of arrest as well as changes in criminal laws and sentencing procedures. For example, the First Step Act of 2018 reduced sentences for those convicted of certain nonviolent offenses, are considered low-risk for repeat offenses, and have served a certain portion of their sentence without incidence of infraction. More recently, home burglaries and drug-related offenses have declined during the COVID-19 pandemic. Changes in citation and arrest procedures for minor offenses during the pandemic are also noteworthy. For example, rather than arresting those suspected of trespassing, petty theft, vandalism, or simple assault or who are in possession of small amounts of marijuana, law enforcement has increasingly followed cite-and-release protocols.

Over 99 percent of those incarcerated in the United States were born in the United States. Roughly 40 percent of all inmates have been convicted of or are awaiting trial for a violent crime, yet the majority are incarcerated for nonviolent offenses. Nearly two-thirds of inmates are held in state facilities including prisons for adults, psychiatric facilities, or juvenile facilities. Another 30 percent are held in local jails and the remainder are in federal facilities. Those involuntarily committed to psychiatric prisons represent less than 1 percent of the total incarcerated population; juveniles account for only around 2 percent of all detainees; those in military jails and prisons constitute less than one-tenth of 1 percent. Nearly 90 percent of inmates identify as cisgender males, but the cisgender female inmate population has increased over 500 percent since 1980. LGBTQIA individuals are overrepresented among inmates. Rates are also disproportionately high among BIPOC populations, although rates of incarceration among whites have increased in the past decade. Those with incomes below the Federal Poverty Level (FPL) constitute over 65 percent of inmates. Each day, nearly half a million people remain incarcerated because they are unable to afford bail.

Physical Environment

Various human right organizations and government entities have reported that America's jails and prisons are in poor condition. Overcrowding has been an increasing concern since the 1980s and remains a serious problem. Prior to the COVID-19 pandemic, the federal prison system and correctional systems in at least fifteen states were operating beyond 100 percent capacity; states such as Arkansas, Nebraska, Delaware, New Hampshire, Wisconsin, and California were at 130 percent or more over capacity. Although responses to the pandemic did initiate some changes that reduced rates of new inmates entering facilities and permitted early release or home confinement for nonviolent offenders who had served a significant portion of their sentence, overcrowding remains an issue, especially in men's facilities. Overcrowding has been linked to increased rates of infectious diseases (especially respiratory and diarrheal), violence, unsanitary conditions, musculoskeletal disorders (e.g., those sustained due to lack of available beds and the resulting requirement that some inmates sleep on the floor), and impaired mental health due to increased stress.

Yet even in facilities where overcrowding is not an issue, the physical conditions of the structures and grounds have been identified as major health concerns. Heating, ventilation, and air conditioning systems are often aged or broken. In some cases, they are inefficient and do not circulate evenly; thus, some parts of the facility may register at typical indoor room temperatures (around 70 degrees Fahrenheit) while others are significantly hotter or cooler. In the Southwest, for example, prison officials have reported heat indexes of nearly 150° F in parts of some correctional facilities. It is anticipated that such extremes will become more common due to climate change. Temperature extremes reduce overall quality of life, increase stress, and diminish mental wellness of inmates. However, extended exposure can cause changes to core body temperature and is associated with hypothermia, heat stroke, pneumonia, reduced cognitive function, loss of consciousness, damage to internal organs, and impaired immune function. Such risks are more pronounced for individuals who are elderly, disabled, or have certain preexisting health conditions. Risks are also greater for those taking medications that impair the body's ability to thermo-regulate or that cause increased sensitivity to temperatures; examples include antidepressants, decongestants, antipsychotics, antihistamines, and antihypertensives. Temperature extremes can also lead to death. Additionally, inadequate ventilation is associated with increased risk of respiratory ailments (especially those related to asthma and allergies) as well as certain types of airborne infectious diseases (e.g., tuberculosis, influenza, the common cold, whooping cough, chickenpox, and COVID-19).

Water and sanitation systems are also an ongoing concern. Polluted wells, eroded and broken pipes, and lack of adequate filtration systems are commonly cited problems. Inmates in some facilities have reported the only water available to them is contaminated with arsenic (known to cause certain types of cancer), bacteria, lead, rust, parasites, and even sewage. Due to inadequate drainage, inmates sometimes experience flooding in their cells during seasonal rains and extreme weather events such as tropical storms and hurricanes. Inmates are typically not evacuated when such conditions arise and, as a result, are at increased risk of health problems due to exposure to mold, bacteria (e.g., *Escherichia coli*, salmonella, and tetanus), viruses (e.g., norovirus and rotavirus), parasites, and vector-borne diseases, particularly those transmitted by mosquitos and rodents. Risks related to contact dermatitis, Staphylococcal infections, necrotizing fasciitis, and other skin issues increase in such conditions.

Inmates may also be exposed to a variety of toxins. Many of these are found in materials used to construct, maintain, repair, and clean jails and prisons. For example, asbestos, lead, formaldehyde, and mercury are commonly used in wood products, PVC, caulk, glue, and other building supplies. Furthermore, volatile organic compounds, short-chain chlorinated paraffins, halogenated flame retardants, and perflourinated compounds are often found in paint, insulation, furniture, mattresses, bedding, and clothing. Such substances increase risk of certain cancers, respiratory ailments, liver disease, nervous system disorders, genetic mutations, and hormonal disorders. In some instances, inmates are exposed to harmful substances due to the actions of other inmates (e.g., smoking cigarettes and the manufacture of illegal drugs). Substances used by guards to punish or control inmates—including pepper spray, tear gas, and other so-called riot control agents—are often toxic and/or cause health issues.

Yet the environment surrounding a correctional facility can also harm the health of inmates. Prisons and jails are often constructed in communities that are environmentally compromised and have existing problems with soil, water, and air quality. Several notable examples include facilities located on or near former mining operations, landfills, or coal ash-dumping sites as well as those constructed near manufacturing plants that release by-products into the air or water. In light of disproportionate rates of arrest, conviction, and incarceration for BIPOC populations, such contamination has been identified as a manifestation of environmental racism. While some inmates have sued state and federal correctional departments for violating their human and constitutional rights by exposing them to harmful substances, many lack the financial resources or knowledge of how to pursue legal action. Others simply do not pursue such action because they fear retaliation by guards or other staff.

Rules and Social Dynamics

Daily life in jails and prisons is governed by formal rules and regulations. These apply to nearly all aspects of inmate life, including conduct; discipline; medical care; daily schedules for meals, exercise, and sleep; visits from family, friends, or attorneys; interactions between inmates; free time; and opportunities for phone calls, leisure, and learning. Established by federal, state, or local governments and enforced by staff, such rules and regulations ostensibly aim to promote the efficient and effective operation of facilities within established legal and budgetary frameworks. Many are also intended to promote safety and health for staff and inmates. Rules that require inmates to remain in quarantine if they have been diagnosed with certain types of highly contagious diseases (e.g., TB, COVID-19, influenza, adenovirus, and hepatitis A and B), for example, aim to limit the spread of such diseases. Yet these rules and regulations can also contribute to impaired health. For instance, the majority of jails and prisons are organized in accordance with cisgender norms and, thus, require that inmates are placed in a facility that aligns with the sex they were assigned at birth. Such practices have been shown to increase gender dysphoria among transgender, nonbinary, and intersex populations and to increase both risk and severity of depression, anxiety, PTSD, and suicidal ideation among these populations. Other commonly cited examples of rules and regulations that are detrimental to inmate well-being include those that require medical co-pays, limit access to preventative care, and permit certain types of punishment such as solitary confinement, denial of exercise, and use of a bland meal replacement commonly known as nutraloaf.

Yet the social dynamics and norms within correctional settings are equally important. Social hierarchies, alliances, and rivalries are prevalent among inmate populations, particularly in state and federal facilities where length of incarceration is typically longer than county and local jails. Status, reputation, and relative power within inmate hierarchies are influenced by a number of factors. Inmates are typically afforded a higher status among their peers if they have been convicted of certain crimes (e.g., killing a police officer or large-scale robberies), demonstrate physical aggression against other inmates or guards, or have connections with organized crime. Due to such status, they enjoy certain privileges that other inmates do not. For example, they are often able to access items that are prohibited or strictly controlled under formal rules and regulations; examples include weapons, illegal drugs, alcohol, prescription medications, cell phones, tattoo equipment, tobacco products, clothing, and certain types of foods. Such items are sometimes used to promote their own comfort, punish other inmates, or retaliate against correctional staff. They are also frequently traded for favors, used to secure alliances among different groups of inmates, or used to bribe guards, administrators, or health-care providers for liberties not afforded to other inmates.

In contrast, individuals who do not endorse or refuse to participate in the social hierarchy generally have low standing among inmate populations and are often targeted for humiliation, physical violence, or bullying. In some cases, they are killed. The same is true for inmates who are convicted of harming vulnerable populations (e.g., children, elderly, or disabled individuals), do not defend themselves against attacks by other inmates or guards, or violate social norms (e.g., sharing information with guards in order to get other inmates into trouble). Homophobia, transphobia, xenophobia, Islamophobia, sexism, and other discriminatory attitudes are prominent among inmates and continue to shape their social dynamics. Thus, individuals are sometimes targeted on the basis of their social identities. Such attitudes have also been noted among many correctional staff and influence their treatment of inmate populations.

In addition, and despite the provisions of the Prison Rape Elimination Act of 2003 and similar measures, sexual violence (e.g., rape, coercion, sexual assault, and sexual harassment) is frequently used to exert power within jails and prisons. Such violence is sometimes used by inmates to control, humiliate, or punish the victim. Other times, inmates demand sexual acts to settle debts or as a form of payment for protection from other inmates or guards. However, staff members are most often the perpetrators of sexual violence against inmates, including in both men's and women's facilities. Those who provide health care, legal assistance, educational instruction, and other forms of support also sometimes perpetrate such abuse. Although all demographic groups may be targeted, LGBTQIA inmates are especially vulnerable to sexual violence. Rates of sexual victimization are also high among incarcerated youth, inmates with cognitive or developmental disabilities, and cisgender women. Sexual violence is associated with a variety of physical health problems including injuries to the genitals and pelvic region, fractures, bruises, muscles strains, and sexually transmitted diseases (STDs). It also impairs psychological well-being and increases risk of anxiety, depression, PTSD, eating disorders, sleep disorders, and suicidal ideation. Among those inmates who are able to become pregnant—including certain transgender and gender nonconforming populations as well as cisgender women of childbearing age—sexual violence increases risk of unintended pregnancy which, in turn, can diminish both physical and mental health. Inmates who become pregnant as a result of sexual violence are at increased risk for miscarriage, stillbirth, preterm labor, and premature delivery.

The rules and social dynamics that govern life in correctional facilities have been associated with a unique type of long-term trauma known as post-incarceration syndrome. It stems from the lack of autonomy and lack of purpose that many prisoners experience during their incarceration as well as social isolation, overcrowding, repeated exposure to violence, and various punitive methods (e.g., solitary confinement, sleep deprivation, physical beatings, and denial of food and water) often used in the US correctional system. Post-incarceration syndrome can impact individuals for months or even years following their release. During the period immediately following their release, formerly incarcerated individuals are at increased risk of death due to drug overdose, unintentional injury, violence, and suicide. Furthermore, post-incarceration syndrome has been linked to increased risk of recidivism and reincarceration.

CHAPTER EIGHT

Indigenous Populations

Descendants of the original inhabitants of and who exercised sovereignty over the geographic area currently known as the contiguous United States and Alaska prior to arrival of and colonization by European settlers are known as Indigenous populations. They are frequently referred to in research and governmental contexts as American Indians and Alaska Natives (AI/AN), Native Americans, Native peoples, or Indigenous Americans. At present, there are nearly six hundred federally recognized Indigenous tribes; two hundred additional tribes are still seeking such recognition. There are approximately 10 million Indigenous individuals in the United States, and they represent just under 3 percent of the total population. Although tribes are dispersed throughout the country, most AI/AN people live in Alaska or in Western states such as Oklahoma, New Mexico, South Dakota, Montana, and Arizona. Approximately 70 percent live in urban or semi-urban areas; one-fifth live on tribal reservations. The largest groups—including the Cherokee, Navajo, Choctaw, Chippewa, Apache, and Blackfeet—have over 100,000 members each. There are also many smaller tribes, including the Augustine Band of Cahuilla Indians which has just over one dozen members. Many tribes that prospered prior to colonization no longer exist due to the combined influences of diseases, warfare, forced migration, and genocide.

This chapter focuses on social determinants of health that influence the health and well-being of AI/AN people. Tribal communities vary significantly regarding customs, cultural norms, language, beliefs, and lifestyle. However, they share a common history that includes loss of political sovereignty and land rights, assimilation, and targeted extermination under governmental policies. Additionally, they share similar experiences due to ongoing social, political, and economic marginalization and related struggles for cultural survival in the twenty-first century. Such marginalization is a core element of the substantial health disparities and health inequities that continue to impact Indigenous populations and that are evident in the poor health, diminished quality of life, and decreased life expectancy that persist among such populations.

CURRENT STATE OF HEALTH

The health disparities that impact AI/AN populations are well documented and evident throughout the lifespan. Whereas the average life expectancy (ALE) at birth in the United States is nearly 79 years overall, it is markedly lower for AI/AN populations; in fact, they have the lowest ALE of all racial and ethnic groups in the United States. On average, AI/AN people live just under 72 years; ALE at birth for cisgender females is approximately 75 years while it is only about 68.5 years for cisgender males. Globally, the ALE for Indigenous populations is consistently lower than for non-Indigenous groups. However, when compared to Canada, New Zealand, and other economically stable countries with large Indigenous populations, the United States has a greater gap in ALE between Indigenous and non-Indigenous groups.

Since the 1980s, the total fertility rate (TFR) among AI/AN populations has declined 20 percent; additionally, and although the overall TFR in the United States increased during the COVID-19 pandemic, it decreased among AI/AN populations during that period. This decrease has been linked to reduced access to sexual and reproductive health care, including prenatal care, treatment for infertility, and family planning services. Although the teen pregnancy rate has declined by over 60 percent among AI/AN populations over the past 30 years, it remains higher than the national average; incidence of unintended pregnancy is also disproportionately high. Similarly, rates of preterm labor, premature birth, miscarriage, stillbirth, and obstetric hemorrhage are higher among Indigenous populations when compared to national averages. However, those with pregnancy-related complications are less likely than individuals of other racial and ethnic groups to have access to surgical delivery options. When compared to non-HLC white populations, rates of maternal mortality are nearly three times higher among AI/AN people. In some cases, such outcomes are the result of preexisting health conditions such as high blood pressure, diabetes, and depression, yet stress—including stress related to poverty, intergenerational trauma, structural and interpersonal violence, and barriers to prenatal health care—is also a contributing factor. In addition, poor pregnancy outcomes among Indigenous populations are a consequence of limited access to culturally competent, affordable health care. Some research indicates that substance use and abuse disorders (SUAD) during pregnancy are more common among AI/AN populations; however, targeted surveillance of such populations has skewed research data. Use and abuse of tobacco, alcohol, and illegal drugs increase health risks during pregnancy. But the criminalization of and associated penalties associated with SUADs during pregnancy discourages many pregnant AI/AN individuals from seeking prenatal care.

Over the past two decades, and even though infant mortality rates have declined overall in the United States and among all other racial and ethnic groups, such rates have held steady among AI/AN populations. At present, Indigenous infants are almost twice as likely as non-HLC whites to die in the first 12 months of life. Despite the health benefits associated with breastfeeding, rates of breastfeeding among Indigenous populations are lower than national averages; among those who do initiate breastfeeding, over 70 percent stop within 6 months of giving birth. The most common causes of death during the first year of life among AI/AN children include birth defects, sudden infant death syndrome (SIDS), accidents, and complications related to pregnancy (e.g., premature birth, infection, oxygen deprivation during delivery, low birth weight, and underdeveloped organs). Rates of certain types of birth defects—including anotia (absence of the outer ear), microtia (abnormally small outer ear), cleft palate, diaphragmatic hernia, gastroschisis (a hole in the abdominal wall), and clubfoot—are disproportionately high among AI/AN newborns. In the 1970s, medical researchers identified fetal alcohol syndrome disorders (FASD) as a major concern among Indigenous populations. Yet recent research indicates that rates of FASD vary significantly by location, maternal age, and income; similarly, current research shows that rates of FASD among AI/AN people are equivalent to and, in some cases, lower than other racial and ethnic groups.

Nearly half of AI/AN youth experience adverse childhood experiences (ACEs). Examples include poverty, food insecurity, housing insecurity, witnessing or being a victim of household violence, incarceration of a parent or close relative, entering the foster care system, lack of adequate infrastructure (e.g., housing, clean water, and sanitation), death of a parent or close family member, bullying, neglect, sexual abuse, discrimination, and intergenerational trauma. They are also more likely than non-Indigenous children to be exposed to violence and to experience multiple ACEs. Consequently, there is an elevated risk of impaired mental health and diminished social well-being for Indigenous children. ACEs contribute to disproportionately high rates of major depressive disorders, self-harming behaviors, and suicide among AI/AN children and adolescents. At present, nearly one-third of deaths among Indigenous youth in the United States are the result of suicide; rates of suicidal ideation and suicide attempts are highest among lesbian, gay, bisexual, transgender, queer (LGBTQ) and two-spirit youth (those who claim a nonbinary gender, sexual, and/or spiritual identity) and among cisgender boys. Those who are victims of bullying (including cyberbullying) are at increased risk of suicidal ideation and attempted suicide. ACEs are also associated with increased risk of certain long-term health problems, especially those associated with high-risk behaviors (e.g., unsafe sex and SUAD). Yet benevolent childhood experiences (BCEs)—such as supportive relationships with friends and teachers—can diminish the impact of ACEs for AI/AN minors.

Physical health remains a concern for AI/AN youth. They experience disproportionately high rates of asthma. Over 40 percent of AI/AN children meet medical guidelines for being overweight or obese by the time they reach their tenth birthday. Rates of chronic conditions such as type 2 diabetes, nonalcoholic fatty liver disease, metabolic syndrome, high blood pressure, and high cholesterol are also higher among certain AIAN children, although these vary by location and tribe. Indigenous youth are also at increased risk of poor oral health—especially dental caries, gum disease, and cracked/broken teeth—and many do not receive regular dental screenings or treatment. Rates of injuries and death due to accidents (e.g., motor vehicle crashes, falls, burns, and drowning) are over twice as high among Indigenous youth when compared to their non-Indigenous populations. In addition, AI/AN youth are more likely to suffer injuries and death due to firearms. Intimate partner violence (IPV), rape, and sexual assault also disproportionately impact AI/AN youth, especially two-spirit and LGBTQ populations as well as cisgender girls.

Among Indigenous adults, chronic diseases increase risk of disability and premature death; approximately three in ten AI/AN adults have a diagnosed disability. Since the late twentieth century, the most common causes of death among this population include heart disease, certain types of cancer (e.g., liver, breast, kidney, stomach, lung, and colorectal), diabetes, liver diseases, and respiratory diseases (e.g., bronchitis, influenza, pneumonia, and chronic obstructive pulmonary disease (COPD)). Although ACEs increase risks of many of these conditions, behavioral factors (e.g., diet, activity levels, and use of tobacco, alcohol, and other drugs) are also significant considerations. Native populations historically engaged in hunting, gathering, fishing, and harvesting to obtain food, yet their contemporary diet is high in processed carbohydrates, sugar, fats, and sodium. At present, nearly half of AI/AN adults meet medical guidelines for obesity and one-fifth are diabetic, including one-third of those over age 64. Rates of metabolic syndrome—sometimes referred to as pre-diabetes and characterized by abnormal blood sugar, blood pressure, and cholesterol levels as well as accumulation of abdominal fat—are unduly high. Although rates vary by tribe and geographic location, recent estimates suggest that one in two AI/AN adults has metabolic syndrome. Nearly half do not participate in any type of moderate or vigorous physical activity on a weekly basis; activity levels are lowest among cisgender women and those over age 40, with low educational attainment, and with lower incomes. Among Indigenous adults, one-fifth smoke cigarettes or other tobacco products regularly. Nearly one-fourth report using illicit drugs or misusing prescription pain relievers; incidence of drug abuse is highest among cisgender men aged 18–34. Rates of alcohol consumption and abuse disorders are higher among AI/AN populations than the general US population. SUADs among AI/AN adults are most common among those who have experienced poverty, cultural marginalization, ACEs, intergenerational trauma, violence, and other types of psychological distress.

Infectious diseases, accidents, and violence contribute to high rates of injury, disability, and premature death among AI/AN adults. Some of the most prominent infectious diseases include tuberculosis, hepatitis C, lower respiratory infections, and certain sexually transmitted diseases (STDs) such as HIV, chlamydia, gonorrhea, and syphilis. During the first 2 years of the COVID-19 pandemic, and when compared to other racial and ethnic groups, Indigenous populations were more likely to be vaccinated; however, they also had disproportionately high rates of infection, hospitalization, and death due to the virus. Rates were especially high among those who lived on tribal reservations. Common causes of serious injuries and death among Indigenous adults include falls, burns, drowning (or near-drowning events), suffocation, poisoning, and assault. However, auto accidents remain the leading cause of unintentional injuries and death. At present, deaths due to auto accidents are 2.5 times higher among AI/AN adults than among the overall US adult population; they are most common at night and when the driver is speeding or pursued by police. Pedestrian deaths due to traffic accidents are also disproportionately high among Indigenous populations; the mortality rate for AI/AN pedestrians struck by a motor vehicle are three times as high as the national average.

Like AI/AN youth, adults have disproportionately high rates of mental health disorders. Most common among these are major depressive disorders, PTSD, and SUAD. Over the past decade, rates of suicide have increased. It is currently the second most common cause of death for cisgender adult males aged 20–44 and the third most common cause of death for cisgender adult females in the same age group. Rates of violent victimization—including assault, homicide, intimate partner violence (IPV), sexual assault, rape, and human trafficking—are two and a half times higher among Native peoples than among the general US population. Yet there are differences by gender. Whereas cisgender men are more likely to be victims of homicide, over 80 percent of cisgender women will experience physical or sexual violence in their lifetimes. In recent years, the scope of missing and murdered Indigenous women and girls has been recognized as a full-fledged crisis. Victimization due to physical and sexual violence is also disproportionately high among native LGBTQ and two-spirit populations. Additionally, and while tribal communities tend to have a good degree of respect and reverence for elders, rates of elder abuse (e.g., neglect, physical harm, coercion, financial exploitation, and sexual abuse) have increased in recent years.

ECONOMIC FACTORS

AI/AN populations experience significant economic challenges including high rates of poverty, limited economic opportunities, and structural barriers to wealth accumulation. Unemployment rates also remain disproportionately high. Those who are employed tend to be concentrated in unskilled, low-wage jobs. Many are unable to meet needs associated with housing, food, and other essentials. Liquid asset poverty, ongoing struggles with land rights, and inadequate resources for retirement are also significant concerns and contribute to both immediate and intergenerational poverty.

Poverty

Nearly one-third of Indigenous people live below the federal poverty level (FPL); this is more than twice as high as the national average. Median household income among such populations is under $25,000 per year; one-fifth of all AI/AN households have incomes under $5,000 annually. Yet rates vary by age, sex, sexual orientation, gender identity, and geographic location. They are highest among AI/AN children under the age of 18, young adults (aged 18–29), and elderly populations (aged 60 and above). Cisgender women are 15 percent more likely to live in poverty than cisgender men. LGBTQ and two-spirit populations also have disproportionately high rates of poverty compared to gender-conforming, heterosexual populations. Rates of poverty are especially high among individuals with disabilities and those over age 60. Additionally, AI/AN populations in rural areas are more likely to have incomes below the FPL than those in more urban areas; this is especially true for those living on tribal reservations. Housing insecurity and food insecurity remain widespread concerns. Rates of homelessness are nearly five times higher among Indigenous populations than among the overall US population. Similarly, AI/AN populations are twice as likely to be food insecure. Resource scarcity is especially common in rural areas; rural populations are also less likely than those in more urban areas to have access to support services including food banks, homeless shelters, health clinics, and public transportation. Programs via the Bureau of Indian Affairs (BIA) do provide some support and resources for low-income populations, yet the BIA has been widely criticized as underfunded, inefficient, and corrupt.

There are variations in poverty rates and overall income between different AI/AN communities. Some have implemented tribal enterprises or tribal economies. Examples include natural resource harvesting and extraction (e.g., timber, mining, and fishing), farming, ranching, gaming, and cultural tourism. Such endeavors can provide much-needed employment and income to community members. Tribes that have implemented casino operations or other forms of gaming (e.g., lottery and bingo) in the decades since the passage of the Indian Gaming Regulatory Act of 1988 typically have higher average household incomes than those without such enterprises. Yet revenues often fluctuate seasonally and in accordance with broader social, economic, and environmental issues (e.g., the Great Recession, the COVID-19 pandemic, and drought). Thus, even among communities with tribal enterprises, poverty remains a problem. Additionally, casinos and other gaming activities often contribute to an increase in alcohol consumption, certain types of crime, and violence. They are also associated with an increase in rates of stress, anxiety disorders, depression, and suicide as well as gambling addiction.

Geographic and environmental factors also influence income. Rates of poverty are disproportionately high on tribal reservations that lack natural resources and/or are plagued by environmental concerns (e.g., poor air and water quality, and lack of fertile land). Reservations that are geographically isolated also have fewer employment opportunities. Both environmental factors and limited access to employment are key factors, for example, in high rates of poverty among the Sioux tribes that reside on reservations in North Dakota and South Dakota. Over 40 percent of households on the Standing Rock, Rosebud, and Pine Ridge reservations have incomes below the FPL. Rates of extreme poverty are also high on these reservations and many residents cannot meet basic needs related to food, water, sanitation, safety, and housing. Resource scarcity increases risk of certain health conditions among AI/AN people including malnutrition, abnormal body weight, diabetes, infectious diseases, skin conditions, and chronic stress. It also contributes to poor mental health, SUADs, and increased risk of suicide.

Employment Patterns

Despite a lengthy history of limited attention by government entities and academic researchers to employment patterns among AI/AN populations, disproportionately high rates of unemployment and underemployment among such populations have been documented since at least the 1950s. Efforts to draw attention to and rectify such issues were central to the American Indian Movement that began in the late 1960s. Yet for the past 50 years, the AI/AN unemployment rate has remained about twice as high as the national average. However, such rates do fluctuate. Due to immediate and lingering impacts of the Great Recession, for example, AI/AN unemployment rates remained at 10 percent or higher for a seven-year period from early 2008 until the end of 2014. From May 2009–February 2011, such rates remained over 12 percent and sometimes exceeded 16 percent. While the overall US unemployment rate also increased during this time, it peaked at 10 percent. The AI/AN workforce was also disproportionately impacted by the COVID-19 pandemic. At the beginning of 2020, the unemployment rate for AI/AN people was 7.5 percent, more than twice as high as the overall US rate of 3.5 percent. By April 2020, unemployment among AI/AN people surged to nearly 30 percent; it did not consistently return to pre-pandemic levels until the end of 2021. Additionally, at the start of 2022, unemployment rates remained higher among AI/AN people than among Black, HLC, APIDA, and white subgroups. Such rates are consistently higher among Indigenous cisgender women than their cisgender male counterparts; such differences reflect inequalities in allocation of family responsibilities as well as ongoing sex discrimination in the workplace. Workplace discrimination also contributes to disproportionately high rates of unemployment among LGBTQ and two-spirit populations.

At least three-fourths of employed Indigenous people work full-time. Those employed in year-round, full-time positions earn an average of 77 cents for each dollar earned by their non-HLC white counterparts. The wage gap is even more pronounced when examining the earnings of AI/AN cisgender women; they earn only 60 cents per dollar earned by non-HLC white males, a difference that translates to an average income deficit of $25,000 per year. Such wage disparities diminish the ability of Indigenous populations to secure basic needs and increases their risk of homeless, food insecurity, and resource scarcity. Indigenous workers are overrepresented in service-related and so-called blue-collar positions including manufacturing, mechanics, construction, maintenance, mining, and transportation/material moving. Such activities are associated with higher-than-average rates of workplace injuries. Native peoples are also overrepresented in pink-collar roles and services industries including sales, health-care support, food preparation, administrative support, and hospitality. Both blue- and pink-collar jobs are associated with limited benefits such as sick leave, flexible spending accounts for health care and childcare, vacation leave, financial planning resources, and flexible or remote work options. Indigenous people remain underrepresented in higher paying white-collar positions; at present, they comprise less than one-half of 1 percent of all those employed in the highest paying professions in the United States including as physicians, attorneys, engineers, surgeons, professional athletes, federal judges, and anesthesiologists. Although they control tribal governments, AI/AN people remain marginalized within the context of non-tribal local governments and among state and federal elected officials. Thus, their ability to implement legislative changes on behalf of their communities remains limited. In 2021, six AI/AN legislators were sworn in as members of the 117th US Congress. It was the highest number of Indigenous leaders to ever serve concurrently but represented only 1 percent of Congressional leaders.

Other Barriers to Economic Stability and Wealth Accumulation

The economic reality of AI/AN populations—both individually and collectively—is profoundly influenced by their disenfranchisement in US society and resulting limited opportunities to accumulate assets, wealth, and other resources. This is evident, for example, in the historic and ongoing control of tribal lands by the federal government. At present, Indigenous persons own only 5 percent of the more than 55 million acres that comprise tribal reservations. As a result of the legal framework established via the US Supreme Court decisions known as the Marshall Trilogy—including *Johnson v. McIntosh (1823), Cherokee Nation v. Georgia (1831)*, and *Worcester v. Georgia (1832)*—the remaining lands are held in trust. Consequently, Indigenous populations cannot buy or sell such lands, nor can they use such lands—including their homes—as collateral to secure lines of credit. Federal control of tribal lands, therefore, continues to exclude many AI/AN peoples from one of the primary mechanisms for wealth accumulation. Furthermore, inability to buy, sell, and/or mortgage tribal lands limits opportunities for AI/AN populations to disrupt the cycle of poverty and to promote intergenerational wealth. Federal legislation also limits the ability of Indigenous communities to make independent decisions about development and use of environmental resources on tribal lands. The bureaucracy created via such legislation—which involves several federal agencies and nearly fifty steps to secure approval—hinders development and investment projects that could promote economic gains for tribal communities.

Indigenous populations tend to have few assets. For each dollar of wealth/assets among non-HLC white households, AI/AN households have less than 10 cents in wealth/assets. Despite the passage of the Indian Home Loan Guarantee Program in 1992—which required only a small down payment to encourage home ownership among AI/AN populations—only about half of Indigenous families own their homes. This is far below the US average of 65 percent for all racial and ethnic groups and lags even further behind the average of 75 percent among non-HLC whites. One in six households headed by Indigenous individuals does not have a savings or checking account; this is the lowest rate among all racial and ethnic groups in the United States. Due to their lower-than-average earnings, AI/AN people also accumulate less in retirement benefits (e.g., pensions, 401(k) plans, and IRA plans) and social security benefits. Consequently, they are at increased risk of poverty in old age; however, limited retirement benefits also result in limited economic resources to bequeath to family members, something that also contributes to high rates of intergenerational poverty. Rates of liquid asset poverty are also high among AI/AN populations. Thus, they tend to have few items of significant value (e.g., art, jewelry, stocks, and automobiles) that can be sold if they have unexpected health expenses due to serious illness or injury, lose their job, or encounter other pressing financial situations.

EDUCATIONAL ACCESS AND QUALITY

Within the context of educational settings, Indigenous populations encounter a variety of obstacles. Rates of school readiness, enrollment, academic achievement, and successful degree completion remain disproportionately low among such populations in K-12 and postsecondary settings. Additionally, issues related to equity and inclusion persist. Some of these issues pertain to representation in the curriculum and among educational professionals. Others stem from implicit and explicit biases that disproportionately target AI/AN students for special education programs and discipline. Finally, educational funding hampers both access to and the quality of education provided to AI/AN students.

Educational Enrollment, Achievement, and Completion Rates

Throughout the United States, K-12 enrollment, high school completion, and postsecondary enrollment rates have steadily increased over the two decades. However, they have stagnated among Indigenous populations; enrollment in K-12 programs decreased by over 10 percent and high school graduation rates have remained virtually unchanged since the start of the twenty-first century. At present, AI/AN students comprise just over 1 percent of all those enrolled in pre-K through grade 12. There are close to two hundred elementary and secondary schools that remain under the control of specific tribes or the Bureau of Indian Education (BIE); less than 10 percent of AI/AN children attend such schools. When compared to non-AI/AN students, Indigenous kindergarteners have lower rates of school readiness; they are less likely to have the cognitive, social, developmental, and behavioral skills necessary to promote learning and academic success. Despite ongoing efforts by the BIE to promote participation in Early Head Start, Head Start, and other pre-K programs, less than half of AI/AN children enroll. This is often due to geographic factors, especially in rural areas and on reservations. However, many parents remain distrustful of programs facilitated by non-AI/AN individuals and, thus, are unwilling to enroll their children. Disproportionately low rates of school readiness among AI/AN children have also been linked to certain health concerns (e.g., low birth weight, preterm birth, being born to a mother with depression, and inadequate access to prenatal health care) as well as poverty and low parental educational attainment.

During elementary, middle, and high school, academic performance among Indigenous students tends to be lower than average. By fourth grade, they average twenty points lower in mathematics and fifteen points lower in reading than national means. On average, AI/AN students in eighth grade earn scores that are seventeen points lower in mathematics and twelve points lower in reading than the overall US student population. Additionally, in 2019, they were the only racial or ethnic group to experience a decrease in average reading and math scores among students in eighth grade when compared to 2017 results. While the achievement gap on standardized exams decreases by the time Indigenous students reach twelfth grade, their mean scores remain fourteen points lower in math and twelve points lower in reading than national averages. Of equal importance, and whereas standardized mathematics scores have increased among APIDA, HLC, and non-HLC white teens since 2000, they have stagnated among AI/AN students. Those residing in rural areas—including on reservations—have limited opportunities for honors or advanced placement (AP) courses or internships and other types of learning opportunities necessary to help them become competitive applicants to high-ranking colleges and universities. Dropout rates remain disproportionately high among Indigenous students, especially cisgender young men. Those who drop out are at increased risk of long-term consequences that diminish lifetime earning potential and decrease ability to meet basic needs. They are also at increased risk of poor physical health, certain types of mental illness (e.g., stress, depressive disorders, and anxiety disorders), disabilities, and premature death. Nationally, 25 percent of AI/AN students do not graduate from high school. However, rates fluctuate considerably; in South Dakota, less than 55 percent of Indigenous students earn a high school diploma while 90 percent or more of those in Alabama, Connecticut, New Jersey, and Tennessee graduate on time.

AI/AN people currently represent only 1 percent of all postsecondary students and earn less than 1 percent of all college degrees including in undergraduate, graduate, and professional programs. Their rates of enrollment have decreased since 2005. Many are first-generation college students. Scores among AI/AN students are over one hundred points lower than the national average for the SAT; since 2000, average scores on the ACT have steadily declined among Indigenous students and they are currently one-fourth lower than the national average. At the time AI/AN students begin postsecondary studies, only one-third meet college-level expectations for language arts, math, science, and other core subjects. Consequently, they are often placed in so-called developmental classes that typically do not count toward degree requirements. Among those who enroll at four-year institutions, only 40 percent earn their degrees within 6 years. Rates of degree completion are higher among AI/AN cisgender women than cisgender men; they are also higher for those who enroll at BIE-controlled institutions. There are currently two BIE universities—Southwestern Indian Polytechnic University and Haskell Indian Nations University. Only one-fourth of all AI/AN people over age 25 have earned a postsecondary degree.

Issues Related to Inclusion and Equity

AI/AN students often feel marginalized and excluded in educational settings. Such feelings are often a consequence of lack of representation in the curriculum. The Native American Languages Act (NALA) of 1990 and Every Student Succeeds Act (ESSA) of 2015 recognized the importance of promoting knowledge of Indigenous cultures, histories, and traditions. Yet over half of US K-12 public schools do not include any attention to AI/AN populations as a required part of educational content. Of those that do, over 80 percent focus on history prior to 1900; that history is often sanitized to diminish or even eliminate attention to the systemic and pervasive injustices Indigenous peoples suffered under the policies of state and federal governments. There is also a tendency to simplify information about Indigenous populations and to ignore the numerous differences between tribes. At the postsecondary level, students are more likely to find Indigenous experiences and voices including in history, art, and literature courses; additionally, some institutions offer certificates or degree minors in Native American studies or Indigenous studies. Yet there are few colleges and universities that allow students to earn a major in such areas; there are even fewer with master's or doctoral programs that focus on AI/AN people and cultures. AI/AN leaders and allies continue to advocate for expanded attention to Indigenous experiences in educational settings, yet ongoing attacks on critical race theory and ethnic studies programs impede such efforts. There is also a paucity of AI/AN representation among educators. They comprise only 1 percent of all K-12 teachers and university professors; their representation among upper-level administrators in educational settings is similarly deficient.

Lack of representation in educational content and among educational leaders contributes to feelings of social marginalization, cultural shame, and lower self-esteem among AI/AN students. It is also associated with increased risk of dropping out of school prior to degree completion. Furthermore, it limits opportunities for culturally informed and responsive pedagogy that can enhance learning outcomes. Lack of representation also contributes to school absenteeism. In K-12 public schools, rates of absenteeism among AI/AN students are twice as high as the average among all student populations. Social dynamics related to marginalization, exclusion, loneliness, bullying, and/or violence are also associated with increased rates of absenteeism among AI/AN students. In addition, Indigenous students who encounter challenges related to transportation, chronic illnesses, undiagnosed learning disabilities, employment, caretaking responsibilities (e.g., for siblings, aging relatives, or ill family members), and/or stress related to academics are among those most likely to be chronically absent and/or to drop out of school.

While AI/AN populations are underrepresented in some aspects of education, they are overrepresented as participants in special education programs (SEP) and as recipients of disciplinary sanctions. During their elementary years, one in seven Indigenous students are placed in SEP; this is 80 percent higher than the average placement rate among all students. Special education programming can provide important forms of support for students with disorders and disabilities that impair cognitive, emotional, physical, and behavioral abilities. Yet recent reach indicates that overrepresentation of Indigenous children in such programs is a consequence of both unconscious and conscious bias among educational professionals. Quite simply, educators may identify greater need for special education services among Indigenous students because they expect such students to have an increased need for such services. Similarly, those behaviors deemed to fall within the range of typical/expected parameters for non-HLC white or APIDA students are more likely to be identified as problems when exhibited by AI/AN students. Additionally, teachers and administrators regularly stereotype Indigenous students as disobedient, delinquents, and even dangerous. AI/AN students are more likely to be disciplined and to receive harsher discipline than students from most other racial and ethnic groups. They are disciplined twice as often as non-HLC white students and APIDA students; they are also more likely to be expelled, even when the infraction is the same. In addition, Indigenous students have unduly high rates of school arrests. Those who are suspended or expelled are at increased risk of dropping out of school before earning their high school diploma. They are also more likely to be incarcerated during their lifetimes and have higher risk of suicide.

Economic aspects of education also figure prominently in the experiences of AI/AN students. Those attending BIE-controlled tribal K-12 schools or rural schools located near reservations regularly encounter problems due to lack of funding. Examples include inferior quality or outdated educational materials and facilities that are in a state of disrepair (e.g., problems with mold, leaking roofs, asbestos, poor ventilation, and inadequate insulation). It is also common for buses that are part of the BIE system to be old and in poor condition. Roads around BIE schools are often inadequately maintained; thus, in rainy or snowy conditions, they can be impassable. In addition, many schools lack adequate computing resources, internet access, and other types of educational technology. They also have difficulty attracting and retaining qualified educators and administrators. While organizations such as Teach for America continue to work to bring skilled educators to BEI schools, many have criticized such efforts as inadequate due to the lack of education-specific training provided to teachers. Overall, BEI schools are among the lowest-performing schools in the nation. When compared to AI/AN students who attend non-BEI controlled schools, those attending BEI schools have worse learning outcomes in core subjects such as math and reading throughout elementary, middle, and high school. Some BEI-controlled schools have graduation rates that hover around 50 percent. At the collegiate level, AI/AN students struggle to afford books, tuition, and other educational expenses. Although some can secure academic or needs-based scholarships or financial assistance through their tribe, such support is often not enough to overcome the economic barriers they encounter. Indeed, economic concerns are one of the primary sources of stress among postsecondary Indigenous students and contribute to the disproportionately high dropout rates among them. In recent years, however, colleges and universities have increasingly opted to offer tuition waivers to those who are members of federally recognized tribes. At present, it is unclear whether such financial support will improve retention and degree completion rates.

HEALTH-CARE ACCESS AND QUALITY

Indigenous people continue to encounter multiple, pervasive barriers to high-quality health care. At present, access to health care for such populations is protected under federal law. Indeed, there are a variety of government entities that are responsible for promoting the health and well-being of AI/AN communities. However, and due to the lengthy history of forced assimilation, relocation, and extermination under government policies, many remain distrustful of government-sponsored health programs. Furthermore, they often find it difficult to access care due to lack of affordability and geographic barriers. Biases in health education programs, clinical research and medical experimentation, health-care practices, and among the health-care workforce also continue to diminish access to and quality of care available to AI/AN populations, including care that is culturally and linguistically appropriate.

Legal Frameworks and the Right to Health Care

Under the legal parameters of various treaties, court decisions, executive orders, and legislation, members of federally recognized tribes are entitled to federally funded health care. However, while some legal actions directed at Native peoples have promoted access to health care and improved health, others have had the opposite result. For example, when the BIA was created in 1824, it promoted assimilation of Native peoples, thereby undermining cultural practices related to education, religion/spirituality, language, dress, and education as well as health, hygiene, and traditional medical practices. In the early part of the twentieth century, the Snyder Act of 1921 authorized the US Congress to dedicate funds to the health of AI/AN people, including for health programs (e.g., vaccinations and health education) and expansion of physician services via the BIA. With the passage of the Transfer Act of 1954, responsibility for health services provided to tribal populations then shifted to the Office of the Surgeon General and were recast as part of broader US public health initiatives. The Transfer Act also promoted a certain degree of autonomy for individual tribes so they could determine for themselves which health practices were culturally acceptable and appropriate. The Indian Health Service (IHS) was established the following year as a division within the US Department of Health and Human Services. The IHS remains the primary federal entity responsible for promoting well-being for tribal populations throughout the nation and for improving access to care that is culturally competent, high quality, comprehensive, and affordable.

However, it wasn't until the passage of the Indian Self-Determination and Education Assistance Act (ISDEAA) of 1975 that tribal communities gained significant autonomy over how health-related funding through the IHS and BIA is allocated. Tribes can exercise such autonomy via 638 contracts—sometimes referred to as a self-determination contracts—that permit them to carry over unused funds from one fiscal year to the next, collect revenue from insurance companies or other third-party entities, and secure certain types of grants that are not otherwise available via the IHS. In 1976, passage of the Indian Health Care Improvement Act (IHCIA) sought to further enhance and expand existing health services to AI/AN populations, specifically by authorizing reimbursement by Medicare and Medicaid to tribal populations receiving care via IHS and tribal health-care facilities. Additionally, the Patient Protection and Affordable Care Act (ACA) of 2010 both reauthorized the IHCIA and expanded health insurance coverage among AI/AN populations, including those previously excluded from coverage because they were not members of federally recognized tribes. Many also qualify for health care through Medicaid, Medicare, and the Children's Health Insurance Program (CHIP). A variety of federal agencies are tasked with promoting access to health care for AI/AN populations; examples include the Office of Minority Health and Health Equity (OMHHE), the Division of Tribal Affairs within the Centers for Medicare and Medicaid Services, the National Institute of Health's division on Minority Health and Health Disparities, and the Federal Office of Rural Health Policy (FORHP), among others. However, due to the lengthy history of governmental policies related to forced assimilation, relocation, and genocide against AI/AN populations, many Indigenous individuals remain distrustful of government agencies and related health programs.

Geographic and Economic Barriers to Care

Despite the legal framework and variety of agencies responsible for fostering access to health care for tribal populations, many continue to experience barriers that impede their access to health care. Geographic barriers remain an issue for many AI/AN populations residing in rural areas. Data from the US Census Bureau indicates that only about one-third of AI/AN populations reside in rural communities. However, critics have argued that such data is inaccurate, particularly due to the use of outdated and conflicting definitions of rural as well as poor data collection techniques. Recent data from Indigenous community leaders as well as nonprofit researchers indicate that approximately two-thirds of Native peoples live in rural communities. Furthermore, tribal lands are overwhelmingly located in rural areas, and over 60 percent of AI/AN populations live on or near tribal lands. Geographic barriers to health care are prominent for such populations, particularly for those who reside in remote rural areas that are located 45 miles or more from a city with a population of at least 20,000. It typically takes an hour or more to travel by car from remote rural areas to the closest city. Some can access health services through local clinics—including tribal clinics—or through mobile health clinics or various public health initiatives. Yet when accidents, serious injuries, or other health crises occur, it can take a considerable amount of time for emergency services to arrive. Thus, there is increased risk of serious complications (e.g., hemorrhage and infection), disability, and death for those living on tribal lands and those residing in remote rural areas.

Economic factors also influence access to health care for AI/AN communities. Access to health insurance is significant in this regard. At present, Indigenous populations have the highest uninsured rates of all racial and ethnic groups in the United States. Among all age groups, 20 percent of AI/AN individuals do not have health insurance. Nearly one in six of those under age 18 and one in three of AI/AN adults aged 18–64 do not have coverage. Native populations who lack insurance often forgo care except in emergency situations, simply because they cannot afford the costs associated with office visits, diagnostic services, and prescriptions. Yet federal funding of health services for AI/AN populations also impedes their access to care. The IHS remains underfunded; recent estimates indicate the IHS receives less than 60 percent of the funding needed to provide adequate care to Native populations. At present, average per capita funding within the IHS system is only around $4,000; in contrast, per capita funding is $8,000 for Medicare recipients and federal prisoners, $10,000 for veterans, and $13,000 for Medicaid recipients.

The unique economic dimensions of health care in rural areas where most AI/AN populations reside are also relevant. Quite simply, and due to lower populations density and corresponding diminished demand for health services, potential for profit is lower in rural areas than in suburban and urban communities; as a result, rural areas that are home to sizeable AI/AN populations have fewer health-care facilities including clinics, hospitals, and pharmacies. Due to lower average pay when compared to more urban settings, rural health facilities often struggle to attract and retain high-quality, qualified providers. Additionally, smaller operating budgets in rural facilities often mean existing equipment is inadequate and outdated; thus, there are limited options for diagnosis and treatment. At such clinics, for example—including tribal clinics—services often include only primary care. Those seeking services at such clinics may be able to secure basic health screenings (e.g., diabetes, STDs, anemia, high cholesterol, and vision), vaccines, and treatment for common health conditions (e.g., influenza, the common cold, arthritis, high blood pressure, ear infections, respiratory infections, rashes, and urinary tract infections). Yet those needing more advanced care (e.g., for cancer, advanced heart disease, kidney disease, high-risk pregnancy, HIV, mental health disorders, behavioral disorders, and endocrine disorders) typically must travel to more urban areas to receive such care. The lack of resources necessary to provide more advanced care to patients also discourages some providers from accepting employment in areas near tribal lands.

Additionally, many clinics do not permit patients to schedule appointments in advance; thus, they must take time off work or school and show up at the clinic early to increase their likelihood of securing an appointment. If they cannot, they must either forgo care or return to the clinic the next day to wait again. Some individuals may seek care outside the IHS system, yet lack of affordability due to co-pays often discourages them from doing so, especially in states that have not opted to expand Medicaid. In the 1970s, the IHS began providing scholarship and loan forgiveness programs to encourage AI/AN students to pursue careers in health care. Nearly 8,000 students have participated in such programs to date. However, nearly one-fourth of positions at IHS health facilities remain vacant. Some communities have attempted to promote improved access by using proceeds from gaming and other tribal enterprises to subsidize health care for their members. However, demand for such support exceeds availability; thus, many go without needed medications and other types of treatment.

Biases in the Health-Care System

Ongoing biases also diminish access to health care and the quality of care provided to Indigenous populations and contribute to the ongoing mistrust that many feel toward the US health-care system. Such biases are sometimes implicit (unintentional) while other times they are deliberate. They have been documented in medical research/experimentation. In the 1970s, details emerged about forced sterilization of Indigenous populations. Such practices reflected eugenics ideology and were supported by policies enacted via the IHS as well as US Department of Health, Education, and Welfare—it was divided into two entities in 1979, including the Department of Education and the Department of Health and Human Services. Similarly, Indigenous children who were forced to attend government-run boarding schools during the nineteenth and twentieth centuries were subjected to nonconsensual medical experiments and treatments. AI/AN populations have also been targeted for unethical experiments involving pharmaceuticals, contraception, and even exposure to nuclear radiation. Such practices violate patient rights related to informed consent, autonomy, beneficial care, and freedom from harmful practices and procedures. Despite the creation of the Native American Research Centers for Health (NARCH) in 2000, Native populations remain underrepresented in biomedical, behavioral, and social health research. At present, approximately two-thirds of clinical trials do not include AI/AN participants.

In clinical settings, biases contribute to limited knowledge about the specific health needs and related cultural health practices of AI/AN populations. They also contribute to delays in diagnosis and treatment as well as miscommunication between health-care providers and patients. Such biases reflect the content and organization of the US health-care system. For example, few advanced health training programs include attention to AI/AN populations, including core cultural values, spirituality, family norms, and traditional practices related to health and healing. When such curriculum is available, it is typically optional and/or included only as a small section within a broader unit (e.g., a unit on patient diversity) rather than as a stand-alone course or series of courses that concentrate on the cultures and health of tribal communities. There is also little attention to AI/AN cultures in continuing education courses providers must complete to maintain their credentials. In addition, there are over 150 Indigenous languages spoken in the United States; some of the most common among these include Navajo, Apache, Ojibwe, Choctaw, and Yupik. One-fifth of AI/AN populations speak a language other than English; elderly individuals are among those most likely to have limited English proficiency (LEP). However, and even though federal law requires translation services for LEP patients, few health facilities have interpreters that are fluent in Indigenous languages. So-called language lines may include some tribal languages as part of their services, yet they typically include only the most common AI/AN languages, and these are often available only via audio interpreting services but not via video services. Consequently, the availability of linguistically and culturally competent care for Indigenous patients remains a rarity. Individuals who live closer to tribally operated clinics typically have better access to such care; however, those who live further from such facilities encounter the most significant barriers in this regard. For example, although AI/AN populations who reside in more urban area typically report fewer geographic barriers to care, they do encounter significant challenges in accessing care that is culturally competent.

Many have argued that increased efforts to recruit and train Indigenous health providers would help rectify existing biases in health care while simultaneously promoting culturally and linguistically care to AI/AN populations. Yet Indigenous populations remain underrepresented in medical schools, health-care leadership, and clinical settings. At present, they constitute only about half of 1 percent of all students who graduate from medical schools and other advanced medical programs such as dental and ophthalmology schools as well as graduate-level nursing programs. They also remain a rarity among faculty and administrators at such schools; this is particularly true for AI/AN cisgender women and two-spirit persons. At present, AI/AN populations represent just over half a percent of the total health-care workforce. Despite ongoing efforts to educate and recruit more Indigenous health professionals, their representation within the US health-care workforce has stagnated over the past 10 years and in some specialties has declined. It remains lowest in neurology, anesthesiology, cardiology, emergency medicine, psychiatry, orthopedic surgery, and clinical pathology. However, representation of AI/AN populations is slightly higher in support roles including as certified nursing assistants (CNAs), home health aides, and technicians. Such roles are among the lowest paying in the health-care field and tend to primarily employ cisgender women. Like other AI/AN workers, those who enter health professions encounter various forms of discrimination. They are less likely to receive promotions and earn less on average than their non-Indigenous co-workers (especially non-HLC white and certain APIDA populations) who are employed in the same jobs. They are also more likely to be victims of bullying, harassment, and other forms of discrimination in the workplace. AI/AN cisgender women and two-spirit populations are at increased risk of sexual harassment and sexual assault from supervisors, co-workers, and patients.

LIVING ENVIRONMENT AND SOCIAL CONTEXT

The current environmental and social factors that influence the health and well-being of Indigenous populations are rooted in their history of forced and coerced relocation. Environmental degradation and climate change disproportionately impact AI/AN populations, including those who live on or near reservations as well as those living in more urban areas. Lack of access to clean water, air, and land are ongoing concerns that impact both physical and mental health. Additionally, they encounter ongoing health issues due to inadequate and poor-quality infrastructure. Finally, the ongoing social marginalization of Indigenous populations is evident in a variety of social institutions and increases their risk of various forms of violence.

A History of Displacement

Coercive measures that led to the displacement and forced relocation of AI/AN people have made them vulnerable to certain environmental risks. For example, under the Indian Removal Act of 1830, tribes from the Southeastern United States (e.g., the Creek, Choctaw, Chickasaw, Seminole, and Cherokee) were forced to leave their ancestral lands and move to reservations in a region that had been dubbed Indian Territory (and later became the state of Oklahoma). In the ensuing years, other Indigenous groups from the Upper Midwest, Northeastern, and Lower Midwest regions of the country—including the Ho-Chunk, Ojibwa, Potawatomi, Sauk, Oneida, and Iowa tribes—were also targeted for removal. The ancestral lands they were forced to leave were fertile areas that supported sustainable agriculture and/or that provided access to forests and waterways (e.g., lakes, rivers, coastal areas, and streams) suitable for husting, fishing, and gathering activities. Yet the reservations were drier and less suitable for growing foods. Reservations also had fewer natural resources, including water as well as the flora and fauna that were central to traditional Indigenous lifeways related to food, spirituality, and medicinal practices. Thus, those who survived the journey encountered ongoing health issues due to the environmental aspects of reservations.

Similarly, the Indian Relocation Act (1956)—sometimes referred to as the Adult Vocational Training Act or the Voluntary Relocation Program—contributed to displacement of AI/AN populations and subjected them to environmentally related health hazards. In what is now widely recognized as a strategy intended to assimilate Indigenous communities into mainstream, white American culture and eliminate tribal reservations, the act stipulated that AI/AN populations who relocated to urban areas would receive financial support as well as vocational training and health insurance. Yet the program was drastically underfunded. Consequently, those who did move to urban areas received minimal support. They also found themselves disconnected from their families and tribal communities—something that has been identified as a key source of trauma for such populations—and living in impoverished neighborhoods of major urban areas (e.g., Chicago, Seattle, and Los Angeles) where they faced significant health risks due to overcrowding, pollution, inferior quality housing, and inadequate services related to health, education, transportation, social welfare, and other basic services.

Living Environment and Infrastructure

At present, health issues related to living environment are significant for Indigenous communities across the country. This is true regardless of whether they live on or near tribal reservations, in rural areas that are distant from reservations, or in more urban settings. Climate change and environmental degradation are key considerations. The poor environmental conditions on reservations are well documented, something Indigenous leaders have linked to environmental racism and limited attention to climate change by political leaders. In recent decades in Alaska, for example, increasing temperatures have contributed to the thawing of permafrost, decreasing sea ice, and alteration of ecosystems. The consequences of such changes have been devastating for Alaska Native (AN) populations. Thawing permafrost has increased risk of exposure to harmful viruses and bacteria. Access to food resources—including native plants, fish, and game—has decreased. There has also been an increase in frequency and severity of flooding, something that has caused widespread erosion. As a result, some coastal tribes have had to leave their ancestral lands; it is likely that many more will need to relocate in the coming years. Although federally recognized tribes are available for disaster-related financial support through the Federal Emergency Management Agency (FEMA), many have criticized such support as inadequate to meet demand. Others have argued that the federal government needs to work toward longer-term, multi-pronged strategies to help mitigate environmental risks to such communities and provide more comprehensive and culturally appropriate support when disasters do occur.

Health concerns related to poor air, soil, and water quality are prominent on reservations throughout the country. Examples include respiratory illnesses (e.g., asthma, bronchitis, and COPD), kidney disease, hypertension, and vector-borne illnesses (e.g., Lyme disease, Rocky Mountain spotted fever, and West Nile virus). Additionally, industries that produce toxic waste are often located near reservations; examples of such industries include mining operations, smelting facilities, manufacturing plants, and nuclear power plants and nuclear storage facilities. From the 1940s through the end of the twentieth century, military test sites for nuclear and chemical weapons were frequently located near AI/AN reservations. Reservations have also been used as dumping sites for waste. As a result, and due to the lengthy half-life of such waste, residents are at increased risk for health problems including cancer, organ failure, neurological disorders, mood disorders, behavioral disorders, endocrine disorders, birth defects, disability, and premature death.

Development projects on or near reservations also threaten the health of Indigenous communities by diminishing access to natural resources. In 2016, for example, members of the Standing Rock Sioux Tribe of North Dakota mounted protests in response to a proposed plan to allow part of the 1,200-mile-long underground Dakota Access Pipeline to run through tribal lands, thereby threatening to contaminate the water supply that serves as the primary source of drinking water to the community. Although construction of the pipeline stopped in December 2016 due to a decision by the US Army Corps of Engineers, that decision was overturned in early 2017 when President Trump ordered expedited review and approval of the project. Since its completion, the pipeline has had numerous leaks. Similarly, hydraulic fracking activities—used to extract oil and gas from beneath rock formations—have led to spills, thereby contaminating water supplies on and near several tribal reservations.

Nearly half of those living on reservations do not have access to indoor plumbing or sanitation/sewage disposal facilities. Existing water and sanitation systems in tribal communities are often outdated or in disrepair. Common problems include rusted pipes, broken pumps, and depleted water aquifers; additionally, existing water sources are often contaminated by human and animal waste, bacteria, viruses, and/or heavy metals. Due to ongoing issues with poor-quality housing, lack of affordable housing, and overcrowding, rates of homelessness and housing insecurity on tribal reservations are nearly five times as high as national averages among all populations. Additionally, problems with inadequate transportation infrastructure on and near reservations—including poor road conditions, lack of sufficient traffic lights and safety lights, and ongoing problems related to snow and ice removal—persist. Such problems diminish access to employment, education, and health services for Indigenous populations. Problems with transportation infrastructure on reservations have been linked to high rates of auto-related injuries and deaths among drivers, passengers, and pedestrians. Such problems also diminish access to health care.

Those residing on and near reservations are at elevated risk for food insecurity; they are four times as likely as non-AI/AN households to be food insecure. Many reservations are food deserts and residents lack adequate access to affordable, fresh, and nutritious foods (e.g., fruits, vegetables, whole grains, and lean proteins). Due to poor soil and water quality and water scarcity, residents often find it difficult—and in some cases impossible—to grow or raise their own food. Additionally, there tend to be few grocery stores on reservations. Consequently, residents may need to travel an hour or more to reach a grocery store to access affordable, healthy food. Convenience stores are more common both on and near reservations, yet food options at such stores tend to be highly processed, lacking in vitamins and minerals, and high in fats, sodium, sugar, and preservatives. Diets that rely heavily on such foods are associated with increased risk of heart disease, diabetes, metabolic syndrome, high blood pressure, dental problems, and cancer. In recent years, and as part of ongoing efforts to rectify food insecurity, there has been a movement among some AI/AN communities to decolonize their diets. This involves reliance on cultural food preparation techniques and consuming native species of plants and animals that are part of precolonial traditions.

Indigenous populations residing in urban areas also encounter a variety of health problems due to environmental factors. As a result of the combination of lower average incomes and ongoing social marginalization of AI/AN populations in the United States, those in urban and suburban communities are more likely to reside in substandard housing that includes poor ventilation, pests (e.g., rodents, insects, and dust mites), overcrowding, temperature extremes, mold, and inferior building materials that expose residents to lead, asbestos, volatile organic compounds, formaldehyde, and other toxins. Low walkability levels and inadequate access to public transportation are also common in such communities. They often lack suitable options for recreation and leisure activities, and existing options are often poorly maintained. Such areas also tend to have a lower concentration of health-care facilities (e.g., clinics, pharmacies, and hospitals) than more affluent areas. Exposure to various forms of urban waste (e.g., household, manufacturing, and commercial), air pollution, water pollution, and noise pollution are significant concerns. Poor-quality living conditions increase risk of physical health issues among urban AI/AN populations; examples include asthma, COPD, and other respiratory health issues; communicable diseases (COVID-19, influenza, colds); and conditions due to chronic exposure to environmental stressors (e.g., insomnia and other sleep disturbances, musculoskeletal issues, hypertension, obesity, heart disease, metabolic syndrome, and diabetes). Inferior quality living conditions are also associated with poor mental health, including mood disorders, anxiety disorders, irritability, persistent feelings of loneliness, SUAD, and suicidal ideation. Mental health issues are exacerbated by the ongoing isolation and discrimination that diminish the quality of life and sense of belonging for many urban AI/AN individuals. In urban and suburban communities, and when compared to non-AI/AN groups, rates of housing insecurity are higher among AI/AN residents; those who are housing insecure are at increased risk of physical and mental health issues due to environmental factors including pollutants, weather and climate, and pests.

Social Marginalization: Representations and Violence

In various social contexts, AI/AN populations encounter ongoing marginalization. This is clear in employment, educational, and health-care settings, as discussed earlier in this chapter; it is also evident in media, news, and popular culture where they remain underrepresented. However, when included, it is typically via well-worn stereotypes. Examples are found in literature, films, children's books, cartoons, and news coverage as well as household décor, sports-related clothing and memorabilia, Halloween costumes, and tourism-related merchandise. Some depict AI/AN populations as primitive, simple-minded, lazy, and uneducated; others portray them as aggressive, greedy, promiscuous, and dangerous. Gender is a key consideration. While common caricatures of Indigenous cisgender women/girls include the controlling matriarch, the princess, the wise elder, and the seductress, those of cisgender men/boys include the medicine man, the alcoholic/drug addict, and the warrior (who is often represented as aggressive both socially and sexually). Such stereotypes are frequently internalized by Indigenous individuals and can diminish their self-esteem and sense of belonging. It is also clear that such stereotypes contribute to the ongoing social marginalization they experience in US society.

The ongoing social marginalization of AI/AN populations increases their risk of violent victimization. When compared to other racial and ethnic groups, they are more likely to be targets of violent crimes, including murder, assault, and rape. Most crimes against Indigenous individuals are committed by non-AI/AN populations. There is a clear gendered component to such crimes. The rate of death due to homicide among AI/AN populations overall is higher than national averages. Among those aged 1–54, homicide is the fifth leading cause of death for cisgender men/boys and the seventh leading cause of death for cisgender women/girls. Additionally, while homicides against cisgender males are typically carried out by a friend or acquaintance and after an argument or some other type of crime has occurred, nearly 90 percent of homicides perpetrated against AI/AN women and girls are carried out by current or former romantic partners. Rates of sexual assault and rape against AI/AN cisgender women and two-spirit individuals are twice as high as national averages; most survivors do not report such crimes due to distrust of police, fear of retaliation by their attacker, or concerns they will be socially ostracized.

Violence against and dehumanization of Indigenous populations is also evident in the US criminal justice system. They are overrepresented as suspects, defendants, detainees, and inmates. They are more likely than non-HLC white populations to be searched during traffic stops. Rates of incarceration are four times higher for AI/AN cisgender men when compared to their non-HLC white counterparts; among cisgender women, rates of incarceration are six times higher for AI/AN populations than for non-HLC whites. In addition, police brutality against Indigenous populations has been documented across the country, including against those who were engaged in peaceful protests related to the Dakota Access Pipeline. They are more likely than all other non-AI/AN populations to be killed by police, yet there remains little media coverage of such killings.

CHAPTER NINE

Low-Income Populations

In plain terms, poverty is a state of monetary and material scarcity that compromises the ability to meet basic needs (e.g., food, shelter, clothing, clean water, and sanitation). Poverty also impairs access to essential services related to education, safety, transportation, and health care. People living in poverty are often referred to as low-income, impoverished, destitute, indigent, needy, poor, or as having low socioeconomic status (SES). Chronic poverty is defined as a period of three years or more in which an individual or household consistently earns income below the Federal Poverty Level (FPL). Chronic poverty is often intergenerational. Yet in other cases, poverty is episodic or situational and may occur unexpectedly due to catastrophic circumstances (e.g., natural disaster, pandemic, and armed conflict); serious illness or injury; job loss; divorce; or death of the primary household wage earner. Episodic poverty is short term (from 2 months to 3 years). However, episodic poverty may develop into chronic poverty. Poverty may also be absolute (below the FPL and lacking basic needs) or relative (when household income is less than 50 percent of the average in a specific community). Extreme poverty or abject poverty—income of less than $1.90 per-day-per-person—is the most persistent and severe form of poverty.

Income has a profound impact on health and well-being. This is true regardless of social identities or geographic location. However, certain populations are overrepresented among those who are impoverished, especially racial and ethnic minorities; the elderly; cisgender women and girls (those whose gender identity aligns with the sex they were assigned at birth); individuals who identify as lesbian, gay, bisexual, transgender, queer, intersex, or asexual (LGBTQIA) or gender nonconforming (GNC); certain immigrant populations; formerly incarcerated individuals; and individuals who are chronically ill or who have disabilities. Although America declared a war on poverty in the mid-1960s, the reality is that rates of poverty have fluctuated significantly over the past 60 years. There are significant differences in rates of poverty from state to state and when comparing rural versus urban areas. Low-income populations are among those Americans most likely to encounter barriers to employment, education, and health care. They are also more likely than wealthier populations to reside in communities that are economically and racially segregated, have poor environmental conditions, and lack or have outdated infrastructure.

Quite simply, impoverished populations have a higher burden of disease for physical and mental conditions; they are also at increased risk of disability and premature death.

CURRENT STATE OF HEALTH

Poverty increases risk, incidence, and severity of illness, injury, and disability. Conversely, poor health increases likelihood and severity of poverty by limiting ability to work, increasing time spent away from work, and increasing health-related expenses. Impoverished populations experience disproportionately high morbidity and mortality rates related to chronic conditions including heart disease, obesity, stroke, chronic obstructive pulmonary disease (COPD), diabetes, and certain types of cancer (e.g., stomach, liver, colorectal, lung, skin, breast, and prostate). Infectious diseases are also a concern. Certain infectious diseases are referred to as diseases of poverty because rates are highest among low-income populations. Examples include hookworm, roundworm, toxoplasmosis, Chagas disease, leishmaniasis, leptospirosis, cytomegalovirus, trench fever, and trichomoniasis. Disability rates among low-income Americans are more than twice as high as among households that are middle class or affluent. Those living in poverty are also disproportionately impacted by weather- and climate-related health conditions, including skin cancer, heat stroke, insect-borne diseases (e.g., West Nile virus, chikungunya, and Lyme disease), and respiratory illnesses (e.g., asthma, allergies, and COPD). Vision impairment and loss are more common among low-income populations. They also encounter disparities in oral health from infancy through old age. They often do not receive regular dental screenings, and untreated cavities are common; they also experience disproportionately high rates of oral cancers and periodontal disease.

Individuals who live in households with total income below the FPL and/or in low-income counties where the average household income is in the bottom twenty-fifth percentile among all US households are more likely to die prematurely. In 2022, the average life expectancy (ALE) for cisgender females in the United States was just over 81 years; it was 76 years for cisgender males. Such figures are marginally lower than most other high-income nations that are part of the Organization for Economic Cooperation and Development (OECD). However, the ALE for low-income Americans is dramatically lower than national averages and is similar to the ALE in middle-income countries. The wealthiest 1 percent of cisgender women in the United States live 15 years longer than the poorest 1 percent of cisgender women; and among poor cisgender men, the ALE is approximately one decade less than among their more affluent counterparts. This is known as the wealth-based mortality gap. It has steadily expanded over the past century and is most pronounced among low-income Indigenous, Black, and LGBTQIA populations.

Children born into low-income families are more likely to be born premature (prior to the thirty-seventh week of pregnancy), at a low birth weight (less than 5.5 pounds), and to have congenital disorders or malformations (often referred to as birth defects). Among the most common are heart defects, neural tube defects (e.g., related to the brain, spinal cord, and nervous system), blood disorders, and Down syndrome (also known as trisomy 21). Congenital anomalies are sometimes hereditary. However, among low-income populations, they are more often a consequence of dietary factors (e.g., when a pregnant individual does not have access to a diet that provides adequate nutrition) and environmental factors (e.g., prenatal exposure to toxic substances in working or living environments or to alcohol, tobacco, medication, or illicit drugs). Prenatal exposure to stress has also emerged as a significant concern. An overabundance of stress hormones during pregnancy affects fetal brain development in ways that are associated with increased likelihood of engagement in high-risk behaviors as well as compromised health status, academic performance, and economic opportunities in childhood and adulthood. Failure to thrive—when weight and height are significantly lower than average for age and sex and/or there is delayed social, physical, and/or cognitive development—is more common among low-income infants and children. Rates of infant and child mortality are also disproportionately high among such populations. Throughout childhood, low-income populations are at increased risk of malnourishment, including being overweight, obese, and underweight; vitamin and mineral deficiencies are also common.

Rates of disabilities are twice as high among impoverished children when compared to those from higher-income families. Such rates have increased by 70 percent among low-income youth over the past two decades; they are highest among low-income Indigenous and Black children and those who belong to more than one racial or ethnic group. Most common among physical disabilities are those related to premature birth. Examples include cerebral palsy, neurological disorders, and issues stemming from malformation or underdevelopment of sensory organs (e.g., vision or hearing impairment or loss) or internal organs (e.g., asthma, bronchopulmonary dysplasia, and necrotizing enterocolitis). Yet cognitive impairments, behavioral disorders, and mental health disorders are also more prevalent among poor children and have been linked to nutritional deficits and inadequate exposure to age-appropriate stimuli (e.g., toys, games, social interactions, preschool and other forms of formal education). However, exposure to traumatic or potentially traumatic experiences is also a contributing factor. Collectively referred to as adverse childhood experiences (ACEs), they trigger an acute stress response in the sympathetic nervous system that can hamper brain development, immune system response, and function of cardiovascular, respiratory, endocrine, and other body systems. ACEs diminish self-esteem, resilience, optimism, and self-control while simultaneously increasing feelings of sadness, fear, anger, guilt, humiliation, and vulnerability. Examples of ACEs include neglect; abuse (physical, emotional, or sexual); bullying; exposure to community violence; living in a household where there is substance abuse, violence, food insecurity, or housing insecurity; having divorced or separated parents; death or serious illness of a close relative; having a parent who is incarcerated. ACEs occur among all demographic groups. However, poverty and other systemic inequities (e.g., racism, homophobia, transphobia, and sexism) are also ACEs and associated with chronic stress. Thus, ACEs are more common among low-income children, especially Black, Indigenous, Hispanic/Latinx/Chicanx (HLC), LGBTQIA, and cisgender female populations.

Children and teens who grow up in poverty are more likely than their more affluent peers to encounter problems with memory and language development. They are also more likely to experience dyslexia, dyscalculia, and autism spectrum disorders as well as various behavioral disorders including attention-deficit hyperactivity disorder (ADHD), oppositional defiant disorder (ODD), impulse control disorder, and conduct disorder. Mental health disorders are also more common, especially anxiety, depression, post-traumatic stress disorder (PTSD), and those associated with emotional dysregulation. Rates of mental illness such as anxiety and major depressive disorder are disproportionately high among low-income adolescents. Suicidal ideation and suicide attempts are more common among poor teens and adults, particularly in counties where incomes are below the national average. Rates are highest among poor cisgender men in rural areas. Low-income teens encounter more physical health problems than their wealthier peers. They are more likely to be overweight or obese, have nutritional deficiencies, and are at increased risk of developing heart disease. Such issues are linked to poor-quality diet as well as low rates of participation in team sports, recreational pursuits, and other types of physical activity. Poor teens are also more likely to smoke cigarettes and use other tobacco products yet less likely to use and abuse alcohol and marijuana. Rates of unintentional injuries due to falls, work activities, and auto accidents are disproportionately high among adolescents from low-income families. They are also more likely to be victims and perpetrators of physical assault and to die in automobile and motorcycle accidents.

Low-income populations are less likely to seek out and receive reproductive and sexual health services than middle-income and wealthy populations. Those with incomes below the FPL and/or who live in areas of concentrated poverty—where 30 percent or more of households live below the FPL—are less likely to use contraception than middle-class Americans. Furthermore, and although rates of certain sexually transmitted infections (STIs)—especially gonorrhea, syphilis, and human papilloma virus (HPV)—have increased overall in the United States in recent years, such increases have been disproportionately high in areas of concentrated poverty, particularly among Black, Indigenous, and HLC populations. Children who grow up in low-income households and impoverished communities typically engage in sexual activity at a younger age—typically, prior to age 15—and are more likely to engage in high-risk sexual behaviors such as having multiple sexual partners and not engaging in safe-sex practices. Rates of adolescent pregnancy are also higher among low-income populations. Overall, birth rates have declined significantly over the past two decades among populations living below the FPL. Yet such rates are 70 percent higher than among those with higher incomes. Low-income pregnant individuals are less likely to receive prenatal care and take prenatal vitamins; they also have higher rates of pregnancy-related complications and poor birth outcomes for both the pregnant individual and offspring. Examples of such outcomes include miscarriage, stillbirth, preterm labor, premature birth, gestational diabetes, and high blood pressure during pregnancy. Low-income populations are also more likely to encounter pregnancy-related complications, require delivery via cesarean section, and die during pregnancy, labor, or delivery.

ECONOMIC FACTORS

Poverty rates in the United States reflect broader economic trends. They are also influenced by the government-funded programs that comprise the social safety net. Yet access to employment that provides a living wage is also an ongoing concern, particularly among those who work in entry-level and low-skilled jobs. In addition, and as the cost of living continues to rise, housing, childcare, food, and other necessities continue to become less affordable.

Poverty Rates and the Safety Net

In the late 1950s when the US Census Bureau first began to record and track the poverty rate, it was at an all-time high of 22 percent. However, the steady increase in labor force participation during the 1960s and throughout the 1970s, combined with overall growth of the US economy as well as expanded social service programs—commonly referred to as the social safety net—implemented via the Economic Opportunity Act of 1964 helped reduce rates of poverty. By the late 1970s, less than 12 percent of Americans lived below the FPL. However, poverty rates fluctuated during the 1980s and 1990s and ranged from 11 to 15 percent; such rates were highest at times when rates of unemployment were also highest. During the 1990s, the Personal Responsibility and Work Opportunities Reconciliation Act of 1996 (PRWORA) overhauled the American welfare system while simultaneously aiming to reduce child poverty. PRWORA resulted in extensive changes to the social safety net. It decreased eligibility for cash assistance, food stamps, and government-sponsored health insurance for poor families. It also placed a strict time limit on receipt of aid. Although welfare caseloads declined in subsequent years, PRWORA did not result in long-term, dramatic reductions in poverty or unemployment. On the contrary, such rates have continued to ebb and flow over the past two decades in response to broader economic, political, and social factors. For example, during the Great Recession (2008–9), rates of home foreclosures and job loss increased across America, especially in low-income communities. Furthermore, low-income populations lost a greater portion of their overall wealth (e.g., savings, property, automobiles, and other items of value) during the Great Recession, and the number of low-income Americans increased by over 20 percent. In response, the US Congress expanded the social safety net via passage of the American Recovery and Reinvestment Act of 2009 (ARRA). Such legislation expanded food stamps and family tax credits. It also increased funds available for cash grants to low-income populations. Yet the time limits imposed by PRWORA rendered some individuals and families ineligible for such benefits.

Similarly, the COVID-19 pandemic disproportionately affected impoverished households. Half of such households experienced reduced earnings during the pandemic due to loss of employment or illness. In 2020, approximately 20 million households were food insecure and over 10 million families were at risk of displacement because they could not afford rent or mortgage payments. Furthermore, increasing demand for certain products (e.g., medications, cleaning products, computers and accessories, packaged foods, and toilet paper) and changes in import and export practices prompted inflation to increase. Thus, purchasing power—what one is able to buy with a specific amount of currency—decreased; while families across the country felt such economic changes, those with the fewest economic resources were most impacted. In the decade prior to the pandemic, the US poverty rate had declined from 15.1 percent in 2010 to 10.5 percent in late 2019. The pandemic reversed such declines. In 2020, the child poverty rate increased by 10 percent. Yet in 2021, poverty rates gradually decreased from the 16.1 percent rate recorded at the end of the first year of the pandemic. This decrease was influenced, in part, by the Coronavirus Aid, Relief, and Economic Security Act (CARES) of 2020 as well as the American Rescue Plan of 2021 (sometimes referred to as the COVID-19 Stimulus Package). These measures included expansion of the Supplemental Nutrition Assistance Program (SNAP), employment benefits, child tax credit, and emergency rental assistance. In addition, cash grants were offered to those with incomes below a certain threshold. The temporary suspension of interest and payment on student loans also helped ease financial woes for low-income Americans during the pandemic.

Employment and a Living Wage

Working adults aged 18–64 represent just over half of all those living in poverty. Approximately 40 percent work for wages while another 18 percent are engaged in household production that involves creating goods for sale (e.g., food, clothing, and agricultural products) or offering services for hire (e.g., childcare, cleaning, laundry, tutoring, carpentry, gardening, elder care, and pet services). One-fourth of low-income adults are either unable to work due to disability or are retired while another 10 percent are students pursuing postsecondary training or education. Thus, less than 10 percent of low-income, able-bodied adults of working age are unemployed and not engaged in education or income-generating activities. There are low-income adults who work part-time. Yet half of low-income households have at least one family member that works full-time for 6 months or more per year, and 25 percent have at least one adult family member who works full-time year-round. Those who are employed yet still living in poverty are known as the working poor. Families with minor children are more likely to be part of the working poor. Furthermore, HLC, Black, and Indigenous populations are two to three times more likely to be employed yet still living in poverty than white and Asian populations.

The percent of Americans who are part of the working poor has increased since 2000. They are concentrated in entry-level jobs that are typically classified as unskilled or low-skilled labor. Such jobs do not involve particularly complex processes or require specialized education, training, knowledge, certification, credentials, or skills prior to employment. In addition, they typically do not provide employees with transferrable job skills and, thus, are often referred to as dead-end jobs. Examples include custodial and janitorial services; food service; warehouse shipping and receiving; agricultural work; sanitation services; taxi driver; receptionist; babysitter; construction; and retail cashier. Average earnings in such jobs, even for full-time employees, typically do not constitute a living wage—that is, they do not provide adequate income for a worker and their family to enjoy a standard of living that meets basic needs. In 2020, the US living wage for a family of four was approximately $70,000. However, there is great variation by state and type of community; the income required to meet basic needs is higher in suburban and urban areas than in rural areas. Cities such as New York, Honolulu, Boston, San Francisco, Los Angeles, Miami, and Washington, DC, have the highest cost of living and, therefore, a higher living wage. Yet most unskilled and low-skill jobs continue to pay only minimum wage. Such compensation varies from state to state. It is $7.25 (as per federal minimum wage law) in twenty states; in seven states plus the District of Columbia, minimum wage is $13.00 or more per hour.

Those who earn $7.25 per hour are not earning a living wage. In fact, an individual who earns such a wage and works 40 hours per week for the entire calendar year will earn just a little over $15,000 before taxes. If that individual lives in Kentucky—the state with the lowest living wage required to meet basic needs—and is unmarried with no dependents, their earnings will represent only a little over half the amount needed to meet typical expenses and basic needs in that state. If they are married and have dependents, the disparity is even greater. The living wage for a family of two adults and one child in the state of Kentucky requires an annual pre-tax income of just over $55,000. Yet if only one parent works at a job that pays minimum wage, household income will be approximately $40,000 short of the amount necessary to meet typical expenses for a family of three. If both parents work full-time and year-round at jobs that pay $7.25 per hour, they will still have earned only about two-thirds of a living wage in Kentucky. The gap between minimum wage and living wage also persists in states with a higher minimum wage. If an individual earns the minimum wage of $10.10 in Hawaii, their annual pre-tax earnings would be just over $21,000. Thus, they would earn only about half of the living wage needed for a single adult with no dependents. Similarly, a person employed full-time in Washington, DC, at $15.20 per hour—the highest minimum wage in the nation—would earn about $11,000 less than the amount needed to meet typical annual expenses for an unmarried individual without children.

Those able to secure higher-paying, skilled labor positions are more likely to earn an income that is commensurate with a living wage. Yet the reality is that low-income populations face significant and persistent barriers to the type of advanced education and training required to secure such positions. Furthermore, not all poor populations work in low-skilled labor positions. In fact, due to increasing inflation as well as the economic devastation that can result from injury, accident, illness, job loss, divorce, natural disasters, or other unexpected circumstances, even skilled workers earning a living wage may struggle to make ends meet. At present, over half of American households lack adequate savings to cover basic living expenses for three months if they become unemployed or unable to work. Similarly, two-thirds of all adults cannot afford a $400 unexpected expense. Populations with incomes below 300 percent of the FPL are also at increased risk of liquid asset poverty; this occurs when overall wealth and assets (e.g., property, stocks, savings, automobiles, and other things of value that can be sold quickly to secure income) are insufficient to cover three months of basic living expenses in the event that the primary wage earner is fired, unemployed, becomes disabled, or dies.

Living Expenses, Housing, and Childcare

Individuals who are employed full-time, live in states where the minimum wage exceeds the federal standard, and/or are employed in skilled labor positions are more likely to earn incomes that exceed the FPL. However, it is common for such individuals and their families to find themselves still unable to afford basic needs. This lack of affordability is, in part, a consequence of rising inflation rates. While inflation has increased globally in recent years, the United States has experienced a disproportionately high increase when compared to other OECD nations. Although such rates have fluctuated since the Great Recession, US inflation surged in 2021 and reached a 40-year high by 2022. As a result, the cost of living increased, especially for items such as food, gas, vehicles, lumber, clothing, personal care products, and certain home items (e.g., furniture and cleaning products). The cost of services also increased, including those related to transportation, pet care, and cleaning and laundry services.

Housing costs have also increased. The subprime mortgage crisis caused housing prices to plummet from 2007 to 2012. However, such prices have increased steadily since 2012, rising twice as fast as inflation. Whereas the median home price in the United States was approximately $211,000 in 2012, it doubled by the end of 2021. Similarly, rental prices have increased dramatically over the past two decades. Whereas median rent for a one-bedroom apartment in the United States was $602 per month in 2000, it surged to just under $1,700 by 2022. Thus, even in locations where the minimum wage is well over the federal minimum, average rental prices are often unaffordable. In Arkansas, where the average fair market rent for housing is well below the national average, an individual earning the state's minimum hourly wage of $11.00 would need to work 43 hours per week to afford average rent of $600 on a one-bedroom apartment and more than 50 hours per week to pay average rent of $750 on a two-bedroom apartment. At present, approximately one-fifth of all United States' employed adults struggle to afford housing. Rates of homelessness and housing insecurity have steadily increased since 2015. At present, up to 4 million individuals in the United States—including both adults and children—are unsheltered for a period of time each year.

Childcare expenses can be similarly challenging. Rates vary by geographic location and are typically lower in rural communities than in more urban areas. Yet for low-income and middle-income households with children under the age of five, childcare constitutes the largest monthly expenditure in most regions of the country. Nationally, the average annual cost of full-time care for a preschool-aged child is $9,400. An individual earning $7.25 per hour would need to work 1,300 hours—more than 32 weeks of full-time labor—to cover this amount. In families with more than one preschool-aged child, childcare expenses often exceed rent or mortgage payments. In those areas where minimum wage is higher, childcare costs also tend to be higher. Therefore, while states in the northeast tend to have higher minimum wages, the cost of childcare in the Northeast is significantly higher than in the Midwest, South, and the West. On average, a family with two children under the age of five and living in the Northeast will have an annual childcare bill of approximately $26,000.

EDUCATIONAL ACCESS AND QUALITY

Students who experience chronic poverty typically lag behind their more affluent peers with regard to academic achievement and completion rates; such disparities have increased in recent decades. Scarcity of resources in public K-12 schools that are located in low-income communities is common; in addition, such schools often struggle to recruit and retain qualified personnel. Despite measures intended to support low-income students, they continue to be marginalized in educational settings.

Primary and Secondary Schooling

Socioeconomic status has a profound influence on educational performance and attainment; this is commonly known as the income achievement gap. Children who experience poverty during infancy and early childhood are less likely than their more affluent peers to be academically and socially ready for school by the time they reach the age of five. It is also common for children from low-income backgrounds to struggle with interpersonal communication, social interactions, self-awareness, resourcefulness, emotional expression, and perseverance. While academic as well as social and emotional skills impact academic performance, they also profoundly influence children's social connections with both peers and teachers. Such skills also impact self-esteem, self-concept, and sense of happiness. The chronic stress associated with living in poverty also impairs cognitive function, memory, and ability to concentrate, especially for children who experience multiple ACEs. Unfortunately, most children who begin school with a deficit in basic skills do not catch up to their peers.

In pre-K, elementary, and middle school, children from impoverished families are significantly less likely than their peers to meet grade-level expectations for reading and math. They are also more likely to underperform on standardized tests that measure verbal ability, reasoning, creativity, critical thinking, and ability to organize and apply information. Children living below the FPL are more likely to lack age-appropriate books in home, preschool, and after-school settings. Their rates of school absenteeism and tardiness are also disproportionately high. Such disparities occur among all racial and ethnic groups; however, they are most pronounced among low-income Black, HLC, and Indigenous populations. By the time they reach high school, low-income students are more than four times more likely to drop out. Such disparities are disproportionately high among low-income cisgender males as well as LGBTQIA, Black, HLC, and Indigenous populations. Students from impoverished families are also significantly less likely to participate in extracurricular activities, including sports, performing arts, visual arts, and civic engagement activities. Unlike their wealthier peers, teenagers from low-income families often have to work in order to contribute to household income. This reduces the time they can devote to homework and to extracurricular or enrichment activities.

Low-income students are slightly more likely to experience certain types of emotional and intellectual disabilities that impact learning and, therefore, to require special education. Yet biases often influence educators' assessment and treatment of low-income students. Educators sometimes expect certain types of cognitive and behavioral problems among low-income students and, therefore, rely on subjective rather than objective analysis when observing and assessing such students. Furthermore, when assessing the academic performance of low-income students, educators frequently mistake vision and hearing impairments as learning disabilities or cognitive impairments. When compared to higher-income students who do not meet grade-level expectations, low-income students are more often funneled into special education programs, especially into separate classrooms. While proponents believe separating students in this manner is appropriate in certain cases or for certain academic subjects, the Individuals with Disabilities Education Act (IDEA) of 1990 promotes inclusive education. Proponents of this model argue that separating students with learning disabilities, cognitive challenges, or behavioral disorders not only diminishes the quality and content of their education but also reinforces normative constructs of ability.

Educators sometimes either implicitly or explicitly equate low-income status with low academic potential; thus, they often have reduced academic expectations for poor students, overlook the academic potential and skills of such students, and do not select them for honors, advanced placement (AP), or gifted-and-talented programs. Low-income students are also more likely than their more affluent peers to be punished or suspended for breaking school rules; this is true even when the infraction is the same. Low-income Indigenous, HLC, and Black students, those with disabilities, and LGBTQIA students are disproportionately impacted by disciplinary actions in school settings. Such actions have minimal impact on reducing undesirable behavior. They do, however, contribute to negative feelings about school and teachers among all student populations; for students who are punished, there are psycho-social and academic consequences. Short term, these include increased feelings of humiliation, resentment, frustration, and marginalization in school settings. Long-term, however, such students are more likely to drop out and to become involved with the criminal justice system. Disparate disciplinary action against poor students has been identified as a key factor in the school-to-prison pipeline.

Funding for public education comes from local, state, and federal governments as well as grants from charitable and corporate entities. However, models used for determining such funding vary by state and school district. About 47 percent of such funding comes from state governments. However, 45 percent comes from local property taxes; therefore, and because schools located in low-income communities have a smaller tax base, they have less funding. Critics argue that the current funding structure of public education in the United States is a form of economic segregation. Schools located in low-income communities have fewer learning resources and often lack adequate computing technology. They are also more likely to receive a failing grade with regard to both the quality of the education they provide and student academic performance. Teachers in low-income school districts are often less experienced and less effective in promoting student learning; furthermore, they may lack training in the range of needs of low-income students. Rates of pay for teachers, administrators, and other staff in low-income communities are typically lower than national averages; thus, high turnover rates are common. Federal funding typically represents 8–10 percent of all funding for public schools; such resources are typically used to promote educational equity by providing support for low-income, disabled, English language learners, or other specific student populations. For example, a school with a high percentage of low-income students may qualify for Title I grants; these can be used to improve curriculum, hire additional teachers, and/or facilitate additional training for staff. Furthermore, the School Breakfast and National School Lunch Program aims to address issues of food insecurity and malnourishment among low-income student populations by providing free and reduced-price lunches and breakfasts. Similarly, the Summer Food Service Program offers nutritional support during the summer months. Additionally, families may qualify for Head Start and Early Head Start programs that aim to promote school readiness among low-income children. A variety of before- and after-school programs and summer programs offered by school districts, community recreation centers, the YMCA, churches, or other charitable organizations also provide academic support, social opportunities, recreational activities, and nutritional support. However, and despite the proven efficacy of such programs, they remain underfunded, and staff turnover remains an ongoing challenge. Furthermore, they have limited capacity, and waiting lists to enroll can be lengthy.

Postsecondary Education and Training

Lower-income students are less likely than their higher-income peers to have the cultural capital and support necessary to successfully navigate the process of researching and applying to colleges as well as securing scholarships or other forms of financial aid for college. Household income is one of the strongest predictors of performance on college admissions exams. On the SAT exam, for example, scores tend to increase as household income increases. Average scores are lowest among students with family incomes below the FPL but significantly higher among middle-class students; scores are consistently highest among students with family incomes above $200,000. Scores on standardized tests are one of the primary tools used to evaluate college readiness and to award competitive scholarships. Yet such exams disadvantage low-income students, particularly in light of the educational disparities they face from pre-K through high school. A number of institutions have incorporated what is known as an adversity score in order to provide a more holistic assessment of students' academic potential. Yet criticisms of the practice have been swift and severe, thus prompting institutions to discontinue the practice. Despite the barriers they face, the percent of low-income students who pursue a college education has increased since 2000. Yet there are disparities by sex. Like their wealthier peers, low-income cisgender females are more likely to enroll in college than their cisgender male peers. Increases in enrollment have been greatest among low-income HLC, Indigenous, and Black populations. Children from families who have experienced intergenerational poverty are less likely to have parents who attended college. Such children are less likely to pursue postsecondary education and training. Over 40 percent of adults who grew up poor have literacy issues and lack the basic skills needed to understand college-level texts.

Postsecondary education and training promote job readiness, particularly in professions that provide a living wage and benefits such as comprehensive health insurance, sick leave, flexible spending accounts for childcare and health, retirement, and vacation leave. Yet among low-income populations who do attend college, income influences not only the type of institution they attend but also their academic performance, persistence, and degree completion rates. Low-income students are underrepresented at all postsecondary institutions, but especially at four-year institutions. They are also less likely to enroll in moderately or highly selective institutions than minimally selective two-year institutions such as private for-profit universities. Importantly, two-year, private, for-profit institutions have the lowest rates of successful degree completion among all types of postsecondary institutions in the United States. Low-income students are approximately 25 percent more likely to drop out during their first year of college. They are only about half as likely as middle-class and wealthy students to earn a college degree within 6 years of completing high school; only about one in five low-income students who enroll will ever earn a degree. Among those who do complete a bachelor's degree, they are less likely than more affluent students to pursue a graduate or professional degree. Additionally, low-income student populations are overrepresented in the social sciences, psychology, and technical trades (e.g., cosmetology, welding, automotive repair, plumbing, paralegal, and dental hygienist). Earning a certification or undergraduate degree in such fields can lead to a rewarding career that includes stable income. Yet job prospects and potential earnings are typically far less in such fields than what is available in STEM (science, technology, engineering, and math) fields. Trades also provide limited potential for career advancement, something that is associated with diminished lifetime earning potential.

Costs associated with tuition, fees, on-campus housing, campus dining services, textbooks, and other necessary expenses have increased over the past 40 years, including at public, private, for-profit, and nonprofit institutions. Such increases have outpaced inflation. In 1980, the average cost of undergraduate tuition and fees at all four-year public universities in the United States was around $800; by 2020, it had increased to over $9,500. At four-year private schools, tuition and fees averaged $3,600 in 1980 but increased to around $33,000 by 2020. In the past 10 years alone, tuition and fees have increased by an average of 25 percent. Most low-income students rely on student financial aid to help meet college costs. Those pursuing an undergraduate degree and whose expected family contribution (EFC) to educational expenses in 2022 is below $5,846 dollars are eligible for a Pell Grant. The maximum amount awarded via a Pell Grant is $6,495. But even those eligible for a Pell Grant or who secure scholarships often find such resources are insufficient to meet total costs associated with tuition, fees, books, and living expenses. This can deter low-income students from pursuing a college degree. Yet others take out student loans. Such loans are an important source of financial support that can help promote access to postsecondary education for low-income students. However, educational loans must be repaid.

The average student loan debt among those completing bachelor's degrees is $37,000; for those with master's degrees, it is twice as high; and for those with doctoral or professional degrees (e.g., law, medicine, and MBA), average student loan debt is over $150,000. Over a million people default on their student loans each year. Loan forgiveness is available via the Public Service Loan Forgiveness (PSLF) program or through programs offered by certain employers. For those who do not qualify for such programs, the average amount of time needed to fully repay students loans is 20 years and the average payment is around $500 per month. Thus, while student loans help make college more affordable in the short term, they have long-term consequences that can impair financial stability. Furthermore, even with various forms of financial aid, students may struggle financially while they are in school. In recent years, rates of housing insecurity and homelessness have increased among student populations. Such rates have been especially high among low-income LGBTQIA students, students with minor children, and racial/ethnic minorities. Approximately 40 percent of all college students had difficulty affording rent, utilities, or other housing-related expenses during 2021. During that same period, over half of college students in the United States struggled to pay for basic needs such as food, clothing, medical care, and transportation. Such challenges are associated with diminished mental health and increased likelihood of engaging in certain high-risk behaviors, including drug and alcohol use. Although some campuses have programs that aim to support students who are housing insecure or food insecure, others do not.

HEALTH-CARE ACCESS AND QUALITY

Health care is more expensive in the United States than in other high-income nations, even for those with health insurance. While various programs that aim to promote access to health care for poor populations do exist, they are often underfunded, understaffed, and provide only limited services. In addition, biases are evident in both the structure of the US health-care system as well as the attitudes and actions of health-care providers. Such biases not only diminish the quality of care provided to low-income populations but can also lead to misdiagnosis, disrespect, and increased health inequities.

The Cost of Health Care

Under the fee-for-service (FFS) model that dominates the US health-care system, patients are charged for each health visit (including both in-person and online), exam, diagnostic test, surgical procedure, or other service rendered. Critics contend that this model encourages unnecessary testing and procedures, promoting economic self-interests of providers over patient health and well-being, contributing to a less efficient health-care system, promoting volume of services over quality, and encouraging treatment rather than prevention. Furthermore, this model is associated with higher health insurance premiums and deductibles. In contrast, a number of other OECD nations rely on bundled-services model wherein all exams, procedures, and treatments are covered via a lump-sum payment; this payment is the same for all individuals. When measured via per person expenditures, average spending for health care in the United States is twice as high as in Canada, France, Germany, the Netherlands, Sweden, and the UK. At present, and despite the fact that preventative health services are associated with reduced overall health-care spending for individuals, health insurance companies, and the government, such services comprise only 3 percent of total health-care expenditures. Another 60 percent is used for inpatient and outpatient treatment; this is about two and a half times the average per person spending for such services in other OECD nations. Per capita, Americans spend 60 percent more on prescription medications (about $1,400) and five times more for health-care administration yet only about half as much on long-term care (e.g., skilled care facilities, and home health services) than other high-income nations.

However, increased spending does not promote improved access to care. Instead, it reflects the reality that average costs of health-care services are higher than in other OECD nations. For example, medications are up to ten times more expensive in the United States. For many Americans, then, health care is simply not affordable. In addition, there are fewer health-care providers, facilities, and pharmacies in low-income neighborhoods, especially in rural areas. Free or reduced-rate health clinics are available in some communities. Low-income populations are the most frequent users of such clinics. During the COVID-19 pandemic, an increasing number of Americans received care at free and reduced-rate clinics. However, such facilities typically rely on donations and volunteer labor; thus, they are chronically underfunded and understaffed and waiting times can be lengthy. Such clinics also tend to offer only primary care. Thus, such clinics often cannot meet the needs of individuals with certain chronic conditions and disabilities, uncommon health issues, or more complex mental health, cognitive, or behavioral disorders.

Health insurance premiums are also higher in the United States than other OECD nations. Over the past decade, health insurance premiums in America have increased at two and a half times the rate of inflation. In 2021, the average cost of employer-sponsored health insurance was $20,000; for an unmarried individual without dependents, such coverage averaged $500 monthly. Although employers assume fiscal responsibility for over 70 percent of health insurance premiums nationally, health insurance can still consume a sizeable portion of monthly resources for employees. Under the Patient Protection and Affordable Care Act (ACA) of 2010, employers are not required to provide health insurance to employees who work less than 30 hours per week. Additionally, employers must only offer health insurance if they have fifty or more full-time employees. In most states, employers must cover at least 50 percent of health insurance premiums for employees; however, they are not required to cover premiums (either in part or total) for family members of employees. ACA did provide additional funding that allowed states to expand Medicaid coverage for low-income populations. In states that opted for such expansion, rates of health insurance coverage and access to health care did improve. However, twelve states chose not to expand Medicaid. Yet even with the expanded coverage and increasing affordability of health care that resulted from ACA, Americans still struggle to pay for health care. Over half of all adults in the United States—including those who are covered by health insurance—delay or simply do not get health care for themselves or their children because they cannot afford it; one-third do not fill prescriptions due to costs. Thirty percent of those with health insurance find it difficult to pay their deductible or to cover out-of-pocket costs and co-pays for medical and dental exams, treatment, or medications. Over a third of all US households find it difficult to afford food, utilities, or other nonmedical necessities due to the cost of health care. Among households earning less than $40,000 annually, nearly one-fifth struggle with unpaid medical debt. Black, Indigenous, and HLC populations as well as those who have disabilities, chronic health conditions, and/or lack health insurance are disproportionately represented among Americans who delay or forego health care and go without medication due to lack of affordability; they also have an unduly high burden of medical debt.

Prescription drug costs are another concern. Prices tend to be higher for drugs used to treat rare diseases. For example, Zokinvy is used to treat Hutchinson-Gilford Progeria, a genetic disorder that causes rapid aging in infants and young children; it costs over $80,000 per month. Yet even for medications used to treat common conditions, monthly costs for a single prescription can be hundreds of dollars. For those who require multiple prescriptions, costs can be almost as high as rent, especially for those who lack health insurance. For example, the out-of-pocket cost for insulin typically ranges from $700 to $1,000 per month for individuals without health insurance; thus, low-income patients with diabetes often skip doses or take only partial doses. While doing so can help reduce their overall health costs, it also jeopardizes their health and puts them at increased risk for erratic blood sugar levels, kidney damage, irregular heartbeat, loss of consciousness, and even death. Certain medications have generic equivalents, yet others do not. Pharmaceutical companies may offer discount programs; health-care companies sometimes provide coupons to help make medication more affordable. Yet patients who have not received information about such options from their provider are more likely to regard their prescriptions as unaffordable and, consequently, are less likely to attempt to fill them.

The Need for Culturally Competent Care

In light of their economic circumstances, low-income populations often have different priorities and perspectives related to well-being and health care than those with higher incomes. For example, while they do not necessarily regard health care as less important than those with higher incomes, those who are poor often must de-prioritize health care so they can pay for other basic necessities. While this strategy has long-term impacts in terms of increased risk of poor health, in the short term it allows them to better meet their needs for food and shelter. However, health-care providers are sometimes simply unaware of the complex and interconnected economic, social, and geographic factors that influence the health of patients who are poor. The stigma associated with poverty diminishes self-esteem and can be a significant source of embarrassment. Low-income patients are, therefore, often reluctant to tell health-care providers about their economic circumstances and its impact on their health and treatment options. When providers are not conscious of such issues, they may simply fail to consider affordability. This is an example of implicit bias. It is evident, for example, when providers automatically choose name-brand drugs rather than generics or fail to provide a range of appropriate treatment options that include those that are more affordable (e.g., herbal treatments or other alternative therapies). Sometimes, however, providers knowingly provide inferior care to low-income populations and/or treat them in ways that marginalize, demean, and exclude them. This is known as explicit bias. Examples include making demeaning of disparaging comments about poor patients, knowingly providing them with inferior care, or refusing to treat them. Regardless of whether biases are implicit or explicit, however, they diminish the quality of care provided to low-income patients and, consequently, are associated with reduced health and well-being for such patients. Biases may also result in health practices that violate laws, medical ethics, and core principles of patient-centered, culturally competent care.

The structure and organization of health care in the United States also make it difficult for poor populations to access health care and diminish the quality of care they receive. While low-income populations may qualify for Medicaid, not all providers accept such insurance. Critics have deemed this a breach of medical ethics. But others have argued that in the profit-driven model upon which the US health-care system is based, such refusal is simply an economic decision for providers, particularly as Medicaid provides reimbursement to providers that is equivalent to only around 80 percent of the amount paid by private insurance. Furthermore, and in light of the profit-and-efficiency-orientation of the US health-care system, providers have little contact with individual patients. Among primary care providers, appointments are typically scheduled every 15–20 minutes; however, actual face-to-face communication between provider and patient is less. As a result, there is little time for providers to develop rapport with patients. Such rapport is essential to promoting trust between patients and providers. It also helps providers better understand the needs, feelings, and life circumstances of patients and to demonstrate respect toward them. Low-income patients who do not trust their providers are more likely to feel disrespected in health-care settings and less likely to communicate openly about how their financial circumstances impact their attitudes about health as well as their understanding of and preferences for treatment. They are also less likely to be satisfied with the care they receive from health professionals and, consequently, less likely to return for subsequent care. In addition, brief appointments promote a single-focus diagnosis wherein the provider identifies and attempts to address the most prominent complaint rather than adopting a more comprehensive understanding of patient health and well-being. As a result, providers are more likely to overlook symptoms and to misdiagnose. During the COVID-19 pandemic, it was common for health clinics to shift to telehealth options. This eliminated the need to travel to clinical settings and, therefore, minimized the amount of time patients needed to be away from work. However, telehealth increased barriers to care for low-income Americans who lack the technology (e.g., computers, smartphones, and broadband internet access) needed to participate in online appointments. In recent years, there has been increased attention to the need for longer appointments and expanded cultural competence in health-care settings. However, in light of the increasing shortage of qualified health-care workers, it seems unlikely that such factors will soon be remedied.

LIVING ENVIRONMENT AND SOCIAL CONTEXT

Low-income populations often reside in communities with low-quality housing. In addition, areas of concentrated poverty tend to have fewer retail options for the purchase of clothing, health care, food, and other basic needs. There are fewer opportunities for recreation and leisure in such communities but increased health risks due to environmental hazards. The perpetuation of stereotypes that depict poor populations as violent, unintelligent, lazy, greedy, and manipulative has a profound impact on social attitudes toward poor populations. Such stereotypes exist in various forms of media and popular culture; they influence legislation as well as social relationships.

Community and Environmental Factors

Communities with a high concentration of residents who live below the FPL have older housing structures. While such housing may be more affordable, it also increases risk of exposure to toxic substances. In the late twentieth century, the US Environmental Protection Agency banned the use of building materials that contain asbestos, lead-based paint, radon, and other toxins due to health risks. Asbestos can cause lung scarring as well as cancers of the lungs, throat, kidneys, gastrointestinal tract, and larynx; lead-based paint can cause anemia, kidney damage, and damage to the nervous system; radon exposure is associated with increased risk of lung cancer. Despite such known risks, many older homes still contain these substances; this is especially true for homes that have not been renovated with newer, more environmentally friendly building materials. In addition, issues such as lack of insulation, inefficient heating and air-conditioning, and doors and windows that are not sealed or fitted properly are common. Energy-inefficient homes make it difficult for residents to maintain adequate indoor temperature and humidity levels, particularly for those with limited incomes. In addition to contributing to stress and disrupting sleep patterns, temperature extremes and abnormal humidity can exacerbate certain physical and mental health conditions. Abnormally high or low indoor temperatures can aggravate chronic health conditions (e.g., diabetes, COPD, arthritis, high blood pressure, immune system disorders, cardiovascular disease, and neurological disorders) and diminish body's ability to maintain appropriate temperature. Heat extremes can also cause dehydration, heat stroke, and increase risk of death, even for those who are in good health. Those exposed to excessively cold indoor temperatures for extended periods may experience hypothermia as well as problems with memory and cognition. When coupled with high humidity, indoor temperature extremes can promote growth of mold and bacteria and, thus, aggravate allergies and asthma and cause fungal infections. Yet such issues are sometimes found in newer apartment buildings, especially those that are constructed with inexpensive, inferior quality materials and have lower average rents.

Areas of concentrated poverty typically have fewer community resources. Of those areas of the United States that have a critical shortfall of essential health services (e.g., clinics, pharmacies, hospitals, and long-term care facilities), nearly 60 percent are in high-poverty communities. Furthermore, such communities tend to be retail deserts; they have fewer retail options and existing stores tend to offer inexpensive but low-quality goods. Additionally, such communities are often food deserts; they have fewer grocery stores per capita than more affluent areas yet have a higher-than-average number of fast-food restaurants and convenience stores. Consequently, residents have limited access to foods that are both affordable and nutritious but have easy access to inexpensive, processed foods that are high in fats, sugar, salt, and calories. Food deserts increase risk of malnutrition, heart disease, obesity, metabolic syndrome, diabetes, stroke, high blood pressure, high cholesterol, and certain cancers. In addition, low-income areas have fewer parks, green spaces, biking trails, and community centers, thereby diminishing opportunities for leisure and recreation and increasing risk of a sedentary lifestyle. Lack of recreational and leisure resources also diminishes opportunities for clubs and teams, thereby contributing to social isolation.

Environmental concerns also disproportionately impact low-income populations. Roughly 20 percent of low-income Americans live in rural areas. Such populations are at increased risk of exposure to pollutants from manufacturing, agriculture, mining, and landfills. Problems with sanitation, poor drainage, deforestation, access to clean and safe drinking water, and extreme weather events are also common. Poor rural populations also have disproportionately high rates of zoonotic diseases such as Zika, West Nile virus, rabies, toxoplasmosis, Lyme disease, avian flu, and Rocky Mountain spotted fever. However, urban areas have the highest rates of poverty; at present, approximately one-fourth of urban residents live in areas of concentrated poverty. Since 2000, the number of urban neighborhoods with concentrated poverty in the United States has more than doubled. The phenomenon of urban heat islands (UHI) has become increasingly common and low-income populations disproportionately reside in UHIs. These areas have higher average temperatures than outlying suburban or rural areas due to a combination of human activities (e.g., transportation, manufacturing, and energy use), minimal vegetation (e.g., trees, gardens, and parks), and wind reduction. Materials used to construct streets often absorb heat; similarly, construction materials reflect light between buildings, thereby increasing temperatures. In addition, the high concentration of tall buildings impedes the flow of wind currents, thereby trapping allergens and other pollutants while also reducing wind-related cooling. Similarly, the greenhouse gases created by transportation and other combustive activities (e.g., heating, cooling, and industry) trap heat and air pollutants. Common health risks associated with UHIs include respiratory ailments, allergies, headaches, dehydration, heat exhaustion, and heat stroke. For those with certain chronic health conditions such as COPD, heart disease, and obesity, living and/or working in a UHI can increase severity of illness as well as risk of death. City planners have attempted to combat the effects of UHIs by promoting the expansion of tree cover, parks, and green spaces as well as the expansion of shade structures and creation of rooftop gardens. Others have added water features. Still others have expanded use of building and paving materials that reflect rather than absorb heat. Yet retrofitting urban areas in an effort to make them more environmentally friendly is often expensive and time-consuming. Furthermore, zoning regulations may limit such options.

Stereotypes and Social Marginalization

Attitudes toward and treatment of poor populations in America contribute to their ongoing marginalization. The poor are underrepresented in movies, television programs (including sitcoms, reality shows, talk shows, and news coverage), and other forms of media and popular culture. However, when they are included, they are often depicted as lazy, unwilling to work, irresponsible, foolish, and/or incompetent. Such stereotypes are reinforced through the use of various caricatures. For example, in the decades leading up to welfare reform in the mid-1990s, news coverage tended to focus on two types of poor cisgender women who received welfare: those who were irresponsible and those who were greedy. Stories that sought to portray welfare recipients as irresponsible relied on well-worn tropes of drug addiction, alcohol use, intimate partner violence, adolescent childbearing, broken families, and absentee fathers. While narratives that relied on the caricature of the irresponsible welfare recipient often suggested that poor cisgender women were deserving of compassion, politicians and taxpayers seized upon the caricature to promote welfare reform, particularly as a measure intended to help poor cisgender women make more responsible choices. Yet other news coverage depicted welfare recipients as greedy, manipulative, and dangerous. This is most obvious in the caricature of the so-called welfare queen, a stereotype formed at the intersection of racial, gendered, and socioeconomic narratives; it depicted poor, Black cisgender women on welfare as defying mainstream norms of gender and family in order to collect a welfare check and other benefits. Thus, they were deemed a threat to American values. This caricature became one of the primary symbols used by those who advocated for legislative reform as a way to punish welfare recipients. Similar stereotypes have been noted in contemporary media and pop culture representations of poor cisgender men. Common representations of irresponsible cisgender men include so-called hillbillies, vagrants, slobs, and rural simpletons. In contrast, stereotypes of such populations as dangerous and manipulative are reinforced via characterizations as drug dealers, perpetrators of interpersonal violence, gang members, and prisoners. Depictions of immigrant, Black, and/or HLC cisgender men who are poor are common. Of equal importance, pop culture and media representations seldom include LGBTQIA populations in depictions of poverty; thus, such representations contribute to the erasure of the pervasive economic marginalization of LGBTQIA populations that persists in American society.

The consequences of such stereotypes are significant. In addition to influencing legislation, as indicated above, they also influence workplace hiring practices, assessment of students in educational settings, and treatment of patients within clinical health settings. Furthermore, such stereotypes perpetuate American notions of meritocracy. This is clear in the myth of the American dream—the notion that anyone can be part of the middle-class and be economically stable if they just work hard enough. Such a notion denies the realities and complexities of class-based ostracism and marginalization in the United States. It also ignores the fact that many low-income populations work hard and yet still cannot make ends meet. Furthermore, the myth of the American dream ignores the fact that the twin forces of capitalism and globalization have created a free market economy that relies on a steady supply of low-wage laborers in order to maintain profits. Stereotypes also influence violence against the poor. This is clearly reflected, for example, in the increasing number of hate crimes that have targeted homeless populations in recent years; such acts have been perpetrated by both civilians and police forces. Stereotypes of poor populations also impact interpersonal relationships, including friendships among both children and adults. Similarly, family and friends of wealthy individuals often discourage them from dating or marrying someone who is poor.

CHAPTER TEN

Rural Populations

A rural area is any area that is not urban and contains a population of less than 2,500 within a defined geographic area (e.g., a county or township). Rural areas vary considerably in regard to weather and climate, topography, economic base, and distance from urban centers. At present, rural areas cover nearly 97 percent of the land mass of the United States and are home to approximately 60 million individuals; one-fifth of all Americans reside in rural areas. Approximately two-thirds of rural residents live east of the Mississippi River and the southeastern United States has the highest proportion of rural residents. However, states such as Wyoming, Montana, North Dakota, Iowa, South Dakota, Maine, New Hampshire, and Vermont and some counties that border Canada and Mexico also have a significant number of rural residents.

Rural residents are diverse in terms of identities and life experiences yet share some common health concerns. They are more likely than urban populations to be in poor health. The gap in health status between urban and rural populations has become more pronounced in the twenty-first century. That gap is due, in part, to diminished economic, educational, and social opportunities as well as barriers to health care that are common in rural areas. Yet health disparities affecting rural populations are also connected to behaviors and lifestyle. Rural populations are more likely than urban and suburban populations to engage in activities that are detrimental to health and simultaneously less likely to engage in behaviors that promote good health. Social norms and social inequities also factor significantly into rural health outcomes and especially impact the elderly, LGBTQIA populations, cisgender women and girls, immigrants, and Black, Indigenous, and People of Color (BIPOC) populations.

CURRENT STATE OF HEALTH

Throughout the lifespan, rural residents tend to be in worse overall health than urban and suburban populations. Although mortality rates in the United States have decreased over the past 20 years, such rates have increased among some rural populations, particularly whites without a college degree. Rates of neonatal, infant, child, and adolescence mortality are also somewhat higher in rural areas. While differences in mortality rates between rural populations when compared to urban populations diminish somewhat for those aged 20–29, they increase again among those aged 30–39; such differences are greatest for those over 39 years of age. The gap in average life expectancy of rural populations as compared to urban US populations has nearly quadrupled since 1970. At present, rural residents live about 2 years less than urban residents. Rural counties have higher rates of premature death (prior to average life expectancy) and consistently rank lower in health outcomes. The Affordable Care Act of 2010 increased the number of rural Americans covered by health insurance, yet they remain less likely to have insurance than urban populations. Furthermore, the Medicaid work requirements implemented in 2020 have been particularly harmful to rural recipients due to limited employment opportunities in rural areas.

Compared to those in urban areas, rural children are more likely to have unmet health needs. They are more likely to be born to mothers who did not receive adequate prenatal care, and rates of premature delivery and infant mortality remain ongoing concerns in rural areas. Such rates are disproportionately high among rural non-Hispanic/Latinx/Chicanx (HLC) Black and Indigenous populations. Furthermore, rural infants are more likely than those born in cities to be low birth weight (less than 5.5 pounds) and to encounter health problems related to underdevelopment of the heart, intestines, lungs, eyes, brain, and immune system. They are also less likely to be breastfed, receive recommended childhood vaccines, undergo well-child visits, and visit a dentist. Rural children are also more likely to rely on government health insurance programs for low-income populations yet less likely than urban children to have any type of health insurance coverage. Poor air and water quality as well as exposure to pesticides and herbicides remain ongoing concerns for children's health in some rural areas. The most common causes of death among rural adolescent populations include unintentional injuries such as automobile accidents, firearms, and drowning. Rural teens are also more likely than urban teens to attempt suicide and nearly twice as likely to die from suicide; rates are even higher among rural LGBTQIA adolescents.

Rural populations are generally older, have a higher proportion of HLC and Indigenous residents, and are less likely to engage in health-seeking behaviors than the US population overall. Rural adults also suffer from higher-than-average rates of depressive disorders, serious mental illness, ongoing mental health disorders, and acute psychological problems. Rates of post-traumatic stress disorder (PTSD) are similar among urban and rural populations, yet rural adults are less likely to seek and receive professional health services for PTSD. Mortality and morbidity rates due to heart disease, cancer, chronic lower respiratory disease, and stroke are disproportionately high in rural areas as are rates of sexually transmitted diseases (STDs) and zoonotic diseases (transmitted via mammals, insects, or other animals). Use and abuse of tobacco, alcohol, and drugs in rural areas have increased in recent years. Adult death rates due to automobile accidents, drug overdoses, drowning, residential fires, and occupational injuries are disproportionately high in rural communities.

Yet health disparities also exist between different rural subpopulations and vary by region. For example, while the obesity rate in rural America is six times higher than in urban communities, rates of rural obesity are highest among rural Black, HLC, and Indigenous cisgender women. Suicide rates are disproportionately high in rural areas, particularly among Indigenous populations, veterans, and men in their 20s and 30s. Diabetes is also a concern in rural communities, but rates are highest in the so-called diabetes belt in the Appalachian Mountains. There are also variations by sex and gender. Among cisgender women, those in rural communities tend to become pregnant at a younger age and have more children than their urban counterparts. Rates of unplanned pregnancy among rural cisgender women and girls are higher than national averages yet they are less likely to terminate such pregnancies. Some have linked this to social norms while others have pointed to limited access to abortion services in rural areas. Rates of intimate partner violence (IPV) are disproportionately high in rural areas; frequency and severity of IPV escalate with increasing rurality. Social isolation, loneliness, and poor social support are linked to poor health in rural communities, especially for LGBTQIA, elderly, disabled, and immigrant populations.

ECONOMIC FACTORS

Economic growth and stability remain ongoing issues in America's rural communities. Rural economies have been hampered due to changes wrought by globalization and technology. Overall, industries in rural areas tend to be much different than those in urban areas; there are also fewer employment opportunities as well as an overconcentration of unskilled and low-skill labor positions in rural areas. In addition, rural populations tend to be poorer than urban and suburban populations and, thus, to experience poverty-related diseases and disorders. They are also more likely to identify cost as a barrier to health care and to rely on government-sponsored health programs for low-income populations.

Rural Economies and Employment

Rates of unemployment tend to be slightly higher in rural than urban areas, and periods of economic recession can devastate rural economies. During the Great Recession (2007–9), rural communities experienced higher rates of job loss and unemployment than urban areas and saw slower return to employment in the ensuing years. Salary increases in rural areas have lagged behind national averages since the recession. Employment opportunities in some rural areas have diversified somewhat in recent years, specifically in retail, service, education, and certain types of manufacturing. There has been a decline in unskilled and low-skill labor positions in rural America in the past three decades. However, entry-level jobs that do not require specialized training, education, or licensure remain disproportionately high in rural areas. Such jobs typically offer part-time employment, hourly wages, and often do not provide employment benefits such as health insurance, flexible spending accounts, or vacation leave.

Among those rural residents who are employed full-time in low-skill and unskilled labor positions, annual earnings are typically below national averages and render such employees part of America's working poor. Such workers face increased risk of certain chronic health conditions (such as diabetes, heart disease, and obesity) as well as poor mental health due to income-related stress and low job satisfaction. Furthermore, many unskilled and low-skill jobs cannot be done remotely. This is especially true in the retail and service sectors as well as manufacturing and agriculture. During the COVID-19 pandemic, for example, rural workers were less likely than those in urban areas to have jobs that permitted remote work. Thus, they were at increased risk for contracting the disease. Overall, rates of infection and death due to COVID-19 have been higher among rural populations. Furthermore, although farming remains a primary source of income for over 2 million American families, approximately half of US farms do not earn a profit that meets or exceeds the Federal Poverty Level (FPL). As a result, many who own and operate farms must work another job, something that can increase stress and limit free time.

At present, approximately one-tenth of rural employees work in agricultural, forestry, mining, gas and oil extraction, and other resource-based activities. Such industries are particularly susceptible to the impacts of environmental degradation, weather patterns, and natural disasters as well as fluctuations in global markets. Agricultural workers—nearly 75 percent of whom are immigrants—are especially vulnerable to certain health risks. These include cuts, broken bones, and amputations due to heavy machinery; injuries and infectious diseases due to contact with animals; suffocation; burns; exposure to toxic substances in herbicides and insecticides; and hypothermia as well as heat-stress due to exposure to weather extremes. Furthermore, agricultural workers often earn incomes below the FPL, and most do not have health insurance. These factors impede their access to health care. Due to fluctuations in work related to seasonal changes, seasonal unemployment is common among agricultural laborers; this increases their financial strain and further diminishes their ability to afford health care.

Poverty in Rural America and Health Impacts

Rates of rural poverty were noted as a significant national concern beginning in the 1960s. Despite a broad range of economic revival strategies in the late twentieth and early twenty-first centuries, rural poverty persists, and areas of concentrated poverty in rural America have become more pronounced. Although the average cost of living in rural areas is lower than in urban communities, average household incomes among rural residents are also generally lower. Rural poverty is disproportionately high in the Southern and Western regions and among Indigenous, Black, and HLC populations as well as households headed by unmarried cisgender women with minor children, especially in parts of Appalachia and the Mississippi Delta. Rural poverty has been linked to limited educational, job training, and employment opportunities as well as disinvestment by some corporations, particularly those that move operations overseas in an effort to reduce expenses. Institutional inequities that perpetuate racism, sexism, and other types of oppression are also key factors in the intergenerational nature of rural poverty.

Rural poverty is often characterized by cycles of debt wherein an individual or household will pawn or sell assets (e.g., vehicles, computers, equipment, or even livestock) or take out so-called payday loans in an attempt to meet basic living expenses or to pay for medical care or prescription medications. Reliance on payday loans among rural populations has become increasingly common. However, payday loans have been deemed a predatory lending practice—sometimes referred to as reverse redlining—that disproportionately targets those who do not have a college degree, are under age 35, identify as Black or HLC, and have incomes below the FPL. Such loans typically must be repaid quickly (within 2–4 weeks) and the average interest on such loans is 20–30 percent. In some cases, interest is over 1,500 percent. Those who default on such loans may face fines, damage to their credit score, and legal action. Thus, these types of short-term economic strategies can push poor rural households further into poverty and diminish mental health due to increased stress, anxiety, and diminished self-esteem.

Chronic poverty in rural America is associated with a higher burden of disease as well as reduced life expectancy and diminished quality of life. Rural residents are more likely than urban dwellers to lack health insurance or be underinsured. At least one-third of rural populations indicate they are unable to afford health care and forgo preventative care and screenings, factors that have been linked to decreased life expectancy. Medical debt is also an ongoing problem. Nearly one-fifth of all rural adults cannot make regular payments on medical debts for themselves or their dependents; among those with incomes below the FPL, the rate is nearly 45 percent. Unpaid medical debt is especially common in poor Southern communities where Republican-led state governments have refused federal funds to expand Medicaid coverage to their citizens. While some nonprofit organizations assist low-income populations with health-care expenses, demand for such resources far exceeds supply. Compared to urban residents, rural populations spend a higher percent of annual income on health-care expenses. This reduces their ability to pay for basic necessities and, thus, increases risk of poor health.

Diseases of poverty are significant concerns in rural America. Such diseases include chronic conditions such as heart disease, hypertension, arthritis, stroke, cancer, obesity, certain respiratory diseases, and malnutrition. Diseases due to parasitic, congenital, and bacterial infections are also disproportionately high among rural populations. Collectively known as infections of poverty, they include trichomoniasis, leptospirosis, hookworm, Chagas disease, leishmaniasis, Dengue fever, toxoplasmosis, and syphilis, among others. Rates are especially high among low-income BIPOC and immigrant populations. Although many of these infections can be treated with antibiotics or anti-parasitic medications, the costs of such medications can be prohibitive. For example, the cost for a full course of pyrimethamine, a generic drug used to treat toxoplasmosis, is just over $20,000 for uninsured patients. For those with insurance, the average cost is nearly $3,500. Medicare does not cover pyrimethamine.

Yet chronic poverty is also associated with increased incidence and severity of stress, anxiety disorders, and depression among rural populations. Such mental health problems can exacerbate existing physical health conditions and cause headaches, digestive disorders, skin rashes, and sleep disturbances. Persistent stress due to long-term financial and material scarcity has been shown to diminish psychological well-being among rural populations and to increase risk of suicidal ideation and suicide attempts. Chronic poverty diminishes physical and mental health of children; it also increases their lifetime risk of poor health. Furthermore, chronic poverty has been linked to various types of abuse in rural communities, including neglect and abuse of children, the elderly, and persons with disabilities as well as gender-based violence (GBV), including sexual assault, rape, intimate partner violence (IPV), and human trafficking.

EDUCATIONAL ACCESS AND QUALITY

In the context of primary and secondary education, US rural students generally perform as well as—and, in some cases, even outperform—their urban peers with regard to standardized tests scores and high school diploma completion rates. Overall, however, rural Americans tend to be less educated than those who live in more urban areas. Such educational outcomes have been linked to diminished overall health status, quality of life, health literacy, and life expectancy as well as lower rates of preventative health screenings and diminished health-seeking behaviors. In recent years, decreased educational attainment has also been linked to rising rates of certain infectious and chronic diseases among rural populations.

Barriers to Educational Attainment

Just over half of all school districts in the United States are located in rural counties. In addition, 20 percent of all students in grades K-12 in the United States reside in rural areas; however, in some states, rural students represent more than one-third of the total K-12 student population. When compared to residents of more urban areas, fewer rural residents complete a high school diploma or earn a GED. In addition, rural students are less likely to attend college or pursue postsecondary job training; additionally, those rural students who do continue their education after high school are less likely to earn their degree. Less than 10 percent of students who graduate from rural high schools successfully complete a bachelor's degree before their twenty-fifth birthday. Like their urban counterparts, rural students whose parents did not attend college are less likely to pursue postsecondary education or vocational training. Such educational disparities are even more pronounced in master's, doctoral, and professional degree programs. Gaps in postsecondary degree attainment are highest among rural Indigenous, Black, and HLC populations.

The reasons for such disparities are complex and include social as well as economic factors. Limited social and cultural capital impede pursuit of postsecondary education among some rural populations. Those without family members or mentors who have attended college and who can guide them through college applications, scholarships, entrance exams, and financial aid are less likely to apply to and enroll in postsecondary institutions. For others, the culture shock of college life can deter them from persisting with educational pursuits. Such culture shock can diminish mental well-being among rural students and contribute to social isolation. Commonly cited aspects of such culture shock include anxiety about not fitting in with other students from more urban areas; stress of living in an unfamiliar and more urban community; feeling anonymous in large classes; and becoming disconnected from family and friends at home. Furthermore, a college education is simply not affordable for many rural students, especially those who experience intergenerational poverty or who cannot secure grants or scholarships. Among those rural students who do pursue postsecondary education, the majority do not return to their rural communities after college but, instead, pursue employment in suburban or urban areas. This phenomenon is known as brain drain and has been linked to limited economic, labor, and human capital resources in rural America.

Yet economic barriers to educational attainment begin long before college. Rates of child poverty—including deep poverty, wherein total household income is less than half of the FPL—are higher in rural than urban areas. Poverty has been identified as an adverse childhood experience (ACE) and is associated with impaired cognitive development and increased incidence of psychological trauma. Children who grow up poor are less likely to earn their high school diploma and more likely to perform poorly in school and to have behavioral issues. Family and community poverty are also associated with diminished overall quality of education institutions, restricted educational opportunities, and decreased support for vulnerable student populations. However, even rural school districts that exist outside of areas of concentrated poverty face unique economic burdens. Rural schools tend to have a lower tax base than urban schools and receive less state funding. Thus, they have smaller operating budgets but also have different costs, including in regard to transportation. While students in more urban areas often live within walking or biking distance of schools or can access public transportation, rural students are generally dispersed over a larger geographic area that may include hundreds of square miles. Thus, rural school districts must transport students to and from school. Over the past two decades, the combination of elevated gas prices, stagnation of state education budgets, and changes to federal accounting procedures have increased the economic burden associated with transporting students in rural districts.

Quality of education is also a concern in rural schools. Rural districts typically offer lower pay and, consequently, have difficulties recruiting and retaining qualified teachers. Because they tend to have fewer students overall than urban school districts, rural districts generally offer a more limited range of courses. This has been noted not only for advanced courses and vocational training for high school students but also for special education, ESL (English as a second language) curriculum, remedial and developmental courses, so-called gifted and talented courses, and academic support services for writing, speaking, and STEM (science, technology, engineering, and math) subjects. Gaps in rural education contribute to decreased health literacy and increased rates of chronic diseases among rural Americans. Additionally, rural students typically have limited options for extracurricular, internship, and service-learning opportunities due to geographic and economic barriers. Given the various ways that such opportunities can promote physical and mental well-being as well as social connections, rural students who lack such opportunities are at increased risk for poor health due to obesity, depression, and social isolation. Furthermore, rural schools often struggle to provide after-school and summer programs. Such programs can increase academic performance, improve school attendance, decrease engagement in high-risk behaviors (including crime, violence, and sexual activity as well as use of drugs, alcohol, and tobacco products), and reduce drop-out rates. Yet due to ongoing challenges with funding, staffing, transportation, and available space, such programs have become increasingly scarce in rural schools.

The Digital Divide in Rural Education

Online and remote learning options can help improve access to a broader range of course offerings, academic support, and flexible learning options for rural students. However, the digital divide—the disparities in access to various types of educational technologies and knowledge of how to use such technologies—remains a significant concern. Due to limited educational budgets, teachers in rural districts often face significant barriers in accessing educational technologies or securing formal training in how to use such technologies. Limited educational technology diminishes quality of educational content; yet it can also deter highly qualified teachers from pursuing employment in rural schools. However, the digital divide is most pronounced in rural "dead zones" that lack broadband access. Rural students from low-income families, BIPOC students, those with disabilities, and limited English proficiency (LEP) student populations are disproportionately affected by the digital divide. Nearly 15 percent of rural US students do not have a home computer or broadband internet access; in some rural school districts, over half of students lack these amenities. Such limitations diminish academic performance and degree completion rates. The digital divide has also been shown to increase school-related stress and decrease students' interest in short- and long-term academic pursuits.

The existing digital divide in rural education has been exacerbated by the COVID-19 pandemic. As schools shifted to online learning in order to comply with social distancing protocols, many rural students were left with limited access to education. Some districts implemented creative measures including by deploying Wi-Fi buses (sometimes referred to as mobile Wi-Fi hubs) to various rural locations so students could sit in parked cars or at public parks in order to access online curriculum. Yet such options were not feasible in all rural districts. Furthermore, students who did not own laptop computers, iPads, or similar devices—or who were unable to obtain one from their school district—were not able to take advantage of mobile Wi-Fi hubs. Some rural students temporarily moved in with family members who had broadband access and, in doing so, were able to access curriculum. In other cases, teachers transferred lectures and course materials to flash drives that were distributed to students who had in-home computers but lacked broadband access. But many rural students did not have such options and, consequently, were forced to make do with printed packets of educational materials and sporadic telephone interactions with teachers. Academic-related stress among rural K-12 students who experienced the digital divide increased significantly during the COVID-19 pandemic. Incidence and severity of anxiety, depression, emotional outbursts, and feelings of low self-worth among such students also increased.

The digital divide also impacts rural students in other ways. Those without access to computers and the internet are more likely to feel socially isolated from and have a difficult time forming and maintaining positive relationships with their peers. They also find it more difficult to obtain support from teachers as well as counselors and other academic partners and, consequently, to feel they are lagging behind their classmates. Among high school students, the digital divide can render them unable to apply to colleges or take standardized tests that are required to advance to the next grade level or for college admission. For students who are stigmatized due to mental health disorders, disabilities, gender expression, or sexual identity, or who encounter abuse within the context of dating or familial relationships, internet access can facilitate access to fundamental support, including social communities (such as online forums for transgender individuals), accurate information about health conditions, and even free helplines for victims of bullying or violence. Yet the digital divide impedes the ability of many rural students to access such resources and, consequently, exacerbates barriers to their health and well-being.

Promoting Well-Being in Rural Schools

In recent years, rural schools have expanded attention to physical, mental, and social health of students. Such efforts have included increased attention to health-related topics in the curriculum, promoting healthy food choices through school nutrition programs, expanding partnerships with public health programs to promote screenings and treatment for common childhood health disorders, and fostering increased physical activity through sports, clubs, and classroom activities. In addition, there has been increased attention to mental health disorders that are common among students as well as how the dynamics of rural settings often contribute to such disorders. Many rural schools use positive behavior intervention supports (PBIS) and social emotional learning (SEL) to promote positive mental health for students. Community health clinics located in rural schools have become increasingly common. Such clinics may provide vaccinations, primary care, reproductive and sexual health services, and treatment for influenza, minor injuries, ear infections, respiratory ailments, and other acute conditions.

There is also an increasing emphasis on holistic support services to students in rural school districts. Such services aim to promote academic skills and healthy social development while also addressing food insecurity, common mental health disorders, bullying, and gender-based violence within the context of adolescent peer groups and dating relationships. Other programs provide support to specific subpopulations of students—including LGBTQIA individuals, immigrants, LEP populations, and those with disabilities—in order to better understand their needs and aid them in navigating their unique academic, social, and health-related challenges. However, the demands for such forms of support far exceed the supply. Furthermore, due to limited budgets and high staff turnover rates that are common in rural school districts, the availability of such services is often inconsistent.

HEALTH-CARE ACCESS AND QUALITY

It has long been recognized that there are fewer health-care facilities in rural than urban and suburban areas. This is true for preventative care, treatment options, and emergency services. Access to and quality of health care in rural communities are also influenced by ongoing shortages in the US health-care workforce as well as biases and inequities within the health-care system.

Barriers to Health Care

Geographic barriers are a significant consideration in rural areas. In general, increased distance from an urban center is associated with decreased access to health-care facilities and services. Rural residents live, on average, twice as far as from primary care services and basic hospital facilities as urban residents. The difference is even greater for those who require tertiary-level care related to obstetrics and gynecology, oncology, neurology, and immunology. Rural areas also tend to have few psychiatric care facilities due to limited revenue potential; consequently, residents must either travel to more urban areas for treatment or simply go without care. Furthermore, rural hospitals have closed at an alarming rate over the past two decades. In 2020, as financial strain on health systems increased due to the COVID-19 pandemic, a record-number of rural hospitals ceased operations. Overall, rural populations have less access to health-care services and are less likely to receive preventative care as well as treatment for acute and chronic conditions. Those with substantive injuries, serious illnesses, disabilities, and unique health conditions (e.g., those caused by congenital abnormalities) face increased risk of complications and death due to limited availability of emergency services. Maldistribution of health facilities is especially pronounced in frontier areas (also known as remote rural areas). Such areas have low population density (less than 6 people per square mile); are isolated from and require considerable travel time (an hour or more) to reach urban population centers; often lack infrastructure such as paved roads, sanitation, electricity, and internet; may be accessible only by helicopter, boat, or snowmobile; and may be inaccessible at times due to heavy rains or snowfall. There are currently over 400 frontier rural counties in America; they are most common in Alaska, New Mexico, Nevada, North Dakota, South Dakota, Montana, and Idaho.

Physical barriers to care are also significant in rural communities and disproportionately impact those with disabilities. At present, nearly one-third of rural adults have a disability that impairs cognition, mobility, communication, or ability to live independently and engage in self-care activities related to hygiene, dressing, and eating. Rural populations are also more likely than urban residents to have multiple disabilities. While the Americans with Disability Act (ADA) requires that health care be available to and accommodates the needs of patients with disabilities, physical barriers (e.g., inaccessible clinical spaces and lack of appropriate ramps, handrails, and other modifications), provider shortages, transportation barriers (including lack of public transportation and limited para-transport services), and cost of care remain significant impediments to health care for those in rural areas.

There is also a chronic shortage of language access services (LAS) in rural communities. Some rural communities have increased efforts to promote culturally and linguistically appropriate services in the past decade. Tele-Health options can help improve access to care for some rural patients, including those with limited English proficiency (LEP) or who have other communication barriers. Yet rural households are less likely than urban households to have a computer, smartphone, or other device necessary to access the internet. This, coupled with limited broadband infrastructure in remote rural areas, limits Tele-Health options for many residents. Furthermore, while limited availability of trained medical translators and multilingual health-care professionals remains a concern throughout the United States, it is especially pronounced in rural areas. Limited LAS has been linked to decreased health-care-seeking behaviors, decreased compliance with treatment plans, and reduced satisfaction among rural LEP patients. Mobile health-care teams that provide in-home services have improved access to care in some rural areas, especially for elderly patients and those with mobility impairments. Yet the costs of establishing and maintaining mobile services can be prohibitive, particularly in communities with a low tax base.

The Rural Health-Care Workforce

Rural America suffers from a chronic shortage of health-care workers, including qualified nurses, primary care physicians, dentists, mental health professionals, pharmacists, surgeons, and allied health professionals (e.g., lab technicians, physical therapists, radiologists, and speech-language pathologists). Health professionals in rural areas tend to have more generalized skills and may, therefore, be unable to diagnose or treat conditions that require specialized care. Thus, patients with certain health issues (e.g., substance abuse disorders, rare diseases, and genetic disorders) are often unable to access care in rural communities. Although some patients may be able to travel to more urban areas to receive care, others cannot due to work schedules, economic factors, or transportation barriers.

Even high-demand services such as palliative care (including hospice) and reproductive health care can be difficult to access in rural communities due to a confluence of economic, geographic, and staffing issues. At present, less than 20 percent of hospice services in the United States are located in rural areas. Nearly half of all rural counties lack an OB-GYN, and 87 percent do not have an abortion provider.

Rural areas have a difficult time recruiting health-care professionals. Under the fee-for-service model that dominates the US health-care system, a health-care facility or provider is paid or reimbursed for each service they provide. Thus, due to the limited number of patients in rural areas and the corresponding limited potential for income, many physicians and surgeons opt to work in more urban areas. Some rural hospitals have offered hiring bonuses as part of recruitment strategies, typically with the stipulation that the new hire remains at the facility for at least 3–5 years. While such bonuses can be effective in the short term, providers may simply relocate once they have fulfilled their contractual obligation. Additionally, such bonuses have been shown to be less effective in recruiting racial and ethnic minorities as well as individuals who grew up in more urban areas.

Low retention rates among health-care providers in rural areas are also a problem. Limited time off from work, long travel distances from home to work, reduced options for childcare and schooling (for those with dependent children), and few opportunities for community engagement beyond the health-care field (e.g., recreational pursuits or civic engagement) are associated with decreased quality of life in rural communities and are commonly cited as reasons why health-care providers leave such areas. Diminished opportunities for professional development are also a concern. Furthermore, many rural health-care professionals indicate that inadequate health-care infrastructure and limited access to new medical technologies hinder their ability to provide optimal care to patients. Staffing shortages often mean that rural providers are required to work overtime and double shifts or to take on responsibilities that are not part of their job description. Such demands contribute to high rates of stress and burnout among rural health-care workers. They also prompt some rural providers to change careers, relocate to more urban areas, or retire early. In rural areas with only one physician or public health nurse, the relocation or retirement of that provider may effectively terminate access to care for residents or, at the very least, exacerbate existing barriers to care.

Bias and Discrimination in Rural Health Care

Structural inequities continue to weaken rural health systems. Such inequities are not natural or inevitable; instead, they reflect the inherent biases within the structure of the US health-care system as they relate to economic and social priorities. Examples include geographic maldistribution of health-care facilities and inadequate health-care workforce, as discussed above. Such biases are also evident in federal and state policies that provide lower reimbursement rates to rural health-care providers than to those working in urban areas. Some rural providers have responded to these lower rates by refusing to accept patients with government-sponsored health insurance. As a result, it is estimated that one-fifth of rural residents who are covered by Medicare, Medicaid, or CHIP are denied care. Limited access to medical interpreters and online translation services in rural areas are further evidence of bias in the US health-care system and have been linked to structural racism and xenophobia.

Biases and inequities are also evident in the attitudes, knowledge, and actions of health-care providers who work in rural areas. The tendency for providers to diminish, dismiss, or otherwise denigrate the lifestyle and health behaviors of rural residents has been noted as an ongoing concern and is especially prominent among providers who did not grow up in rural areas. Stereotypes that depict rural populations as simple-minded, radically different from urban populations, and as homogenous—both in regard to their identities and their health-related needs—continue to inform the practice of some health-care workers. Such stereotypes have been noted in provider-to-patient communication, assessment of patient symptoms, and derogatory statements made by providers to co-workers. Clinical care that relies on stereotypes violates core principles of medical ethics and patient-centered care, thereby exacerbating systemic inequities that continue to disadvantage BIPOC populations, sexual minorities, immigrants, the poor, and other marginalized groups. Some medical training programs have found that engaging their students in outreach in rural areas helps to dispel such stereotypes and fosters more culturally competent health practice. However, many rural health facilities have been slow to implement diversity and cultural competency training, citing budget constraints and already overworked staff to explain their hesitancy.

LIVING ENVIRONMENT AND SOCIAL CONTEXT

Rural areas vary considerably with regard to natural environment, infrastructure, and social institutions. The demographics of different rural populations also vary as do their beliefs, values, political views, religious affiliations, and other cultural norms. Despite such differences, it is clear that environmental and social factors have a significant influence on the health and well-being of rural Americans. In some rural areas, such factors promote good health; in other areas, they exacerbate existing health conditions, especially for vulnerable populations.

Environmental Factors

There are great variations in natural features, climate, and weather patterns in rural areas throughout the United States. Despite such differences, it is clear that the natural elements of rural environments impact the health and well-being of those who live and work in such areas. Many rural residents depend on natural resources to earn a living, especially in industries such as food production, animal husbandry, mining, forestry, fishing, and certain types of tourism. Yet rural residents also rely on natural resources to help meet their basic needs as well as for leisure and recreational pursuits. Consequently, the health of rural residents is fundamentally influenced by environmental factors, including climate and temperatures; quality of air, water, and soil; and availability of various natural resources.

Rural communities are vulnerable to climate change and its consequences. In recent years, there has been an increase in frequency and severity of extreme weather events (including floods, hurricanes, tornadoes, wildfires, tropical storms, hailstorms, droughts, extreme winds, and heatwaves) in rural America. Such weather events, coupled with rising average temperatures and changes in the amounts and frequency of precipitation, pose significant health risks and have put an additional strain on rural health systems. Extreme weather events have been shown to aggravate chronic health conditions and to increase incidence and severity of traumatic injuries, respiratory ailments, and certain types of mental health disorders, especially anxiety and PTSD. Children, elderly populations, and those with preexisting health conditions as well as those who work outdoors or who spend extended time outdoors for recreation or leisure activities are most at risk for heat-related exhaustion, stroke, and death. Weather-related health problems are highest among rural poor, Indigenous, and Black populations.

Changing weather and temperature patterns also impact rural health in other ways. For example, rising temperatures and the associated changes with ecosystems have expanded the geographic range and otherwise altered movement patterns of various animal species that can transmit diseases to humans. Examples of vector-borne diseases (those transmitted by insects) include Lyme disease, Rocky Mountain spotted fever, West Nile virus, Zika, Heartland virus, and chikungunya. Since 2000, cases of vector-borne diseases have nearly doubled in the United States, with the most significant increases occurring in rural counties. Furthermore, as natural ecosystems decline, wild animals increasingly come into direct contact with human populations, livestock, and pets. Consequently, there is increased risk of injuries (e.g., bites or scratches) as well as transmission of certain diseases (e.g., rabies, *E. coli*, and leptospirosis) and parasites (e.g., hookworms, roundworms, and tapeworms). However, zoonotic diseases can also be transmitted indirectly such as when animal urine or fecal matter is present on plants (e.g., fruits and vegetables), in soil, or enters rivers, lakes, or ponds used for swimming, fishing, or recreation. Some zoonotic diseases can be transmitted via groundwater used for irrigation, livestock, and drinking water. Over 90 percent of rural Americans rely on groundwater (including private wells) as their primary source of drinking water.

Furthermore, climate change has contributed to desertification, a process wherein formerly fertile land becomes increasingly arid. It is especially a concern in the Great Plains and Southwest. Desertification has been linked to increasing food insecurity, decreased quality and availability of water, and respiratory diseases due to increased pollutants, particulate matter, and allergens in the air. Desertification also raises the temperature and salinity of natural water sources, thereby creating ideal conditions for the growth of cyanobacteria, also known as blue-green algae. Such algae produce toxins that are harmful to those who come into contact with affected water sources (by swimming, for example) or who eat fish or drink water from such sources. Exposure to cyanobacteria can cause irritation of the skin, eyes, nose, and throat; gastrointestinal problems; neurological problems; and death.

Transportation, Housing, and Sanitation

A number of problems persist with regard to infrastructure, housing, and sanitation in rural America. Rural residents often must travel long distances to work or school or to obtain health care, food, or other essential services. Options for public transportation in rural areas are limited and, therefore, those who do not own vehicles face increased risk of social isolation, limited options for employment and education, and difficulty meeting basic needs. Many rural roads are plagued by uneven surfaces, age-related deterioration, or can become obstructed or unsafe due to inclement weather; it is also common for them to be narrow, unpaved, have sharp turns or steep inclines, and lack adequate signage and safety features. Rural roads often lack bike lanes, a paved shoulder, or a sidewalk; thus, they can be dangerous for pedestrians or cyclists. Nearly 40 percent of rural roads and half of rural bridges are not in good condition; 10 percent of rural bridges are structurally deficient. Quite simply, rural transportation routes are dangerous: over half of all vehicle accidents and fatalities occur on rural roads.

Problems with rural roadways also exacerbate geographic barriers to employment, education, and health care. Furthermore, deficiencies in transportation infrastructure increase response time for police, fire, and ambulance services, thereby contributing to increased risk of poor health outcomes and death in emergency situations. Such deficiencies also contribute to food insecurity in rural communities. Nearly one-fifth of rural counties are classified as food deserts; thus, residents have limited access to fresh, nutritious food. In some rural communities, residents must travel more than an hour to reach the nearest supermarket. Low-income and BIPOC populations are among those rural populations most likely to be food insecure and, therefore, are at increased risk of malnutrition, obesity, certain chronic diseases (e.g., heart disease, high blood pressure, and type 2 diabetes), and reduced life expectancy.

Housing is a problem in many rural areas. A disproportionate percent of inhabited housing structures that do not meet minimum standards for health and safety are located in rural areas. Some of the most common problems with housing include presence of lead-based paint, inadequate insulation, and lack of or inefficient heating, cooling, and air filtration systems. Furthermore, much of rural housing is old and in need of significant repair, maintenance, or replacement. Overcrowding is also a problem in many rural areas and is associated with increased rates of mental health disorders, certain infectious diseases, and infant and child mortality due to respiratory conditions and accidents. During the COVID-19 pandemic, overcrowding was identified as a key factor in the transmission of disease in rural households where available space prohibited safe social-distancing practices. Rural populations most at risk for health problems due to inadequate housing include those with incomes below the FPL, the elderly, Black populations, and those with disabilities. In addition, homelessness is becoming increasingly common in rural areas, particularly among LGBTQIA youth and individuals with PTSD or drug addiction. While programs facilitated by nonprofit organizations and the US Department of Agriculture aim to rectify the lack of availability of safe, affordable, and structurally sound housing in rural America, economic resources for such programs have decreased in recent years.

In addition, improved water and sanitation infrastructure are lacking in many rural areas and disproportionately affect Black and Indigenous populations. Thus, many critics have linked such problems to systemic racism. While municipal water systems must comply with the provisions of the Safe Drinking Water Act and standards established by the Environmental Protection Agency, the private wells and small water systems in rural areas are not subject to such regulations. Furthermore, due to manufacturing waste, agricultural runoff, and biological and chemical contaminants (such as algae, metals, salts, bacteria, and parasites), many rural water sources are not suitable for human consumption. Inadequate or failing sanitation systems in rural communities can cause untreated sewage to pool near homes or enter streams, ponds, and other water sources or to back up into homes, schools, and other buildings, thereby increasing risk of exposure to parasites, bacteria, and viruses.

Social Dynamics

In the past decade, rural populations have become somewhat more diverse, particularly as an increasing percent of Black and HLC populations have moved to rural areas.

Yet rural communities tend to be less racially and ethnically diverse than urban areas. BIPOC populations constitute less than one-fourth of rural Americans, and rural Indigenous populations have decreased in recent years. Furthermore, many rural areas remain segregated by race, ethnicity, income, and religion. Consequently, while there is some degree of diversity among rural Americans overall, specific rural communities are often rather homogenous and tend to have an overrepresentation of whites. Although there has been a marginal increase in the number of urban residents relocating to rural areas since 2015, the majority of rural residents were born in rural communities. Most rural adults marry during their lifetimes. Despite the fact that contraceptive use rates are somewhat higher in rural than urban areas, rural cisgender women tend to have their first child earlier than urban cisgender women; they are also more likely to be unmarried mothers. Although birth rates are higher in rural than urban areas, the US rural population continues to decline.

Rural populations are as likely as urban populations to identify economic matters, health care, and environmental concerns as political priorities. Yet due to their social dynamics, rural communities are often characterized as both socially tight-knit and exclusionary. It is common for residents to take pride in their rural heritage. This is especially common among rural farming families who have lived in the same community for generations. Typically, there is a strong emphasis on kinship ties, family lineage, and taking care of one's family and a strong sense of interdependence among extended families and neighbors and it is common for rural populations to share resources with one another, including vehicles, tools and equipment, or food resources (e.g., meat obtained via hunting or fishing, produce, and eggs). Religion is also a significant factor in rural America; although rural populations are not more likely than their urban counterparts to affiliate with a particular religious tradition, they are more likely to attend church services at least once per week and to participate in church-related social activities. Churches often function as a social hub in rural areas. It is also common for them to organize fund-raisers, food banks, clothing drives, and to collect school supplies for low-income populations. Rural churches often provide physical space for health clinics, voting, ESL classes, and sports or other recreational activities. They can also be a primary point of social engagement for newcomers who share the same religious traditions.

However, the social dynamics of rural communities can also marginalize or exclude certain populations, including individuals who do not conform to social norms and beliefs as well as those who relocate from other areas. Long-term rural residents tend to be more politically conservative and are more likely to identify as Republican. Therefore, those who hold more liberal political views may face harsh criticism or be socially ostracized. In addition, rural populations tend to be older and more strongly endorse traditional gender norms as they pertain to social roles, marriage, and family. Furthermore, rural residents may be distrustful of individuals who were not born in their communities and regard them as social outsiders. This is true even when such outsiders support the local economy (e.g., tourists) or provide necessary labor in industries such as agriculture, education, manufacturing, or health care. Rural populations also tend to be less tolerant and welcoming to those they perceive as different from them. Thus, racial and ethnic minorities, immigrants, and LGBTQIA populations are especially vulnerable to discrimination in rural areas. Such discrimination takes a variety of forms including social exclusion and economic marginalization, thereby contributing to loneliness, isolation, chronic stress, depression, and anxiety.

Rural social dynamics have also been identified as key contributors to various forms of violence as well as use and abuse of alcohol, tobacco, and illegal drugs. Rates of sexual victimization (including both rape and sexual assault) as well as intimate partner violence (IPV) are higher in rural than urban areas, especially in remote rural communities. Such forms of abuse disproportionately affect cisgender women and girls, Indigenous, LGBTQIA, and LEP populations. In addition, human trafficking, child abuse, and elder abuse are serious problems in rural America. Victims may refrain from reporting such abuse because they fear that doing so will result in loss of privacy or contribute to or aggravate social stigma and ostracization. Furthermore, and given the prevalence of gun ownership among many rural families, victims may not report abuse because they fear doing so will escalate the violence. In other cases, victims who file complaints find they are dismissed or not taken seriously when law enforcement officers or judges are friends, relatives, or neighbors of the perpetrator. The limited availability of domestic violence shelters in rural America also discourages victims from leaving their abusers, particularly as doing so may render them and their children homeless. Rates of peer, family, and community acceptance of alcohol and tobacco use are also a significant concern in rural communities. Easy access to alcohol at social functions and family gatherings is common. Rural adolescents begin using alcohol and tobacco products at a younger age than urban teens and are more likely to incorporate such substances into social activities. Rates of substance abuse, addiction, and death due to overdose from methamphetamines and opioids continue to rise among rural populations. Yet due to limited health-care infrastructure and the high cost of treatment for addiction, those who abuse controlled substances may find it nearly impossible to obtain comprehensive treatment.

CHAPTER ELEVEN

Sexual and Gender Minority Populations

The social construction of sex and gender remains a defining feature of US culture and is rooted in patriarchal ideologies, specifically heteronormativity and cisnormativity. These ideologies falsely posit that sex and gender are synonymous and, consequently, presume heterosexuality while also normalizing the alignment of biological sex, gender identity, sexuality, and gender roles into simplistic and binary categories of female/feminine/woman and male/masculine/man. Consequently, individuals who identify as both cisgender and heterosexual (cishet)—that is, those whose gender identity aligns with the sex they are assigned at time of birth, and who are romantically and sexually attracted to and/or engage in sexual behavior with individuals of the other sex—are accepted, celebrated, and even rewarded. However, those who do not conform to sex/gender norms—and who are often collectively referred to as sexual and gender minorities (SGM) or sexual and gender diverse groups (SDG)—encounter ongoing discrimination, vilification, ostracism, and even violence. SGM groups are often represented by the acronym LGBTQIA to denote lesbian, gay, bisexual, transgender, queer, intersex, and asexual populations. It is common for such populations to be discussed collectively, particularly as a means of addressing the common needs, experiences, and challenges among them.

Yet significant differences also exist. Lesbian and gay populations are emotionally, physically, and/or sexually attracted to individuals of the same sex. Bisexual populations—who may sometimes identify as pansexual—are attracted to individuals of diverse sexual and gender identities. For transgender individuals, their gender identity and/or gender expression does not align with the sex assigned to them at birth; some have a decidedly masculine or feminine gender identity, yet others do not and, thus, they may identify as gender nonbinary (GNB or Enby), gender nonconforming (GNC), bigender, or genderqueer. Some cultural groups have distinct terms for SGM populations; for example, some Native American/First Nations groups use the term “Two Spirit,” and it denotes a unique degree of respect. Historically, the term queer was used to ridicule and stigmatize lesbian, gay, bisexual, transgender, and pansexual populations. In recent decades, however, many SGM proudly claim queerness as both a social and political identity. "Intersex" is a term used to describe a broad range of variations in hormones, chromosomes, internal sex organs, external genitalia, and secondary sex characteristics that do not align with normative medical categories of female and male. Most individuals with intersex traits identify as girl/woman, boy/man, or GNB, but some do claim intersex as their gender identity. Asexual (or Ace) individuals often have limited interest in sexual activities but many desire emotional and romantic intimacy. Gender and sexual identities are not mutually exclusive; thus, an individual who identifies as a gender minority may also identify as a sexual minority. Furthermore, gender and sexual identity/expression are not fixed; both can and do change over time. Changes in gender identity/expression are known as gender fluidity while changes in sexual identity/expression are referred to as sexual fluidity.

This chapter focuses on the health and well-being of SGM populations in the United States. It is grounded in the minority stress model, a theoretical approach that acknowledges the unique stressors that impact members of the LGBTQIA community and posits that such stressors are intricately intertwined with the psychological, physical, and social well-being of such populations. Regardless of whether they openly share their identities or not, SGM populations continue to suffer significant health disparities.

CURRENT STATE OF HEALTH

SGM populations are less likely than cishet population to be in good or excellent physical health; they are also more likely to rate their own health as poor and to have certain acute and chronic health conditions. Rates of chronic diseases are highest among SGM elderly, low-income, and Black, Indigenous, and People of Color (BIPOC) subgroups. Yet there are some differences among subgroups. For example, when compared to other SGM subgroups, those with intersex traits are twice as likely to be in poor physical health. Cardiovascular diseases (CVD)—for example, heart attack, stroke, peripheral artery disease, coronary heart disease, and high blood pressure—are a common concern among SGM populations, particularly among cisgender gay, lesbian, and bisexual groups as well as transgender groups. Like cishet men, cisgender gay and bisexual men tend to have high rates of CVD; they typically develop such diseases at a younger age than cisgender women. Although cisgender bisexual (cisbi) women are less likely to develop CVD than cisbi men, they do have higher rates of such diseases than cishet women. High allostatic load—specifically the chronic and repeat stress associated with living in a cisnormative and heteronormative society—is a key contributor to CVD among SGM populations. Gender-affirming hormone therapy may increase risk of CVD in transgender, GNB, and intersex populations. Overall, SGM populations tend to experience physical disabilities at a younger age than non-SGM populations. They are also at increased risk for chronic illnesses and disabilities—especially as they age—as well as premature death. Average life expectancy (ALE) of those living in communities where they feel welcomed and supported is comparable to non-SGM populations; for those living in areas with pervasive anti-SGM prejudice, however, ALE is a decade less than the national average among all populations.

Cancer is also a concern. Recent reports suggest that transgender, GNB, and intersex populations receiving hormone therapies—either as part of gender-affirming health care or as part of treatment for endocrine disorders or other health conditions—are at increased risk of developing cancer, yet research in this area remains scarce. Furthermore, existing research indicates that cancer rates among cisgender lesbian, gay, and bisexual subgroups are often higher than national averages among cishet populations. For example, rates of breast cancer are disproportionately high among cisbi and cisgender lesbian women. However, among cisgender gay and cisbi men, rates of prostate and testicular cancer are on par with national averages. Cancer rates among SGM people may be linked to certain behavioral factors such as physical activity levels, nutrition, smoking, and alcohol consumption. Yet childbearing patterns and certain infectious diseases (e.g., human papilloma virus (HPV)) may also be contributing factors. For example, cisbi and cisgender gay men have higher rates of colon, rectal, and anal cancer; this has been linked to increased incidence of anal HPV infections among such populations. However, disparities in health insurance coverage, systemic barriers to regular cancer screenings and cancer treatment, and the lack of consistent collection of data pertaining to both sexual identity and gender identity in national cancer registries continue to limit a full and accurate understanding of cancer among LGBTQIA populations. Those who openly share their identities—including with health-care providers—have lower rates of cancer and related mortality than those who conceal their sexual and/or gender identity.

Physical fitness, activity levels, and rates of obesity vary among SGM populations. Cisgender lesbian, gay, and bisexual subgroups are more likely than heterosexual populations to meet federal guidelines for physical activity and physical fitness. Over 70 percent of cisbi adults meet such guidelines; this is higher than among cisgender lesbian and gay populations. While cisgender lesbians have slightly higher average rates of aerobic physical activity (e.g., walking, running, biking, and using stationary exercise machines) than cishet women, they are more likely to be overweight or obese. Among lesbians, rates of obesity are highest for those who reside in rural areas, are over age 40, and have sedentary jobs. Cisgender gay men tend to be more physically active and to have lower average body weight than cishet men. In contrast, cisbi men are more likely to be overweight or obese than cishet men while cisbi women are more likely to be underweight when compared to both cisgender lesbian and cishet women. Additionally, bisexual, GNB, and transgender adolescents and adults are more likely to have abnormal body weight—being either underweight or overweight—than cishet populations. While there is a paucity of research on those with intersex traits, evidence suggests abnormal body weight is also an issue among such populations.

Eating disorders are a concern among some SGM subgroups. Cisgender gay men are more likely than cishet men, lesbians, and cisbi populations to develop an eating disorder, especially anorexia nervosa or bulimia. At present, one-tenth of all SGM teens and young adults have a diagnosed eating disorder while another 20 percent engage in disorder eating patterns but have not yet received a clinical diagnosis. Among all SGM subgroups, rates of eating disorders are highest among transgender, GNB, and intersex populations. Various social-emotional-psychological factors influence such rates; examples include gender dysphoria (the distress that occurs when an individual's gender identity does not correspond with the sex they were assigned at birth), trauma, and ongoing stress due to marginalization in US society. SGM individuals who engage in restrictive eating practices are at increased risk for nutritional deficiencies and related physical and mental health issues. Cisgender lesbians and cisbi women and girls who are Black or white are more likely to have a higher body mass index (BMI) than their cishet counterparts; in contrast, lesbian and bisexual women who are Asian and Hispanic/Latinx/Chicanx (HLC) are more likely to be underweight. Cisgender gay and cisbi Black men and boys are more likely to be obese than cisgender men and boys of other racial and ethnic groups. Abnormal body weight is more common among low-income SGM groups. Being overweight or obese increases risk of heart disease, diabetes, fatty liver disease, osteoarthritis, and high blood pressure. Those with low body weight may also suffer from impaired immune function, skin ailments, dental problems, nutrient deficiencies, and heart irregularities.

SGM persons are more likely than cishet populations to use tobacco products, consume alcohol on a regular basis, engage in excessive alcohol consumption, and abuse drugs. They typically begin to use such substances at a younger age than their cishet counterparts and have higher risk of substance use and abuse disorders (SUAD) throughout the lifespan. Use and abuse of such substances are often a response to the stress associated with living in a cisnormative and heteronormative society. However, marketing is also a factor. Since the late twentieth century, tobacco and alcohol companies have increasingly targeted SGM populations via both print and electronic marketing campaigns, including via sponsorship of Pride Month activities. LGBTQIA youth are nearly four times as likely as their cishet peers to use tobacco products; rates of use are especially high among GNB and transgender subgroups. SGM teens are also less likely than their cishet peers to believe that e-cigarettes pose risks to their health and well-being. Among adult populations, cisgender lesbian, gay, and bisexual subgroups are 30 percent more likely than cishet populations to smoke cigarettes while transgender adults are more than twice as likely to do so. Use of tobacco products has been identified as a key factor in rates of lung cancer, oral cancer, and respiratory illnesses (e.g., asthma, chronic obstructive pulmonary disease (COPD), bronchitis, and emphysema) among SGM populations. Similarly, such populations are more likely than cishet populations to use alcohol at a younger age, drink to excess, and develop an alcohol use disorder; such disorders increase risk and severity of liver problems, certain types of cancer, accidental injuries, neurological problems, depression, sleep disorders, impaired immune function, and gastrointestinal problems. Alcohol use disorders are most common among Black and HLC subgroups, those residing in states with anti-LGBTQIA legislation, and individuals who feel rejected by family and friends. Use and abuse of illegal and prescription substances are also unduly high among SGM populations; research indicates drug abuse is especially common among those with chronic physical or mental health conditions.

Certain types of communicable diseases also disproportionately impact the SGM community. In recent years, for example, outbreaks of infectious diseases including meningitis, antibiotic resistant Shigella, and monkeypox have disproportionately impacted cisgender gay men, especially younger, low-income, Black, and HLC populations. During the pandemic, sexual and gender minorities experienced higher rates of COVID-19 infection than non-SGM populations. They were also more likely to become seriously ill, be hospitalized, and die from the virus. Greater incidence of certain underlying health conditions (e.g., asthma, COPD, cancer, CVD, and kidney disease) among SGM populations has been linked to increased morbidity and mortality rates among those who contracted COVID-19. The pandemic also negatively impacted mental well-being and social connectedness among SGM populations, regardless of whether they contracted the virus or not. Interestingly, LGBTQIA people tended to have more positive attitudes toward vaccines against COVID than cishet groups; they were also more likely to believe that obtaining such vaccines was part of their responsibility to protect the health of others. Yet many encountered barriers that made it difficult to obtain vaccines.

Reproductive and sexual health concerns vary among SGM subgroups. Overall, such populations tend to have markedly lower rates of childbearing than non-SGM populations. However, some do pursue parenthood. Sometimes, this occurs in the context of a heterosexual relationship such as a marriage, nonmarital partnership, or even an informal arrangement (e.g., between friends) created with the explicit intent of having offspring. Rates of miscarriage, stillbirth, preterm births, and low-birth weight infants are slightly higher among cisgender lesbians than cishet women but are markedly higher among GNB, transgender, and intersex pregnant individuals, especially BIPOC and low-income subgroups. Others pursue parenthood via formal surrogacy arrangements, adoption (including foster-to-adopt), and/or the use of assisted reproductive technologies (e.g., in-vitro fertilization and intra-uterine insemination). Same-sex couples are four to five times as likely as heterosexual couples to adopt a child. However, given the costs associated with adoption, surrogacy, and reproductive technologies, such avenues to parenthood are often not accessible to low-income SGM populations. Additionally, some states permit foster and adoption agencies to use religious beliefs as a basis for refusing services to LGBTQIA populations. Overall, rates of unintended pregnancy among SGM teens are on par with such rates among non-SGM teens; however, cisbi girls are more than three times as likely to become pregnant before age 20 than cishet girls.

Rates of sexually transmitted infections (STI) in the United States have increased in recent years, including among most LGBTQIA populations. However, rates and types of infections vary among SGM subgroups. Cisgender men who have sex only with other men (MSM) have higher-than-average rates of HIV, Hepatitis A, Hepatitis B, chlamydia, gonorrhea, and syphilis while STI rates are much lower among cisgender lesbians and cisgender asexual populations. When compared to cishet men, transgender populations as well as cisgender gay and cisbi men have higher rates of syphilis, gonorrhea, HIV, and chlamydia; rates are highest among low-income, Black, and HLC populations and those who are housing insecure. Among SGM populations, STI rates are lowest among those in monogamous and consensual relationships, who consistently use condoms and/or dental dams, and who have good access to comprehensive sexual and reproductive health care. Sexual behaviors have been linked to other health conditions in certain subgroups. For example, bacterial vaginosis—an imbalance of vaginal bacteria—is twice as common among cisgender lesbians when compared to cishet women. Although BV is not an STI, cisgender women can transmit it to one another during sexual activities; incidence is highest among those who have multiple sexual partners. Untreated BV increases risk of STI, miscarriage, premature birth, and pelvic inflammatory disease. In addition, and like cishet women and others who engage in receptive anal intercourse (RAI), cisgender gay and cisbi men have disproportionately high rates of inflammatory bowel disease, ulcerative colitis, and Crohn's disease. Rates are particularly high among those who do not use condoms or otherwise follow safe-sex practices and may be a consequence of HPV infection.

Timing and pace of identity development vary among SGM subgroups; such development is a key component of mental well-being. Children born with intersex traits are sometimes subjected to medically unnecessary surgeries and hormonal treatments to bring their bodies into alignment with medically defined binary categories of sex. Such procedures can lead to physical complications (e.g., infection, pain, impaired sexual function, and infertility) and can impair sexual and gender identity development, thereby increasing risk of poor mental health. Among transgender and GNB populations, gender dysphoria is typically present in early childhood; nearly 80 percent experience it prior to their seventh birthday. However, many wait until their 20s before sharing their gender identity with others and starting their process of social transition (i.e., to begin living openly as transgender or GNB). It is common to wait even longer to begin gender-affirming medical care, including hormone and surgical therapies. Those with access to such therapies enjoy greater mental wellness than those who do not. Cisgender lesbians are typically aware of their sexual identity at a younger age than cisbi girls. Yet lesbians typically experience their first romantic relationships and first sexual encounter at a slightly later age than cishet women. Lesbians generally experience higher rates of acceptance from social networks than cisgender gay men and boys but take longer to move from awareness of same-sex attraction to self-identification and then coming out to social networks. On average, cisgender gay boys experience their first same-sex sexual attraction at age 11; this is two and a half years earlier than among cisgender lesbians. Cisgender gay men and boys also tend to self-identify at a younger age than lesbian populations. Among all SGM subgroups, those born since the mid-1970s tend to self-identify and share gender and/or sexual identity with others at a younger age than previous generations.

Mental health disorders are disproportionately high among SGM groups, including from childhood through old age. Some of the most common mental health concerns include anxiety disorders, feelings of social isolation and exclusion, depression, eating disorders, substance use and abuse disorders (SUAD), post-traumatic stress disorders (PTSD), self-harming behaviors, and suicidal ideation. Two-thirds of LGBTQIA teens experience generalized anxiety disorder, depression, and/or another mental health disorder; nearly half engage in non-suicidal self-harming behaviors. Rates are highest among transgender and nonbinary adolescents. Suicidal ideation and suicide attempts are four times as common among SGM youth when compared to their non-SGM peers. Teens who are subjected to conversion therapy—interventions that attempt to force SGM individuals to conform to normative gender and sexual identities/roles—are at increased lifetime risk of suicide. Rates of depression, stress, social isolation, loneliness, SUAD, and suicidality are also disproportionately high among SGM adults, and rates of certain mental health issues (e.g., depression and loneliness) increase with age.

SGM groups also bear an undue burden as victims of exploitation and violence. Examples of such violence include child abuse and neglect, verbal abuse, bullying, threats, financial abuse, physical attacks, trafficking, intimate partner violence (IPV), hazing, stalking, sexual harassment, sexual assault, rape, and elder abuse. Cisgender lesbian women and girls of all age groups are more likely to be victims of IPV than cishet women and girls. Over 40 percent of lesbians experience some type of IPV during their lifetimes. Half of transgender and GNB individuals experience IPV; this is more than three times as high as among cisgender populations. SGM populations are also four times as likely as cishet populations to be victims of non-IPV violent crime; perpetrators are typically known to the victim (e.g., a family member, classmate, co-worker, friend, or neighbor). Compared to national averages among all populations, LGBTQIA individuals are twice as likely to be victims of gun violence. One-fifth of all hate crimes in the United States are perpetrated against SGM individuals. Violent victimization is associated with increased rates and severity of trauma-related disorders including PTSD, adjustment disorders, acute stress disorder, and dissociative identity disorder. It also diminishes physical well-being and increases risk of SUAD, self-harming behaviors, suicidal ideation, and suicide attempts. However, SGM victims often do not report such violence to the police. Homocide rates involving SGM victims are higher than national averages; most victims are BIPOC.

ECONOMIC FACTORS

LGBTQIA populations fare worse economically than cishet groups. They have higher-than-average rates of poverty and debt but are less likely than cishet populations to have the resources necessary to meet basic needs and to cover emergency expenses. Rates of unemployment and underemployment are disproportionately high among SGM populations; they are overrepresented in entry-level jobs yet remain marginalized in jobs that offer higher wages, benefits, and opportunities for advancement. Persistent discrimination continues to shape the experiences of SGM workers in the United States, thereby diminishing job satisfaction as well as health.

Poverty and Its Consequences

Rates of poverty among SGM populations are disproportionately high when compared to national averages among all populations. LGBTQIA groups are about one-third more likely than cishet populations to live in households with incomes below the Federal Poverty Level (FPL). At present, one in five of all adult SGM individuals lives below the FPL. However, poverty rates vary considerably among subgroups; they are highest among BIPOC and elderly populations. Additionally, and whereas transgender individuals and cisbi women have disproportionately high rates of poverty, such rates are significantly lower among cisgender lesbians and cisbi men. Cisgender gay men have the lowest poverty rates among all SGM subgroups; the average household income of gay married couples is comparable to that of heterosexual married couples. However, same-sex married couples raising children are two-thirds more likely than their cishet counterparts to live below the FPL. Poverty increases risk of certain infectious and chronic diseases. It also increases risk of food insecurity and health conditions related to nutrient deficiencies and abnormal body weight. At least one-third of all SGM youth—including half of Black and Indigenous populations—are food insecure. During the first two years of the COVID-19 pandemic, rates of food insecurity among SGM adults were nearly twice as high as among cishet adults; such rates were highest among those over age 65 as well as transgender, GNB, and bisexual populations.

SGM populations are also at increased risk for homelessness and housing insecurity; this is especially true for transgender, BIPOC, elderly, and adolescent/young adult subgroups. Among adults, only half own their own homes; this is one-third lower than among non-SGM adults. When compared to their cishet peers, LGBTQIA populations are twice as likely to be homeless or housing insecure. Thus, they are at increased risk for certain communicable diseases (e.g., hepatitis, tuberculosis, and influenza), skin diseases, injuries, and mental health conditions—including SUAD—associated with chronic stress. Exposure to temperature and weather extremes also contributes to poor physical and mental health among housing insecure individuals. They are also at increased risk for violence, including physical assault, sexual assault, rape, trafficking, and homicide. Risk of such violence is especially pronounced among housing insecure SGM minors who are estranged from their parents and/or who are unaccompanied by an adult who cares for them and affirms their sexual and/or gender identity. Additionally, those who engage in what is commonly referred to as survival sex (e.g., participating in sexual activities in exchange for food, shelter, clothing, and other basic needs) are at increased risk for unintended pregnancy, STIs, and sexual violence. Half of all homeless LGBTQIA teens and young adults under age 25 engage in survival sex.

Employment, Income, and Wealth

Systemic inequities continue to shape employment, income, and wealth accumulation among LGBTQIA populations. In all types of jobs, such populations remain underrepresented; this is especially pronounced in higher-paying, skilled labor, and leadership positions including as mid- and upper-level managers, chief executive officers, chief fiscal officers, board members, and in elected positions within local, state, and federal governments. At present, less than 1 percent of such positions are held by SGM women, while only 3 percent are held by SGM men. This underrepresentation is often referred to as the lavender ceiling, a concept that refers to the persistent social barriers that diminish career opportunities and advancement for SGM individuals. Such barriers are especially pronounced at the intersection of gender, sexuality, race, ethnicity, and disability status. Consequently, SGM populations tend to be overrepresented in jobs that do not require advanced education or training; such jobs are associated with lower wages, fewer opportunities for advancement, and fewer benefits such as health insurance, paid sick leave, vacation leave, and retirement options. The employment rate among SGM groups, collectively, is about 7 percent lower than among cishet populations. Yet employment varies significantly among SGM subgroups. From 2000 through 2019, unemployment rates among bisexual populations, cisgender gay men, and cisgender lesbians declined steadily. During this period, unemployment rates were lowest among white and Asian cisgender gay men but markedly higher among transgender and GNB populations. Prior to the pandemic, nearly one-third of transgender and GNB populations were actively seeking but unable to secure employment. Additionally, among cisgender gay, lesbian, and bisexual populations, those who are not married are more likely to be unemployed than those who are married. During the COVID-19 pandemic, LGBTQIA adolescents and adults who were actively seeking paid employment were 25 percent more likely than cishet populations to be unemployed; job recovery rates in both public and private sectors have been slower among SGM populations. Rates of underemployment—wherein an individual works in a job that does not allow them to make full use of their skills and/or they are seeking a full-time job but can only secure part-time work—are also disproportionately high, particularly among transgender and GNB subgroups.

SGM populations are employed in a variety of industries but have somewhat unique patterns of employment. Cisgender lesbian women are less likely than cishet women to be employed in female-dominated industries (e.g., elementary school teachers, nurses, childcare workers, and administrative assistants) while cisgender gay men are less likely than cishet men to be employed in male-dominated industries (e.g., construction, plumbing and electrical work, and manufacturing). While certain industries such as real estate, finance, information technology, and legal services tend to be rated as more SGM-friendly when compared to other industries, cishet workers consistently report higher rates of job satisfaction than LGBTQIA workers across all industries. Since the late twentieth century, it has become increasingly common for SGM individuals to own their own businesses. However, they are less likely than cishet populations to receive business loans and are more likely to encounter financial challenges that threaten their ability to remain in business. During the COVID-19 pandemic, financial losses among LGBTQIA-owned businesses were 50 percent higher than cishet-owned businesses.

The wage gap also influences the well-being of SGM populations. Full-time SGM employees earn only about 90 percent of average wages earned by cishet populations in similar jobs. This diminishes their ability to meet basic needs—including as related to health care—and to accumulate wealth and assets, including savings, life insurance, retirement funds, real estate, and investment accounts. They are also less likely than non-SGM groups to have savings adequate to cover living expenses in the event of serious illness or injury, job loss, or other another emergency. Thus, the wage gap influences both short- and long-term financial stability of SGM individuals and their families. However, wages vary among SGM subgroups. For example, average earnings among cisgender gay and cisbi men are nearly the same as their cishet counterparts; in contrast, average wages are 13 percent less among cisgender lesbian and cisbi women when compared to cishet women. The wage gap is even greater for gender minorities—nonbinary individuals and transgender men are paid 30 percent less than gender-conforming employees while transgender women are paid 40 percent less than cishet workers. Average wages among Asian and white SGM populations are comparable to those earned by cishet groups. However, they are decidedly lower for other groups: HLC workers earn 10 percent less than cishet workers, while Black workers earn 20 percent less. Among Indigenous SGM populations, the wage gap is 30 percent. The gap is even greater for SGM cisgender and transgender BIPOC women, especially those over 40 years of age. Debt is also an ongoing concern for many members of the LGBTQIA community. Collectively, such populations tend to have a higher debt-to-earnings ratio and lower credit score than non-SGM populations.

Workplace Discrimination

Since the 1970s, various advocacy groups (e.g., Lambda Legal, GLAAD, Human Rights Campaign, and Out & Equal) have worked to promote workplace equity for LGBTQIA populations. However, measures to guarantee such equity have been slow, often inadequate, and subject to significant opposition. For example, in 1982, Wisconsin passed the first statewide law prohibiting workplace discrimination against sexual minorities; however, such legislation did not include protections for transgender, GNB, or other gender minorities. It wasn't until eleven years later, with the passage of the Human Rights Act in 1993, that Minnesota became the first state to provide legal protection to both sexual minority and gender minority populations. During that same year, President Clinton signed the "Don't Ask, Don't Tell" (DADT) policy; it legally permitted gay, lesbian, and bisexual individuals to join the military. However, they could only do so if they did not make their sexual identity known to their military peers or supervisors. In 2010, DADT was repealed under the Obama Administration, thereby allowing sexual minorities to openly serve in the armed forces. Yet it took until 2016 for the military ban on transgender and GNB populations to be lifted; the following year, bolstered by support from conservative religious organizations, the Trump administration attempted to reinstate such bans. In 2020, however, in a 6–3 decision in *Bostock v. Clayton County*, the Supreme Court of the United States (SCOTUS) declared that discrimination against SGM populations in employment violates Title VII of the Civil Rights Act of 1964. To date, the *Bostock* decision has garnered the most comprehensive protection for SGM employees.

Yet practices and attitudes that discriminate against and contribute to an unwelcoming work environment for SGM populations continue to be documented in all industries, including governmental, private, and nonprofit organizations. Applicants who are open about their gender identity or sexual identity are less likely to get a job interview and less likely to receive an offer of employment than cishet applicants. SGM employees are frequently paid less than their cishet peers who have similar education, training, and work experience. In addition, they are less likely that cishet employees to be promoted or offered other opportunities for advancement yet are more likely to be disciplined, demoted, or fired. Workplace harassment also remains common. More than one-third of SGM employees experience verbal harassment (e.g., name-calling, yelling, use of derogatory language, or anti-LGBTQIA slurs) in the workplace while another 20 percent are targets of physical harassment (e.g., hitting, pushing, tripping, kicking, and/or destruction of personal property) by supervisors, co-workers, or customers. One in four also experiences sexual harassment including nonconsensual sexual touching, sexual jokes, requests for sexual favors in exchange for career advancement, questions about their sexual history, explicit communications (e.g., emails, texts, and phone calls), sexual assault, and rape. Rates of such victimization are highest among BIPOC women, transgender, and GNB subgroups. Nearly half of SGM workers do not come out to colleagues or supervisors for fear of being harassed, fired, demoted, or otherwise penalized and victimized.

Harassment in the workplace is associated with increased incidence and severity of physical ailments including headaches, stress, irregular sleep patterns, musculoskeletal pains, and gastrointestinal upset. Workplace harassment also impairs mental well-being and can contribute to depression, anxiety, SUAD, suicidal ideation, and PTSD. Many victims do not report such harassment because they fear their claims will not be taken seriously. Others believe reporting with result in increased harassment or that they will lose their jobs. Those employed in workplaces that are unwelcoming to LGBTQIA populations may go to great lengths to conceal their identities. They may alter appearance, refuse to talk about their personal life, avoid work-related holiday celebrations and other social events, and refrain from using workplace bathrooms. Nearly 50 percent of SGM employees do not share their sexual and/or gender identity with their supervisors out of fear that doing so will lead to harassment or other types of discriminatory treatment. Individuals who are subjected to harassment and other forms of discrimination tend to feel isolated and have low rates of job satisfaction; they also take more sick leave and are more likely to quit than those in LGBTQIA-friendly workplaces.

EDUCATIONAL ACCESS AND QUALITY

Most public and private K-12 schools, colleges, universities, and other education and training programs in the United States do not collect information on gender identity, sexual identity, or about the experiences of SGM student populations. Critics have argued that failure to do so reflects the ongoing presumption of heterosexuality and cisnormativity in most educational institutions. In recent decades, however, research in this realm has expanded. SGM students tend to thrive in educational settings that are welcoming and affirming. However, those who feel marginalized, ostracized, and excluded are less likely to do well academically and to graduate than their non-SGM peers; they are also more likely to be socially marginalized, in poor physical health, and suffer from acute and chronic mental health conditions.

Attendance, Academic Achievement, and Degree Completion

Approximately 6 percent of all middle school students identify as sexual minorities and/or gender minorities; rates are twice as high among high schoolers. Among all students enrolled in postsecondary education and training programs, nearly one-fifth identify as members of the LGBTQIA community. At all levels of education, and when compared to non-SGM populations, SGM students have higher rates of absenteeism and are more likely to be chronically absent, something that hinders their academic performance and is associated with decreased likelihood of degree completion. Yet absenteeism also diminishes health and social well-being. Those who are chronically absent are more likely to fall behind in their studies, fail to meet grade-level expectations in core subjects including reading, math, and science, and have a lower grade point average (GPA) than students who attend school regularly. Such struggles have been linked to increased incidence and severity of academic-related stress and anxiety. Chronically absent students are also more likely to be estranged from their age-group peers and to lack supportive relationships with teachers, counselors, and other school professionals. Thus, they are at increased risk for loneliness, depression, anxiety, and similar conditions.

Those who are chronically absent are also more likely to drop out of school before completing a high school degree. Dropout rates are disproportionately high among SGM students. Nearly one-third of all SGM students drop out of school during middle school or high school; this is three times higher than the national average among non-SGM populations. Individuals who drop out are more likely to live in poverty as adults; they are also more likely to be incarcerated during adolescence and adulthood. Some who drop out may later attend so-called alternative educational programs or participate in online schooling. Others pursue a General Educational Development (GED) diploma. Such options can increase likelihood of degree completion for some SGM students. However, many alternative and online programs are underfunded, provide substandard instruction, and have low degree completion rates when compared to traditional brick-and-mortar high schools. Students who complete their high school education via alternative, online, or GED options are less likely to pursue college than those who earn a degree from a traditional school. Consequently, such options decrease the lifetime earning potential of SGM students and, in turn, increase their risk of living below the FPL during adulthood.

At the postsecondary level, one-third of SGM students choose a college that is far from home as a strategy for finding a more welcoming and inclusive environment. Indeed, they are four times as likely as cishet students to choose a college far from home and family. However, for low-income SGM students, this is often not an option due to the additional expenses associated with travel and out-of-state tuition. Although nearly one-fifth of all students enrolled in postsecondary education self-identify as part of the LGBTQIA community, there remains little nationwide, systemic attention to retention rates among such students. However, they are at increased risk of dropping out of college, with rates of attrition highest among BIPOC, transgender, GNB, and low-income subgroups. Interestingly, cisgender lesbian, gay, and bisexual student populations are more likely to attend college and to earn an undergraduate degree than their non-SGM peers. Within graduate and professional programs, however, degree completion rates vary among SGM subgroups. Graduate degree attainment rates among cisgender lesbians, cisbi women, and cisbi men are comparable to rates among cishet populations yet. However, cisgender gay men are nearly 50 percent more likely earn a graduate or professional degree than cishet men. Among cisgender gay and cisbi men, rates of successful degree completion in graduate and professional programs are highest among Asian men. In contrast, cisgender lesbian and cisbi women are less likely to earn a graduate or professional degree; graduate and professional degree attainment is more common among those who identify as white but significantly lower among cisgender lesbian and bisexual BIPOC women. Data on college and graduate/professional degree attainment among transgender, GNB, intersex, and asexual populations is sparse. Yet recent research suggests that postsecondary degree completion rates among transgender and GNB adults who become aware of and begin living openly in accordance with their gender identity at a younger-than-average age and who do so within the context of a supportive familial and social environment are equivalent to and, in some cases, slightly higher than among cishet adults.

Barriers to Inclusion and Equity

One of the most significant factors in shaping the educational experiences and attainment of SGM students is institutional climate. This refers to the core beliefs, values, and attitudes found in academic settings, specifically as they relate to inclusion and equity. Climate is reflected in institutional policies, programming, and practices; however, the attitudes and behaviors of various social actors (e.g., administrators, teachers, volunteers, counselors, coaches, tutors, students, and parents) are also contributing factors. At the primary, secondary, and postsecondary levels, SGM students attending schools with anti-discrimination and anti-harassment policies that are clearly defined and consistently enforced have markedly higher self-esteem, perform better academically, and feel a stronger sense of social belonging than those attending schools where such policies are lacking, ambiguous, and/or poorly applied. But there are other factors that contribute to climate and shape the experiences of SGM students. Quite simply, many SGM students do not feel welcomed in educational settings. Much of this is due to bullying and harassment. Although such behavior occurs at all levels of education, it is most prominent in middle school and high school contexts. While attending school, over 90 percent of SGM students in grades 6 through 12 are subjected to negative and disparaging comments about sexual minorities and/or gender minorities. Such comments reinforce stereotypes about SGM populations. Additionally, in schools where such comments are commonplace, SGM students are more likely to be victims of physical attacks. Three-fourths of SGM middle and high school students are targets of verbal harassment by peers; at least one-third are also physically harassed or physically assaulted. Moreover, rates of IPV (e.g., dating violence, stalking, sexual assault, and rape) that victimize SGM students aged 12–18 are unduly high.

The climate in K-12 settings is also shaped by anti-SGM legislation. In 2022 alone, proposal and passage of such legislation were linked to increases in social marginalization and exclusion, bullying, physical attacks, and other types of violence against SGM students both in and out of school settings. Some laws have banned books by LGBTQIA authors and/or those that focus on the lives and experiences of SGM individuals (including fiction and nonfiction). Many laws prohibit attention to gender identity and sexual identity as part of the educational content including in history, science, and literature courses. Furthermore, there is a consistent lack of attention to SGM populations in health classes, particularly in sex education and curricula related to healthy relationships. Only one-third of states offer inclusive sex education that explicitly includes LGBTQIA populations; yet within those states, not all schools are required to offer such education. And only six states require that sex education be both inclusive and medically accurate.

Yet the influence of such laws extends well beyond curricula. In some contexts, student clubs and organizations (e.g., Gay-Straight Alliance, Pride, and Association for Queer Students) that primarily serve and/or include attention to SGM groups have been effectively banned. Some districts have barred teachers from using gender neutral or preferred pronouns for transgender and GNB students; instead, teachers must use the pronouns that correspond with the students' sex assigned at birth. So-called bathroom bills and fairness in sports bills rely on binary, normative categories to prohibit transgender and GNB students from using the restroom that aligns with their gender identity and to exclude such students from participating in school-sponsored sports teams. Some laws have also designated educational professionals as mandatory reporters; thus, if a student comes out to them as a sexual minority or gender minority, teachers and administrators are required to notify the students' parents. Even display of the rainbow flag and other symbols associated with LGBTQIA pride is prohibited in some districts. In educational settings where such measures are in place, SGM students report high rates of social marginalization and isolation. Those enrolled in unwelcoming and unsupportive school environments are three times more likely than their non-SGM peers to suffer from depression, anxiety disorders, and physical ailments related to chronic stress (e.g., headaches, digestive disorders, sleep disturbances, muscle aches and pains, and abnormal body weight). They are also at increased risk for PTSD, non-suicidal self-harming behaviors, suicidal ideation, and suicide attempts. SGM teens are four times more likely than their cishet peers to attempt suicide; rates are highest among BIPOC bisexual, transgender, GNB, intersex, and asexual youth.

Recent research suggests that an increasing number of educational professionals are committed to and trained to help promote diverse, equitable, and inclusive educational environments. They do this by incorporating LGBTQIA-related content into curricula, promoting inclusive policies in their districts, forming mentoring relationships with individual students, and planning and facilitating events such as lavender prom, lavender graduation, and Pride celebrations. However, this is not always the case. In fact, some educators remain unaware of the unique needs of SGM students—including, for example, the disproportionately high rates of housing insecurity, food insecurity, familial estrangement, and mental health disorders among them—due to inadequate professional development and training. Yet others knowingly engage in discriminatory behaviors that contribute to an unwelcoming and, in some cases, a hostile climate for SGM students. This type of explicit bias is obvious, for example, in settings where educators use discriminatory language, refuse to use preferred pronouns, or do not enforce anti-bullying and anti-discrimination policies. Yet it is also clear in disciplinary practices. SGM students—especially BIPOC, homeless, and low-income groups—in pre-K through twelfth grade are more likely to be punished and to receive harsher punishment for the same behavioral infraction than their cishet peers. Such disparities in discipline contribute to school absenteeism, poor academic performance, diminished mental health, and increased feelings of social isolation among SGM students. They also increase the likelihood that such students will drop out of school and become involved in the juvenile justice system; such involvement, in turn, makes it more likely such students will be incarcerated during adulthood.

In many postsecondary institutions, the climate is somewhat more welcoming and supportive for SGM students. Yet disparities persist. SGM undergraduate and graduate students are nearly twice as likely as their cishet peers to be victims of harassment and bullying (including both in-person and online) as well as physical attacks; SGM students are also at least three times as likely as non-SGM students to be sexually harassed on college and university campuses and to be victims of IPV and sexual violence while attending college. Such victimization is most common in university-sponsored on-campus housing. At present, there are over two hundred campuses throughout the nation with active LGBTQIA centers that aim to provide targeted support and services for SGM students; however, many are underfunded and, consequently, services are often inadequate to meet demand. Nearly two-thirds of SGM students attending postsecondary institutions have not come out to professors or other educational professionals, and 40 percent are not out to their peers. For many, this is due to a perceived lack of a genuinely welcoming and supportive climate at the school they are attending. And for others, it is due to the social, academic, and personal risks of openly sharing their sexual and/or gender identify in such contexts. Those who have come out are twice as likely as cishet students to report unfair treatment by professors, staff, and administrators. Poor mental health is an ongoing issue for many SGM college students; rates of anxiety disorders, depressive disorders, PTSD, and suicidality are disproportionately high among such students. However, less than one-third of colleges and universities provide counseling services that are culturally competent and are both aware of and responsive to the unique needs of SGM populations. Although certain colleges and universities have been lauded for their ongoing efforts to create a more welcoming and inclusive campus climate, others seem to go out of their way to create a hostile environment for such students. Many rely on a Title IX religious-based exemption to exclude SGM populations from their campuses. Yet others implement campus-wide bans on same-sex relationships, bar student organizations that include attention to SGM groups, and promote conversion therapy.

HEALTH-CARE ACCESS AND QUALITY

SGM populations are less likely than cishet groups to have health insurance. In addition, historical ideologies that deemed LGBTQIA populations abnormal continue to shape scientific research. Such ideologies also influence the actions and attitudes of many health-care professionals. SGM populations remain underrepresented as members of the health-care workforce. Collectively, such factors diminish the quality of care provided to SGM patients; they also reinforce barriers to affordable and affirming care.

Health Insurance Coverage

The Patient Protection and Affordable Care Act (ACA) of 2010 aimed to expand access to health insurance and health care for all Americans. Drawing on antidiscrimination language from the Civil Rights Act of 1964 as well as Title IX of the Educational Amendments of 1972, Section 1557 of ACA prohibited discrimination in insurance coverage based on race, color, national origin, age, and disability as well as sex. Within Section 1557, sex was defined broadly. Thus, ACA effectively rendered it illegal to deny health insurance coverage to SGM populations or to otherwise discriminate against such populations in health-care settings, including by denying care or providing inferior care. However, the law was challenged repeatedly on religious grounds, including in the case of *Franciscan Alliance, Inc., v. Azar (2016)*. The Trump administration attempted to narrow ACA's definition of sex to include only binary biological categories of female and male and to eliminate sexual and gender identity/expression altogether. However, in the 2020 *Bostock* decision, SCOTUS asserted that "sex" is a broad category that includes both sexual and gender identity. Thus, when the US Department of Health and Human Services (HHS) issued a final ruling only weeks after the court's decision, it affirmed that SGM populations are protected under the parameters of Section 1557. The US Department of Justice (DOJ) expressed similar sentiments in a memorandum issued in early 2021. And in 2022, the Office for Civil Rights (OCR) division of the HHS issued a proposed ruling specifying that discrimination based on gender identity, sex-related characteristics, and/or sexual orientation is prohibited under the law. Prior to the *Bostock* ruling, however, SCOTUS decisions in *United States v. Windsor (2013)* and *Obergefell v. Hodges (2015)* had expanded health insurance coverage to legally married same-sex couples.

The impact of the ACA and the SCOTUS decisions described above has promoted increased access to health insurance for LGBTQIA populations. Since 2010, uninsured rates among such populations have been reduced by nearly half; rates of Medicaid coverage for SGM individuals have nearly doubled. Over half of LGBTQIA populations currently receiving Medicaid work part-time or full-time; one-third are unable to work due to injury, chronic health conditions, or disabilities. In recent years, there have been other changes to health insurance coverage among SGM populations. For example, employer-provided insurance has increasingly included transgender coverage, specifically as related to gender-affirming hormonal and surgical therapies. Whereas no Fortune 500 companies included such coverage in 2000, approximately 70 percent of such companies included it in their standard health-care insurance in 2021. Despite such changes in public and private health insurance, it is estimated that one-tenth of SGM populations currently do not have health insurance coverage; uninsured rates are highest among BIPOC groups, immigrants, those who are unemployed, and individuals with disabilities. One-third of SGM living below the FPL lack insurance; rates of coverage are lowest in states that did not expand Medicaid coverage (e.g., Wyoming, Wisconsin, North Carolina, and Kansas as well as most Gulf States and those in the so-called Deep South). During the first year of the COVID-19 pandemic, insurance coverage decreased among SGM populations due largely to disproportionately high rates of job loss among them.

At present, SGM populations have slightly lower rates of insurance coverage than cishet populations. They are also less likely to have employer-sponsored health insurance and are more likely to rely on government-sponsored health insurance for low-income populations. However, there are differences in health insurance coverage among different SGM populations. For example, those who are legally married or in legally recognized domestic partnerships are more likely to be insured. Additionally, those living in Washington, DC, Puerto Rico, and the twenty-two states—the majority of which are located on the west coast, in the northeast, or in the upper Midwest—that have passed legislation prohibiting discrimination based on sexual identity and/or gender identity are more likely to be insured. Yet over half of SGM populations live in states or territories that do not provide such protections. At present, fifteen states have explicitly banned gender-affirming care from health benefits provided to state employees and nine states exclude such care for Medicaid recipients. The Equality Act, introduced in the US House of Representatives in early 2021, prohibits discrimination based on sex, sexual orientation, and gender identity, thereby promoting improved access to health insurance and health care for SGMs. While the legislation had broad-based support and was passed by the house, it has yet to receive senate approval.

Biases in the US Health-Care System

There is a lengthy history of discrimination against LGBTQIA populations within the US health-care system. From the colonial period and well into the mid-twentieth century, and due to the influences of varying religious, philosophical, and scientific ideologies, individuals whose identities did not align with cishet norms were dubbed monsters, sexual perverts, unnatural, and even subhuman. Consequently, they were socially marginalized and subjected to widespread scorn, ridicule, and violence. Yet such ideologies were also used to justify medical experimentation on SGM populations. Examples included surgeries and hormonal treatments to modify the physical appearance (e.g., genitals, body hair, fat distribution, and breast development) of individuals with intersex traits; psychological counseling in an attempt to rid lesbian, gay, and bisexual populations of same-sex attraction; and the use of lobotomies, electroshock treatments, hypnosis, and toxic substances to try to force gay, lesbian, bisexual, transgender, queer, and GNB populations to conform to heterosexual and cisgender norms. Although such practices have drawn increasing scrutiny since the 1960s due to enhanced attention to ethics, informed consent, and patient's rights both within medical research and clinical health-care settings, such practices persist. Examples include conversion therapy, genital "normalizing" surgery on infants and children with intersex traits, and refusal of affirming care to gender diverse populations, including adolescents.

The Sexual & Gender Minority Research Office (SGMRO), established in 2015 as a unique entity within the National Institutes of Health (NIH), aims to promote inclusion of SGM populations in all health-care settings. Yet there remains a significant lack of attention to such populations in clinical research and scholarship. They continue to be largely excluded from clinical trials related to cancer, aging processes, diabetes, heart disease, non-sexually transmitted infectious diseases, acute conditions, health behaviors, disabilities, infertility, and sexual function. For example, many studies assume cishet identities among research participants, something that is clearly reflected in the language used in such studies (e.g., reliance on gender-specific pronouns; wording that conflates sex and gender). When researchers do make a concerted effort to include SGM groups in clinical research, it is typically for studies that specifically pertain to sexual behaviors, sexually transmitted diseases, gender-affirming care, and gender dysphoria. Thus, the relative importance of SGM populations in research is reduced to their gender and/or sexual identities, expressions, and/or behaviors while the other aspects of their identities, experiences, and/or behaviors are rendered irrelevant. Such a reductionist approach fails to accurately acknowledge the diversity that exists among SGM populations; of equal importance, it contributes to their ongoing stigmatization and marginalization, both within the US health-care system and more broadly in US society. Such research also yields outcomes with diminished scientific merit, accuracy, and applicability.

Although guidelines issued by the NIH, HHS, and CDC encourage health-care providers to collect information on sexual and gender identity/expression/behavior among all patient populations, there remains insufficient attention to the collection of such data in many clinical settings, particularly those in which heteronormativity and cisnormativity are reflected in policies and practices (e.g., documents used for intake, health history, informed consent, and authorization for access to medical data; hiring and promotion of health-care personnel). When such data is gathered, it is often done in a simplistic manner that conflates sex and gender, fails to accurately represent a diverse range of sexual and gender identities/expressions/behaviors, and/or fails to collect data in a manner that adheres to key principles of culturally competent care (e.g., by using disparaging terms, and prioritizing one aspect of identity over others). Thus, problems with data collection in clinical settings contribute to the ongoing lack of awareness and understanding of SGM populations and their health needs.

Yet explicit bias is also a factor. Nearly 70 percent of SGM populations report encountering discrimination when seeking health-care services; however, many advocacy groups suggest that actual rates are likely higher due to underreporting and the fact that such populations remain understudied. Those with intersex traits and those who identify as transgender, GNB, bigender, and genderqueer are most likely to be targets of such prejudice. Common examples of such discrimination include using language that dismisses, denigrates, stereotypes, or is otherwise disrespectful; purposefully misgendering someone verbally and/or on patient paperwork; refusing to use a patient's preferred name and/or pronouns; and using anti-SGM slurs or monikers to other members of the health-care team, other patients, or SGM patients, themselves. Other times, individuals are denied medical appointments, exams, medications, and surgical procedures based on their sexual and/or gender identity/expression. Additionally, some providers demonstrate an inappropriate hyper-fixation with gender and sexuality when they are not relevant to the health issue at hand (e.g., when a patient is receiving a routine vaccination or a refill for asthma medication). In other cases, SGM populations encounter physical violence from members of the health-care team including rough physical exams, physical assault, and being unnecessarily restrained. Nearly a third of SGM patient report being sexually assaulted by a health-care professional; examples include unnecessary gynecological exams, nonconsensual touching, and rape. Research indicates that rates of such victimization occur among all SGM subgroups but are highest among racial and ethnic minorities, low-income, and homeless/housing insecure populations as well as those with limited English fluency and proficiency. Rates are also disproportionately high among SGM individuals with disabilities. Those who encounter discrimination in health-care settings are less likely to seek health services in the future. Recent studies indicate that one-third to one-half of adult SGM populations have avoided seeking care due to previous experiences of discrimination in clinical settings.

Availability of Affordable and Culturally Competent Care

Limited availability of health care remains one of the most widespread and pervasive barriers to well-being for sexual minorities and gender minorities. Given disparities in health insurance coverage as well as average incomes, as discussed above, SGM populations are more likely to face financial barriers to care. They are significantly more likely than non-SGM populations to delay or forego health care due to lack of affordability. They are also less likely than heterosexual and gender-conforming populations to lack a regular primary health-care provider due to costs; consequently, they typically have greater need for reduced-cost and free health services, including those available through community-sponsored clinics. However, clinics for low-income populations often lack providers with expertise pertaining to the unique health needs of sexual and gender minority patients. For many LGBTQIA individuals, the costs associated with prescription medications are also a burden. Among cisgender gay and lesbian populations, nearly one in seven delays or goes without prescriptions each year due to lack of affordability; among cisbi populations, the rate is nearly one in four; and among GNB populations, it is one in three. Such differences are due, in part, to income disparities among SGM populations, particularly as GNB and cisbi subgroups have lower average incomes than cisgender gay and lesbian subgroups.

However, for GNB patients, access to health care is often hampered by the fact that many insurance plans do not cover hormonal treatments, surgical procedures, voice/communication therapy, mental health services, fertility treatments, and other health services related to gender-affirming care. Such exclusions are found in some employer-provided insurance plans as well as those offered in certain states under state-specific Medicaid policies. As of late 2022, only Maine and Illinois provided explicit coverage of all gender-affirming health services to Medicaid recipients; another twenty-nine states covered some gender-affirming health services but excluded others; and Texas and Alabama specifically excluded coverage of gender-affirming care for Medicaid recipients. Additionally, some private insurance plans—including those provided by employers as well as those purchased by individuals—have exclusionary policies. For those without insurance, costs associated with gender-affirming hormonal therapy can range from \$30 to nearly \$250 per month, not including the costs associated with office visits or laboratory tests. For gender-affirming surgeries, average costs range for \$10,000 to \$30,000 depending on the procedure; many transitioning individuals have multiple surgeries and, thus, may accrue cumulative costs that are much higher. Therefore, exclusionary policies pose additional and often insurmountable barriers to care for those needing gender-affirming care. Some health clinics offer lower-cost options for such care and a few nonprofit organizations provide grants that cover a portion of care that is both affirming and culturally competent. Yet for those who are unaware of or do not live near such services, such care often remains unaffordable. Geographic barriers to care also remain an issue across LGBTQIA populations; however, they are especially pronounced for those seeking gender-affirming care and for individuals with intersex traits. Although increased representation of SGM populations among health-care providers would likely help combat such barriers, they remain underrepresented as members of the health-care workforce.

LIVING ENVIRONMENT AND SOCIAL CONTEXT

The United States currently ranks twelfth on the worldwide LGBT Equality Index, a designation that suggests it is an overall welcoming and supportive country for SGM populations. However, SGM populations remain marginalized and systemically disadvantaged in US society. This is evident in employment, educational, and health-care settings as discussed earlier in this chapter. Yet it is equally clear in governmental, judicial, and social contexts as well as in media and popular culture.

Governmental and Judicial Systems

Despite decades of efforts from SGM activists and allies who have called for increasing attention to such populations, the needs and experiences of LGBTQIA populations—both collectively and via collection and analysis of disaggregated data—continue to be largely ignored by the federal government and most politicians. There remains a persistent lack of attention to SGM populations in government-sponsored research and data collection. For example, it has been less than 15 years since data pertaining to sexual identity and/or gender identity was first collected as part of the nationwide High School Longitudinal Survey. Similarly, it wasn't until 2016 that certain household surveys sponsored by the federal government—including, for example, the National Crime Victimization Survey, the National Health Interview Survey, and the National Survey on Drug Use and Health—began to collect such data. Via the Census and the American Community Survey, the US Census Bureau does gather data on sex—specifically defining sex via biomedical, cisnormative constructs. However, questions specific to sexual identity and gender identity are not included. Additionally, when the US Census Bureau implemented the Household Pulse Survey (HPS) in 2020 to measure the economic impacts of the COVID-19 pandemic, sexual identity and gender identity were excluded. Such identities were later added to the HPS in July 2021, thus representing the first time in history that the US Census Bureau systematically gathered and analyzed data on LGBTQIA populations. This does not necessarily mean, however, that the bureau will continue to do so. After all, while the Federal Reserve included questions on sexual identity and gender identity as part of the Survey of Household Economic Decisionmaking (SHED) in 2019, such questions were eliminated from SHED surveys in 2020.

Some current governmental surveys include questions related to marital status and/or living arrangements (e.g., cohabitating with a partner); thus, they do provide some insight into the experiences of some same-sex couples. However, over 80 percent of SGM populations—including unmarried and noncohabitating cisgender lesbian, gay, and bisexual individuals as well as those who identify as intersex, asexual, or transgender—remain largely obscured. Similar patterns reflecting a lack of attention to SGM populations by state and local governments have been noted. Some nongovernmental organizations, nonprofit entities, and academic researchers actively promote increased attention to LGBTQIA populations via data collection and analysis. However, the lack of attention to such populations within government-sponsored general population surveys continues to hinder understanding of both their experiences and their needs. Furthermore, SGM populations remain underrepresented among elected officials; although such representation has increased in recent years, they currently represent less than one-half of 1 percent of all elected officials in the United States, including at local, state, and federal levels. Furthermore, many politicians fail to provide adequate attention to SGM constituents and their needs. This is clear, for example, not only in the lack of proposed legislation to safeguard and expand the rights of such populations but also in the increasing proposal and passage of what is commonly referred to as anti-LGTBQIA legislation that seeks to limit the rights of and to allow discrimination against SGM populations.

Within the US criminal justice system, SGM populations also remain marginalized. Historically, and due largely to the influence of conservative religious ideology, such populations were vilified and targeted for arrest, prosecution, and incarceration. In the early Colonial Era, for example, same-sex sexual activities were punishable by death. Laws prohibiting such activities were implemented in the post-Revolutionary Era. From the late nineteenth century through the mid-twentieth century, support for such laws came from social reformers, eugenicists, and psychologists. Additionally, there is a lengthy history of arrest and prosecution of individuals who wear clothing that does not align with mainstream gender norms. Legal measures that permitted the forced sterilization of SGM populations were also widespread and persisted throughout the twentieth century. In the wake of the Stonewall Riots in 1969, however, LGBTQIA populations increasingly advocated for equal rights. As part of such efforts, same-sex couples sought the right to legally marry, yet their applications for marriage licenses were routinely denied by the courts; some states even passed legislation that explicitly banned same-sex unions. In 1996, President Clinton signed the Defense of Marriage Act (DOMA), defining marriage as a legal union between cishet couples; it also allowed both federal and state governments to refuse to recognize same-sex marriages performed elsewhere (e.g., in another state or another country). In subsequent years, over thirty states passed legislation banning same-sex unions. DOMA also permitted states to deny parental rights to nonbiological parents in same-sex relationships, thus rendering such parents unable to adopt children, take leave to care for a sick child, or petition for visitation, custody, or child support if their relationship with their partner ended. Following the precedent established by DOMA, many states banned SGM populations from adopting children. Beginning in 2004, however, other states began to pass legislation that legally recognized same-sex unions. Yet the most significant changes in terms of expanding legal rights for LGBTQIA populations have come at the federal level. In the SCOTUS decision in *Lawrence v. Texas (2003)*, so-called sodomy laws were deemed unconstitutional. In *United States v. Windsor (2013)*, the court found that DOMA's narrow definition of marriage violated the Fifth Amendment's equal protection clause. Then, in *Obergefell v. Hodges (2015)*, the constitutional right of same-sex couples to legally marry was established. The 2020 decision in *Bostock*, discussed above, has helped expand civil rights for SGM populations in employment, educational, and health-care settings. And in December 2022, the Respect for Marriage Act was signed into law, effectively overturning DOMA.

Yet SGM populations remain marginalized within the US judicial and corrections systems. For example, the legal process for transgender and GNB individuals to change their name can be time-consuming and costly. Additionally, some states require that those seeking to change their gender marker on government-issued documents (e.g., driver's license and passport) provide documentation from a health-care provider to indicate that they have undergone gender-affirming surgical therapy and that their gender transition is complete. Furthermore, while those unfamiliar with the process of changing such documents may be able to get guidance from friends or community organizations, individuals without such support can find it confusing. Yet even those who are well supported often feel intimidated by the judicial system due to its lengthy history of marginalizing SGM populations as well as the unwelcoming attitudes they often encounter from judges, clerks, attorneys, and other judicial representatives. At present, less than half of states offer the option of selecting "X" as a gender-neutral identity marker on driver's licenses. Even fewer allow parents to select a nonbinary designation on the birth certificate of their children or permit the amendment of birth certificates to include a gender-neutral identity marker. Some states—including Montana, Oklahoma, Tennessee, and West Virginia—explicitly prohibit changes to gender designation on official documents. In April of 2022, however, the US State Department began allowing citizens to select a gender-neutral option on passports and to do so without medical proof of transition.

Within the criminal justice system, SGM populations are overrepresented. As adolescents, they are twice as likely as their cishet peers to enter the juvenile justice system. Among adults, rates of arrest among cisgender lesbian, gay, and bisexual populations are more than twice as high as among cishet groups. Rates of arrest are especially high among cisgender lesbian women; they are more than four times as likely as cishet women to be arrested during their lifetimes. Similar disparities exist in conviction rates and incarceration rates. In addition, ongoing discrimination by police and corrections officers against members of the LGBTQIA community is well documented; examples include unlawful surveillance (also known as profiling), entrapment, physical violence, use of excessive force, verbal insults, sexual harassment, and sexual assault. BIPOC transgender and GNB populations are especially vulnerable. While such actions diminish both the physical and mental health of victims, they also create a climate of fear that diminishes the likelihood that SGM individuals will seek police support when they are victims of other crimes. Lack of appropriate training for police officers, coupled with the cishet normative policies that continue to dominate the criminal justice system, typically means that transgender, GNB, and intersex inmates are often denied placement in facilities and access to clothing that corresponds with their gender identity. This can harm to mental health and dramatically increases their risk of suicidal ideation and suicide attempts. It also increases their risk of being attacked by other incarcerated individuals as well as correctional officers. In addition, and although the right of all populations—including inmates—to access culturally competent health care was established by the Civil Rights Act of 1964 and affirmed by subsequent legislation, most jails and prisons fail to provide such care to SGM populations.

Social Norms and Attitudes

Since the start of the twenty-first century, there has been a dramatic increase in the number of Americans who self-identify as members of the LGBTQIA community. In 2000, 2 percent of all adults in the United States identified as SGM. Such rates increased to 3.5 percent in 2012; by 2022, there were at least 20 million individuals aged 18 and over who openly identified as SGM. Rates of self-identification are lowest among adults over age 54 and are highest among those born after 1980. At present, 20 percent of those born between 1997 and 2012 self-identify as SGM. Increasing self-identification suggests growing acceptance of and support for LGBTQIA populations. Yet there are millions more who conceal their identities. The decision to share or conceal one's identity is influenced by numerous social, political, and economic factors. While some may be open with close friends and family, others are not; some are out only to those closest to them but remain closeted in employment, academic, and other settings.

There has been some evidence of increasing social acceptance of and support for SGM populations in the United States. However, they continue to be socially marginalized in both obvious and subtle ways. While strong family support can serve as a protective factor that reduces risk of certain health issues (e.g., depression, anxiety, SUAD, and suicidality) among SGM populations, many remain ostracized and marginalized within their families. Upon coming out, some youth and young adults are rejected by their parents and forced to leave their parents' homes. Others may find that their parents withdraw financial support, are less loving and affectionate with them, and/or become abusive. SGM minors are nearly four times as likely as their cishet peers to be victims of emotional, physical, and/or sexual abuse from parents and other family members. Additionally, SGM children and adults are often marginalized and ridiculed by members of their extended families. They are often excluded from family gatherings (e.g., holiday celebrations, weddings, and birthday parties). Family members sometimes refuse to acknowledge and affirm their sexual and/or gender identity. They may also dismiss same-sex relationships as "not legitimate" or use birth name rather than chosen name of a transgender individual (known as dead-naming).

Marginalization of SGM populations is also clear in other social contexts. The Fair Housing Act prohibits discrimination in the sale and rental of housing. Despite this, housing discrimination against SGM populations persists; it has been identified as a key factor in disproportionately high rates of homeless and housing insecurity among such populations. Additionally, while some retailers have adopted policies and practices to promote inclusion, others have not. In fact, some private businesses actively refuse service to SGM populations. While such refusal violates state laws in some parts of the United States, it remains legal in many states. At the federal level, there is currently no consensus concerning whether private businesses have the right to refuse service to SGM customers. Yet that changed in 2023 when SCOTUS issued its ruling in *303 Creative LLC v. Elenis*, a case in which a website designer cited religious beliefs as the basis for refusing to create a wedding website for a same-sex couple.

Media and popular culture influence social acceptance of and support for LGBTQIA populations. Even though the inclusion of SGM groups in film, television, news, advertisements, and commercials has increased markedly in the twenty-first century, they remain underrepresented. In mainstream network, cable, and streaming series, less than 12 percent of all characters with recurring roles (including both leading and supporting roles) are identified as SGM; most are cisgender lesbian, gay, or bisexual. Representations of transgender and GNB characters remain scarce, and characters who identify as asexual or intersex are virtually nonexistent. Representation of BIPOC sexual minorities and gender minorities has steadily increased over the past 15 years and they currently comprise about half of all SGM characters in mainstream television programs. However, there are few characters who are elderly or who have disabilities. In addition, tokenism (wherein LGBTQIA characters are represented but have no significant role in the plot) and queer baiting (the inclusion of scenes or dialogue that suggest a character may be a SGM yet there is no further exploration of their identity) have become increasingly common, something that critics have argued is a marketing strategy.

Positive representations of SGM populations in media and popular culture are associated with improved mental health and self-esteem among LGBTQIA populations, especially adolescents and young adults. Such representations can also help combat negative social attitudes toward SGM populations, foster increased awareness of their needs, and increase social acceptance of and support for such populations. However, dominant representations continue to rely on and reinforce well-worn stereotypes. Some of the most prominent among such stereotypes include the depiction of SGM populations as criminals (e.g., serial killers and pedophiles), mentally ill, victims of IPV, obsessed with sex and romantic relationships, and/or as buffoons who are irresponsible, infantilized, and continually the butt of jokes. Such representations diminish the complexities of life for SGM populations living in a cisnormative and heteronormative society. Of equal importance, they have negative social and political impacts. Stereotypical depictions have been linked to diminished mental and physical health among SGM populations. They also diminish support for such populations in familial, employment, educational, legislative, and health-care contexts. Additionally, such representations have been linked to violence against SGM populations, including bullying and IPV as well as gun violence (e.g., armed assault, certain hate crimes, and mass shootings). In recent years, the expansion of social media has influenced social acceptance of and support for SGM populations; however, such influence has been mixed. On the one hand, social media platforms can be sources of support for those who have not yet come out, are engaged in the coming-out process, and/or have tense or unsupportive relationships with family. In fact, virtual communities can promote information sharing, help foster meaningful social connections, and enhance a sense of belonging. However, social media can also be a platform for sharing of misinformation, bullying, and exploitation.

CHAPTER TWELVE

Veterans

Individuals who are former members of the US military forces but are no longer serving in such a capacity are known as veterans. Some were employed in full-time active duty in the Army, Navy, Air Force, Marine Corps, or Coast Guard. Others held part-time roles as members of the military reserve, maintaining a full-time civilian job while also training with a unit of the armed forces on a regular basis—typically one weekend per month plus several weeks of additional training per year—and participating in active duty deployment on-demand. Reserve options within the US military include the Coast Guard Reserve, Army National Guard, Marine Reserve Corps, Air Force Reserve, Air National Guard, Navy Reserve, and Army Reserve. Both full- and part-time military personnel can serve in combat (e.g., infantry, special forces, pilots, and artillery crew) or noncombat roles (e.g., engineering, communications, health care, computing, mechanics, intelligence, transportation, maintenance, and human resources). Although many veterans served in conflict zones, about 40 percent never participated in combat operations.

Legislation that provides health care and other support services for veterans who received honorable discharge from US military service can be traced back to the mid-nineteenth century with the establishment of the National Asylum for Disabled Volunteer Soldiers. Such support was expanded at the start of the First World War and again following the Second World War with the establishment of what was originally known as the Veterans Bureau. It then transformed into the Veterans Administration (VA), a federal entity charged with assessing the needs of and coordinating services for veterans. Many services offered through the VA relate to health—including disability compensation, rehabilitation, medical research, hospitalization, and long-term treatment—but there are also economic and educational programs. Historically, health-related programs for veterans have tended to focus on physical health issues. Yet from the late twentieth century to present, there has been increasing attention to the mental and social well-being of veterans. At present, it is clear that veterans encounter a variety of health issues that are unique to their involvement with the armed forces; some issues are more common among those who served in combat operations. Yet even veterans who never traveled to conflict zones may encounter certain health conditions that are linked to their military experiences, particularly as such experiences are shaped by the rigid military hierarchy and by the various forms of systemic discrimination documented within the US military. Some of these conditions impair physical health and have been linked to higher rates of illness, injury, and disability as well as increased risk of premature death. Yet others diminish mental health and can impair the ability of veterans to work, learn, and maintain meaningful social connections.

CURRENT STATE OF HEALTH

Combat service increases risk of physical injuries including lacerations, gunshot wounds, burns, broken bones, nerve damage, and paralysis. Hearing loss is also common and often results from heavy artillery such as guns, explosives, and the military vehicles used in both combat and noncombat operations. Vision loss is also a concern for many veterans; it may stem from injuries sustained during combat or training exercises but can also occur due to age-related macular degeneration, diabetic retinopathy, and glaucoma. Prolonged stress endured during military service increases risk of physical health issues such as chronic pain, high blood pressure, migraine headaches, heart disease, stroke, osteoarthritis, respiratory problems, diabetes, gastrointestinal problems (e.g., chronic heartburn and irritable bowel syndrome), accelerated aging, disability, and premature death. Stress has also been identified as a key factor in post-traumatic stress disorder (PTSD), depression, anxiety, suicidal ideation, and substance use and abuse disorders (SUAD)—including abuse of alcohol, tobacco, prescriptions, and illicit substances—among veterans. Mental health disorders are twice as common among veterans as the general US population and are highest among veterans who participated in combat operations. Additionally, the stress endured during military service can diminish ability to manage emotions—especially anger, sadness, and grief—and, thus, can hinder both personal and professional relationships. Yet half of veterans experience poor mental health as a consequence of the difficulties they encounter adjusting to post-military life. Some find civilian life to be disorienting, particularly when compared with the more organized and predictable routine of the military. For others, poor mental health is exacerbated by economic problems, uncertainty about the post-military employment, or feeling disconnected from friends, families, or co-workers who do not understand or respect their military experiences.

Injuries sustained during combat operations can cause long-term problems. Shrapnel injuries are some of the most common; shrapnel refers to the small, sharp fragments of metal, plastic, or other materials that are created when an explosive device detonates. Such fragments may be parts of the explosive device itself or may be from other objects (e.g., vehicles, structures, or equipment) that are propelled by the force of an explosion. These fragments can pierce and/or become lodged in the body of individuals within close range. Although shrapnel sometimes causes only superficial injuries such as lacerations and bruising, it can also penetrate deeper into the body and become embedded in muscle tissue; damage internal organs; break bones; and sever nerves, tendons, or major structures of the circulatory system. While even superficial shrapnel wounds increase risk of uncontrolled bleeding, infection, and necrosis of bodily tissue, such risks are greater with more extensive shrapnel injuries and can lead to disability and death. Some shrapnel may be surgically removed; other times, risk of surgical removal is too great, or fragments are not detected until months or years after they enter the body. Shrapnel that remains in the body may cause toxic embedded injuries, specifically when fragments release metal ions into the blood stream and cause chronic health problems (typically referred to as shrapnel sickness). Lead-based embedded shrapnel can contribute to anemia, muscle weakness, joint pain, kidney damage, high blood pressure, brain damage, hallucinations, seizures, cognitive and memory decline, and impaired reproductive health (e.g., miscarriage, stillbirth, and infertility). Other metals found in shrapnel include nickel, iron, cadmium, copper, uranium, arsenic, tungsten, chromium, aluminum, steel, and brass. Such metals increase risk of various types of cancer and can impair respiratory, neurological, gastrointestinal, circulatory, reproductive, and cardiovascular function. Shrapnel sickness increases risk of disability and premature death.

Trauma to the head and spinal cord is also common. These are often caused by explosive devices (e.g., grenades, rockets, and land mines), bullet wounds, shrapnel, collisions, falls, physical assaults, vehicle crashes, and other combat-related events. Yet even those who do not serve in active combat may experience such injuries due to incidents involving machinery and equipment used in military training, humanitarian campaigns, and equipment testing. Head trauma is associated with increased risk of traumatic brain injury (TBI), a condition characterized by brain dysfunction. In the past decade, nearly half a million veterans have been diagnosed with TBI. Mild cases are also known as concussions, and symptoms typically include headaches, impaired physical balance, dizziness, memory loss, sleepiness, sensitivity to light and/or sound, brief loss of consciousness, confusion, nausea, and irritability. Approximately 90 percent of veterans with TBI experience mild symptoms. However, others suffer from moderate or severe TBI; typically symptoms include persistent headaches, convulsions, seizure, muscle weakness, numbness in limbs, slurred speech, confusion, lasting memory loss, aggression, and mood instability. In some cases, TBI causes coma or death. Symptoms of TBI can last for months, years, or be permanent. Medication may relieve pain and minimize swelling of brain tissues. In some cases, a decompressive craniotomy may be performed; this involves surgical removal of part of the skull in order to relieve pressure on the brain. Surgery may also be used to remove fragments of bone, shrapnel, or blood clots in the brain or to remove severely damaged or dead cerebral tissue. Therapy may help improve memory, cognitive function, and physical health; yet severe TBI renders some veterans permanently disabled. For veterans with spinal cord injuries, common health problems include persistent pain, headaches, numbness of extremities (hands, feet, fingers, toes), impaired reflexes, weakness, coordination issues, impaired balance, loss of bladder or bowel control, impaired breathing, muscle spasms, difficulties maintaining balance, and sexual dysfunction. In severe cases, spinal cord damage can lead to permanent paralysis of the legs (paraplegia) or arms and legs (quadriplegia).

Due to the violent nature of armed conflict and the types of weapons used in contemporary military operations, injury to (such as burns and lacerations) and loss of fingers, toes, hands, feet, arms, and legs are common. During the military conflicts in Iraq and Afghanistan (2001–6), major limb amputations constituted 5 percent of all serious injuries. Most were due to traumatic severing of extremities (e.g., limb loss due to an explosion). However, some were surgical amputations and done to minimize risks of infection and blood loss when serious injuries occurred. Veterans with limb amputations are typically treated with physical therapy and many receive prosthetic devices. Prosthetics are intended to replace the amputated limb and help the individual regain function. However, problems with fit, comfort, function, and weight of prosthetic devices often discourage veterans from wearing them. Limb amputation is associated with increased risk of major depressive disorders, anxiety disorders, PTSD, suicidal ideation, poor self-esteem, emotional dysregulation related to anger and grief, and diminished quality of life. Additionally, many veterans experience phantom limb pain (PLP), a condition characterized by the sensation of pain in a body part that has been amputated. PLP often results from nerve damage at the amputation site but may also result from infection, inflammation, circulatory problems, poor-fitting prosthetics, changes in the weather, other health conditions (e.g., shingles or angina), or lifestyle factors (e.g., smoking and alcohol use). PLP can range in intensity from mild to severe; it increases risk of depression, suicidal ideation, low self-esteem, and SUAD.

Health conditions among veterans vary to some degree by service history, particularly as the living conditions associated with one military campaign may differ greatly than those used in another. Those who served in the First World War (1914–18) and the Vietnam War (1961–73) often suffered from a condition known as trench foot (sometimes referred to as jungle rot). This occurred when soldiers were in wet conditions for extended periods and unable to keep their feet dry. In the short term, this caused open sores, blisters, fungal growth, bacterial infections, and the peeling of outer layers of the skin on the feet. Over extended periods, it caused nerve damage, decreased blood flow, and led to death of skin, muscle, and other tissues. Some veterans had toes or feet amputated due to untreated trench foot. In contrast, those who participated in the Persian Gulf War (1990–91)—including both Operation Desert Shield and Operation Desert Storm—were exposed to high concentrations of airborne particulate matter (PM) due to the combination of weather conditions (e.g., arid climate and strong winds), exhaust from military and civilian vehicles, and oil well fires. Common PM-related health problems during deployment included irritation of the skin, sinuses, eyes, and respiratory tract. Yet there have also been long-term health problems for veterans, including heart problems, diminished lung function, and premature death.

Health risks associated with exposure to radiation, chemicals, and other toxins also differ among veterans based on service history. Many veterans who were exposed to the chemical defoliant known as Agent Orange during the Vietnam War continue to experience a variety of immune system disorders, high rates of cancer (e.g., lung, bone, bladder, testicular, breast, brain, kidney, pancreatic, and others), neurological disorders, respiratory disorders, dementia, gastrointestinal diseases, and endocrine disorders. Additionally, reproductive health problems—including high rates of infertility, miscarriage, stillbirth, birth defects, and preterm delivery—have been linked to Agent Orange exposure. Data demonstrate that the health impacts of Agent Orange are intergenerational—abnormalities of the reproductive tract and birth defects have been noted in both children and grandchildren of Vietnam veterans. In contrast, veterans of military campaigns in Afghanistan, the Persian Gulf, and Iraq have abnormally high rates of cancers of the lungs, kidneys, liver, bone, lymphatic system, and brain. Such maladies have been linked to long-term exposure to uranium dust. In other cases, veterans suffer from poor health due to infectious diseases encountered in combat zones or due to the vaccines they were required to receive during specific military campaigns. Among veterans who served in Afghanistan, for example, health problems related to infection with latent mycobacterium tuberculosis, Shigella, and visceral leishmaniasis remain a concern. Similarly, the chronic health problems collectively known as Gulf War Illness (GWI) have been linked to the vaccines for anthrax and botulism military personnel were required to receive prior to deployment.

Yet military activities can also lead to long-term injuries and disabilities for veterans who did not participate in combat. Examples include injuries and diseases sustained from operating or repairing military vehicles, electronics, and other equipment; exposure to environmental hazards; and injuries due to overuse or trauma (e.g., stress fractures, tendinitis, bursitis, strains, sprains, herniated disks, nerve damage, and joint deterioration) that occur during training or other military-related activities. Although some occupational hazards are found in many different types of military activities, others are more prominent in certain types of job roles or specific to location. Noncombat injuries that lead to musculoskeletal injuries (MSKI) involving the back, neck, and lower extremities are often sustained in physical training exercises or from job responsibilities associated with transportation, equipment maintenance, or heavy lifting. Noncombat MSKI are most common among cisgender females and those over age 40. In the short term, such injuries are associated with increased rates of limited duty days, delayed deployment, non-deployable status, and medical discharge. However, they also increase incidence of chronic pain, limited function, and disability among veterans. Furthermore, while certain environmental health hazards are common for those with specific military job responsibilities (e.g., those who work with paints or chemicals), others are specific to location. Veterans who were stationed at Camp Lejeune or Marine Corps Air Station New River in North Carolina between 1953 and 1987, for example, continue to have health problems related to consumption of contaminated drinking water at those military bases. Most common among such problems are leukemia, aplastic anemia, cancer (esp. of the bladder, kidney, liver, or lymphatic system), and Parkinson's disease. Similarly, at numerous military bases throughout the United States, chemicals containing perfluoroalkyl and polyfluoroalkyl-based compounds (collectively known as PFAS) were used in fire-fighting training exercises that incorporated Aqueous Film-Forming Foam (AFFF). PFAS do not break down over time. They have been detected in the surface water, ground water, and soil as well as in the bodily tissues of aquatic and mammal species that live in areas around military bases where AFFF was used. PFAS have been linked to certain types of cancer (e.g., ovarian, prostate, testicular, and breast), ulcerative colitis, impaired immune function, infertility, and increased risk of asthma, thyroid disease, and high cholesterol in veteran populations.

Discrimination within the US military has been deemed a significant problem. Many have pointed to the hierarchical organization and the insular culture of the armed forces as perpetuating the types of power imbalances that are at the core of systemic inequities. Historically, differential treatment was permitted under military policies, specifically those that segregated combat units and assignment of duties by race and gender and that prohibited gay, lesbian, and transgender populations from joining the military. At present, behaviors such as bullying, hazing, harassment, and other forms of discrimination are explicitly forbidden under policies of the Department of Defense (DoD), specifically as defined by article 93, "Cruelty and Maltreatment," and article 128, "Assault." In addition, various branches of the military, federal laws (e.g., the Civil Rights Acts of 1964 and 1991, the Pregnancy Discrimination Act of 1978, and the Americans with Disabilities Act of 1990), Executive Orders (e.g., EO 14004, "Enabling All Qualified Americans to Serve Their Country in Uniform"), and state laws prohibit such practices. Yet such behaviors remain more prominent among military forces than civilian populations. They have been documented among active duty and reserve forces, including in combat zones, on military bases, and off military property. Discrimination occurs within all branches of service, although the majority of complaints are initiated within the Marine Corps. In 2015, and in response to evidence that the DoD had not taken adequate measures to collect data on, prevent, or respond to incidents of hazing, harassment, and other forms of discrimination, the US Congress called for an independent review of such behaviors. It also expanded anti-discrimination training for military forces and required the DoD to establish a system for collecting data on incidents of discrimination in the military, submit annual reports of such data to Congress, and fill Military Equal Opportunity (MEO) positions with highly qualified personnel.

Despite such efforts, discrimination in the US military persists. It is evident in a variety of behaviors that target military service members on the basis of gender identity and expression, sex, race, ethnicity, disability, religion, age, or other aspects of identity. Documented examples include verbal harassment, threats, emotional abuse, battery, bullying, assault, forced prostitution, sexual harassment, stalking, and homicide. Furthermore, military sexual trauma (MST)—including sexual harassment, sexual assault, and rape—remains a problem. Discriminatory behaviors are associated with a variety of health consequences for military personnel. In the short term, victims may experience elevated blood pressure, changes in mood, increased incidence and severity of headaches and gastrointestinal problems, stress, anxiety, depression, sleep disorders, social isolation, diminished self-esteem, decreased feelings of belonging, panic disorders, PTSD, and increased risk of suicidal ideation. However, those who witness such behaviors often experience similar health issues. For both victims and witnesses, health problems can persist for years and even decades, including long after they complete their military service. They are also at increased risk for decreased job performance and job satisfaction; thus, some victims request a transfer to another division or leave the military altogether. This is particularly true for those who experience ongoing bullying, hazing, or harassment; who file complaints only to find that their concerns are dismissed; and/or who encounter retaliation from colleagues or commanding officers after filing complaints.

ECONOMIC FACTORS

Veterans often experience financial hardship. Many are unemployed or underemployed. Such concerns are most pronounced among veterans who are younger; have less military experience; and/or have physical disabilities, PTSD, and SUAD. Rates of housing insecurity and food insecurity are disproportionately high among veterans; many are unable to meet other basic needs and/or have significant debt. Various factors including relatively low wages, limited financial literacy, and military recruiting tactics that disproportionately target low-income populations have been linked to financial concerns among veterans.

Employment and Income

Experience, knowledge, and skills gained in the military can help individuals secure employment once they leave the armed forces. At present, veterans comprise approximately 5.5 percent of the total US workforce; thus, nearly 9,000,000 veterans are civilian employees. Nine out of ten employed veterans are cisgender males, something that reflects the reality that cisgender women, transgender individuals, and gender nonbinary (GNB) populations remain underrepresented in the military. Veterans are concentrated in certain employment sectors, specifically those related to management, finances, and other professional occupations as well as jobs related to maintenance, installation, equipment repair, and transportation that involves the moving of material goods. Yet there are some differences by sex. Although cisgender female veterans are as likely to be employed in managerial, business, and financial sectors as cisgender male veterans, they are more likely to be employed in professional, service sector, and administrative support positions than their male peers. However, cisgender female veterans are less likely to work in construction, production, transportation, maintenance, repair, and installation.

Under the provisions of the Veterans' Preference Act of 1944 (VPA) as well as corresponding state laws, veterans who received either a general or honorable discharge, served during specific campaigns, were disabled during their military service, and meet other requirements are provided with special consideration over nonveteran applicants when seeking federal or state jobs. This assists some in making the transition from military life to civilian employment, yet not all veterans qualify for employment preference. Furthermore, discriminatory practices during the hiring process and in the workplace continue to hamper many veterans. Although illegal under the Uniformed Services Employment and Reemployment Rights Act of 1994 (USERRA), such discrimination persists; it is especially pronounced for veterans with disabilities and those dishonorably discharged from military service. Consequently, many veterans remain unemployed. Others are underemployed and relegated to low-skill, entry-level jobs that do not enable them to use their full range of skills. Such jobs typically do not provide an adequate living wage, health benefits, or other benefits such as paid sick leave, vacation leave, flexible spending accounts, and flex time. Lack of employment-related health insurance for veterans who do not qualify for VA health benefits is associated with increased incidence and severity of both acute and chronic health conditions.

Historical data demonstrates that veterans are, in general, less likely than nonveterans to be unemployed. Yet in recent years the gap between rates of unemployment among veterans and nonveterans has decreased. At present, only one-fourth of veterans have a job waiting for them when they leave the military. Rates of unemployment are disproportionately high among veterans who suffer from military-related mental and physical health problems, especially PTSD and physical disabilities. Such rates are also impacted by broader economic issues as well as individual factors including length of time since discharge from the armed forces, age, and specific military campaigns in which they participated. While unemployment rates increased overall among the American workforce during both the Great Recession (2007–9) and the COVID-19 pandemic, increases in unemployment were more pronounced among veterans, especially in rural areas. Yet employment rates rebounded for veterans more quickly than for nonveterans during these periods. Overall, those recently discharged from military service tend to have higher rates of unemployment than the general US population, yet such rates are lower among veterans whose military service ended more than 6 years ago. Unemployment rates among veterans of all racial and ethnic groups are lowest for those aged 35 to 65. Such rates do, however, vary based on military experience. Those collectively known as Gulf War-era II veterans—in active duty in Iraq and/or Afghanistan at any point since September 2001—have disproportionately high rates of unemployment compared to other veterans and the nonveteran workforce. Incidence and severity of service-related disabilities and other health issues among Gulf War-era II veterans may help explain such trends.

Economic Challenges among Veterans

Many veterans are at increased risk of housing insecurity, food insecurity, and inability to pay bills. Such financial problems are often related to poor health, especially for those with disabilities and mental illnesses. However, financial problems also exacerbate risk of poor mental and physical health. Veterans are among those demographic groups most likely to be housing insecure. While the number of homeless and unsheltered veterans has decreased substantially in recent decades—a change that reflects expanded governmental and nongovernmental support for such populations—on any given night in the United States, there are between 40,000 and 70,000 veterans who lack safe, affordable, permanent shelter. Veterans represent 10 to 15 percent of all homeless and unsheltered Americans; they are more likely to experience chronic homelessness than other demographic groups. Veterans who lack shelter are at increased risk for various physical health issues (e.g., infections, communicable diseases, musculoskeletal problems, vector-borne illnesses, and exposure to weather and climate) as well as poor mental health due to chronic stress. Veterans are also among those groups of Americans who are most likely to experience food insecurity and to lack access to adequate, affordable, and nutritious food. On a typical day, at least one-tenth of veterans skip meals or go without food due to lack of affordability. Rates of food insecurity are highest among veterans who are cisgender women, have disabilities, live in rural areas, and were recently discharged from service. One-third of veterans have difficulty paying for other basic needs, including health care. Over a million veterans have unpaid medical debt that exceeds their disposable income. Mental health issues (e.g., PTSD, major depressive disorders, and SUAD), social isolation, and difficulties adjusting to post-military life increase risk of economic insecurity. However, increasing costs of housing, food, and other goods as well as the lack of timely and comprehensive health services for those with disabilities, mental health disorders, SUAD, and other health concerns are also factors. Education and wealth are also important to consider. Whereas veterans tended to be more educated and have more wealth than nonveterans during the latter half of the twentieth century, by 2010 such trends had reversed, thereby contributing to increased economic vulnerability for veteran populations.

Yet for many veterans, long-term financial challenges can be traced to the low wages they earn and financial decisions they make while in the military. Among full-time junior military personnel (e.g., private, corporal, recruit, first class, and apprentice), base pay is generally less than $25,000 per year. While there are some annual bonuses and monthly stipends provided to those with particular skills or credentials (e.g., fluency in multiple languages; degrees in nursing, pharmacy, or optometry) or who pursue particular roles (e.g., aviation, diving, and submarine duty), the earnings of many military personnel still do not constitute a living wage, particularly for those with dependents. Expenses related to relocation and deployment can also be burdensome. Such factors, combined with the limited financial literacy among many service members, can lead to significant debt. Veterans are more likely than nonveterans to have a bad credit score; they are also eight times more likely to be delinquent or to default on loans than they were prior to entering the military. For some veterans, however, their economic woes started long before they entered the military. Research indicates that military recruiters disproportionately target low-income adolescents—especially Black, Hispanic/Latinx/Chicanx (HLC), and Indigenous populations as well as those who lack permanent, legal citizenship—by presenting the military as a path out of poverty. Benefits related to health care, education, and retirement for veterans who served in the military for at least 20 years or received a medical discharge can help them meet financial obligations. Yet it is widely recognized that most veterans are unable to live off of such benefits and, thus, must have other sources of income. Various nonprofit entities and politicians continue to advocate for increased financial support to help relieve the debt burden of veterans and help cover their living, health care, and educational expenses.

EDUCATIONAL ACCESS AND QUALITY

Those who enter the US military tend to be better educated than their peers. Furthermore, military personnel are provided with unique education and training opportunities within the context of the various branches of the armed services, including so-called soft skills as well as specialized knowledge in certain technical fields. Yet there are also a variety of options for who wish to pursue postsecondary education and training. These include financial support at both the federal and state levels. Additionally, many colleges and universities have created unique programs and offices dedicated to supporting student-veterans. However, many veterans encounter significant challenges within the unique context of higher education. Such challenges are associated with lowered academic performance, increased risk of dropping out, and diminished social and mental well-being.

Education Prior to and during Military Service

Ninety eight percent of military personnel have earned a high school diploma; in contrast, only about 87 percent of adults in the general US adult population have earned such credentials. While it is possible to join the military without a diploma—specifically by successfully completing the General Educational Development (GED) exam—military policies permit no more than 10 percent of all new inductees to have a GED; different branches of the armed services may further restrict participation for those who hold a GED. In practice, then, less than 5 percent of military inductees lack a high school diploma. Individuals who wish to enter the military must also take the Armed Services Vocational Aptitude Battery (ASVAB) and earn a score that ranks in the top two-thirds of all test-takers. Although some have likened the ASVAB to a basic IQ test, in reality it assesses math, verbal, technical, spatial, and science competencies, specifically as they are related to military service. The ASVAB is an accurate predictor of performance on standardized college admissions exams (e.g., the ACT and the SAT). However, unlike the ACT and SAT which ask test-takers to solve problems and apply knowledge, the ASVAB assesses prior knowledge; it does not include a problem-solving component.

Among military officers, a bachelor's degree is required; most have earned such a degree prior to joining the military but some earn it while serving. This may be done through military academies (e.g., the United States Military Academy in West Point, New York; the United States Air Force Academy in Colorado Springs, Colorado; and the Citadel Military College of South Carolina) or Reserve Officer Training Corps (ROTC) programs. Available at more than 1,500 colleges and universities across the United States, ROTC includes undergraduate and graduate educational opportunities. ROTC college programs are competitive. Some provide scholarships that cover tuition, books, and student fees; some scholarship recipients may also receive a monthly living stipend. Scholarships are sometimes awarded for academic performance and involvement with Junior ROTC programs during high school. Yet most recipients apply for and earn such scholarships after they have completed some postsecondary education. ROTC scholarship recipients must serve a minimum of 8 years as a commissioned officer in the armed services. However, not all ROTC participants receive scholarships. The demands of ROTC programs are substantial. Participants must meet minimum GPA requirements; depending on the branch of the military they have joined, ROTC cadets may also be restricted to majors such as engineering, leadership, communication, and technology. They must also devote time to ROTC training, events, and even volunteering. Furthermore, they are required to maintain physical fitness, complete military field exercises, and participate in summer training programs. Cadets may be terminated from the ROTC program if they use illegal drugs or otherwise violate legal codes or military codes. Those who are terminated from or voluntarily quit must repay any ROTC scholarships received. Individuals who are medically classified as overweight or obese, have certain disabilities (e.g., cognitive impairments, deafness, mobility impairments, and epilepsy) or have health conditions (e.g., diabetes, arthritis, endometriosis, coronary heart disease, and mental illness) are not able to join ROTC.

A variety of educational and job training opportunities are also available while serving in the military. These can help prepare individuals for civilian careers after they leave the armed services. For example, there are nearly 150 occupational specialties within the various branches of the armed forces. Examples include aviation, computing, health care, construction and maintenance (including fields such as plumbing, electrical, and welding), police services, media, and intelligence. Those who gain experience and credentials in such areas during their military service typically find themselves well prepared for civilian careers once they are discharged from the armed forces. Yet even those who do not earn experience or credentials in such specialties often find that the military provides on-the-job training in so-called soft skills such as teamwork, leadership, problem-solving, flexibility, and ability to work independently. Such skills are transferrable to a variety of civilian fields.

Support for Veterans Pursuing Postsecondary Education and Training

Those veterans who served at least 90 days of active duty and ended their military service with a general discharge or honorable discharge are typically entitled to educational benefits. Some veterans qualify for educational support through the GI Bill (GIB). Originally known as the Servicemen's Readjustment Act of 1944, there are currently two types of GIBs: the Montgomery GIB and the post-9/11 GIB. Both offer financial support for up to 36 months for postsecondary degree programs, noncollege vocational programs (including those that lead to trade certifications), and certain internships and apprenticeships. Individuals who are eligible for both programs may receive up to 48 months of education-related financial support. The Montgomery GIB provides a monthly educational stipend of just over $2,000 for active duty military and approximately $400 for members of the reserves and National Guard. Stipends are paid directly to the student and intended to cover tuition and fees only; the program does not include a stipend for housing, books, or other educational expenses. In contrast, the post-9/11 GIB covers tuition for qualified veterans—including the full cost at in-state universities and approximately $26,400 at private institutions for the 2022–3 academic year—and makes payments directly to postsecondary institutions. It also provides a book stipend, monthly housing stipend, and up to $1,000 in relocation costs. Benefits offered via the post-9/11 GIB can be transferred to dependents.

Prior to the end of calendar year 2012, veterans were required to use their GIB educational benefits within 15 years of being discharged from the military. However, with passage of the Henry W. Colmery Veterans Educational Assistance Act of 2017—also known as the Forever GI Bill—time limits on such benefits were removed for veterans as well as dependents. Certain veterans may qualify for the Yellow Ribbon Program; it is intended to help veterans access those universities with higher tuition rates, including private or out-of-state institutions. A component of the GI Bill, the Yellow Ribbon Program allows postsecondary institutions to waive up to $10,000 in tuition for veterans; the VA matches the total amount waived by colleges and universities (for a total tuition waiver of up to $20,000 per student-veteran). The Yellow Ribbon Program can be combined with the post-9/11 GIB. However, not all postsecondary institutions participate in the Yellow Ribbon Program; furthermore, not all participating institutions provide the full tuition waiver allotted by the program. At least 20 states also provide free tuition for veterans pursuing an undergraduate degree and who meet certain requirements (e.g., received the Purple Heart, Medal of Honor, Distinguished Service Medal, or other notable honors; were honorably discharged; served in the military for a minimum of one year; and meet residency requirements). Such requirements vary considerably from state to state. Veterans who earn their undergraduate degrees through state-sponsored programs can then use their GIB benefits to pursue graduate studies. Of those veterans pursuing college degrees, however, only one-fifth are enrolled in graduate-level programs. Veterans who meet established income guidelines are eligible for Pell Grants to help pay for education-related expenses; GIB benefits do not count as income when calculating eligibility for such grants.

Some postsecondary institutions permit veterans to receive academic credit for military service; this is known as military transfer credit (MTC). This option, however, depends on the academic degree program a veteran is pursuing. While the American Council on Education makes recommendation about what types of military experience can count toward college credit, individual colleges and universities set their own policies for awarding MTCs. Thus, what might be accepted as MTC at one institution might be rejected at another. Furthermore, MTCs are typically only applicable to lower-level coursework or electives; they are generally not an option for upper-level courses. MTC is more likely to be awarded at institutions that have active programs and support services for student-veterans. Examples of such programs and services include an established Office of Student Veterans Services; ongoing Green Zone Ally Training (to help faculty and staff better understand and support the needs of students who are veterans); regular events to acknowledge and honor the contributions of veterans who are members of the campus community; and student organizations specifically for veterans.

Challenges within Educational Settings

Despite these various sources of support, many veterans still encounter difficulties within the context of postsecondary institutions. Financial concerns are common, particularly among veterans with dependents. Yet like many nonveteran students, even those without spouses or children may find it difficult to pay for living expenses while attending college. Such financial challenges are often connected to broader economic concerns such as increasing inflation and the increasing costs of housing, food, and other necessities, including childcare. Yet some veterans encounter financial difficulties when they cannot complete their degree programs within the time limits of the GIB. This is common among those who are not enrolled in classes full time, especially veterans who are employed full-time while pursuing a college degree and/or who have family responsibilities that include caring for young children or aging family members. Sometimes, veterans must repeat courses; this extends the time required to complete their degrees and can exceed the parameters of the GIB. Veterans with disabilities are also more likely than nondisabled veterans to enroll part-time and may require time away from school to address medical needs including undergoing surgical procedures or other forms of treatment. Thus, they are more likely than nondisabled veteran populations to require more than 36 months to earn their degrees. In addition, the GIB does not cover tuition for courses that are not related to major. Such benefits may also be used only for one academic major and do not cover academic minors. Therefore, if an enrolled veteran pursues a second major or a minor or takes courses that are unrelated to their primary major, they must find other ways to pay for them. At present, nearly half of all veterans enrolled in undergraduate degree programs do not use GIB educational benefits. Many do not understand how to access such benefits; research indicates that bureaucratic red tape encountered at the VA and/or at postsecondary institutions is also a common deterrent. Some veterans enroll in postsecondary education immediately after leaving the military and yet struggle to adjust to civilian life, including to the unique structure and expectations of postsecondary education. Such struggles are especially common for veterans with PTSD and other mental health conditions, physical disabilities, and other chronic health issues. Consequently, those affected are more likely to demonstrate substandard academic performance and, consequently, to have to retake courses. They are also more likely to exhaust their educational benefits before completing their degree.

Nearly 30 percent of veterans enrolled in college borrow student loans. Whereas a typical nonveteran undergraduate student attending a public, 4-year institution averages around $7,500 in student loans each year, veterans average just over $8,000 annually. This may be due to the fact that veterans are typically older than traditional, nonveteran student populations; thus, they are more likely to have dependents and to be financially independent than students who are not veterans. Those veterans who attend private, 4-year institutions typically borrow 25 percent more in student loans each year than veterans attending public institutions. Veterans enrolled in for-profit institutions are more likely than those attending public schools to incur student loan debt. By the time they complete a bachelor's degree, the average veteran who attended a public institution has accumulated over $25,000 in student debt. While veterans with certain disabilities can qualify for cancellation of student debt through what is commonly referred to as a total and permanent disability discharge, many disabled veterans are not aware of this option. Less than one-fourth of those eligible have applied for loan forgiveness through this program. Over half of veterans eligible for disability-related student loan forgiveness are currently in default on repayment of their student loans. Yet even those who make on-time payments may find that fully repaying their student loans can take a decade or more. Consequently, such payments can consume a significant portion of household income, threaten financial stability, and be an ongoing source of stress. Student loan debt can also make it more difficult for veterans to afford basic needs such as food, housing, and health care.

Many veterans also struggle with the organizational aspects of higher education. Schedules in higher education are typically much more flexible than those that dictate military life. For example, although college courses are offered on a regular schedule, they typically only meet a few times per week and for only an hour or two at a time; even students who are enrolled full-time generally have scheduled class meetings for only 12 to 15 hours per week. Thus, postsecondary students often have significant periods of unscheduled time. Such time allows students to study, work for wages, volunteer, socialize, exercise, relax, or tend to personal and familial responsibilities. However, some veterans find it difficult to adapt to the relative abundance of unstructured time afforded most college students. This is most common among veterans who are unmarried and do not have children, those who are not employed, and veterans with certain mental health concerns, including anxiety disorders, depression, attention deficit/hyperactivity disorder (ADHD), PTSD, and SUAD. Yet other veterans have different time-related challenges, particularly those who are attempting to balance education, employment, and family responsibilities. They generally have less free time. They are also more likely to not get adequate sleep than their more traditional-aged, nonveteran student peers and to encounter stress due to competing demands on their time. Such issues can diminish their academic performance and increase their risk of degree non-completion. Some student organizations and campus veteran services offices have incorporated workshops on effective time management and stress-reduction techniques. Student counseling services and student wellness centers can also provide individual counseling, support groups, and other services to help promote mental wellness and stress reduction for student-veterans.

Social dynamics within postsecondary settings can also be difficult for veterans. Many struggle to form significant and meaningful social connections with their nonveteran peers. This may be due to the fact that veterans tend to be somewhat older than the nonveteran student population. Yet student-veterans are also more likely to live off-campus; this diminishes the amount of time they are physically present on campus and reduces their likelihood of participating in study groups, internships, sports and recreational activities, and various campus events (e.g., guest speakers, celebrations, and films). Social isolation is especially common among student-veterans with physical, behavioral, cognitive, and emotional disorders or disabilities. Veterans attending college may also find that other students, faculty, and staff lack understanding about military experiences; in some cases, they encounter anti-military attitudes. These dynamics increase risk of social isolation for student-veterans and can even leave them feeling personally attacked. Additionally, social isolation is associated with increased risk of substance abuse, poor mental health, and suicidal ideation among veterans attending college. Rates of housing insecurity and food insecurity are disproportionately high among student-veteran populations and can increase feelings of social isolation, diminish mental and physical health, and create significant barriers to academic success.

HEALTH-CARE ACCESS AND QUALITY

Most veterans are entitled to health-care service through the VA. For those with significant military-related injuries, illnesses, or disabilities, such care may be provided free of charge. However, those who receive care under the TRICARE health insurance program are charged co-pays. Issues with quality of care and access to care have plagued the VA health system for decades; such issues received considerable attention during the VA scandal in 2014. In recent decades, administrative and legislative changes have aimed to promote improved health-care services for veterans. Such changes have been bolstered by judicial decisions as well as federal approval for certain medical procedures. However, it is clear that many veterans continue to lack access to high-quality, convenient, and affordable health care.

Health Services and Benefits for Veterans

Veterans who served in active duty for at least two years—or, in the case, of reservists, completed their full term of active duty—and received either a general or honorable discharge are entitled to health-care benefits through the VA. Such benefits are also available to spouses and dependents. However, this does not mean that health care provided through the VA is necessarily free. Within the VA system, veterans are assigned to different priority groups. Those with extensive service-related disabilities (30 percent or more disabled), who are former prisoners of war, are unable to work due to a service-related disability, and/or received either the Purple Heart or the Medal of Honor (MOH), are given highest priority rankings (groups 1–4). Veterans with less extensive disabilities, who do not have disabilities, are receiving Medicaid benefits and/or a military pension, were discharged from military service less than 5 years ago, and/or whose household income exceeds poverty guidelines, are assigned lower rankings (groups 5–8).

Individual VA-related health costs are dependent upon priority group ranking. For example, a veteran assigned to priority group 1 must have service-related disability that renders them unable to work, reduces typical physical or cognitive function by at least 50 percent, and/or have received the MOH for exceptional bravery and self-sacrifice during combat. The VA provides free health care—including for physical, mental, and dental health—to veterans in priority group 1. Veterans receiving a military pension and are classified as low-income may also receive free health care through the VA. In addition, veterans in all priority groups are entitled to free care for any health condition related to their military service. Yet those in groups 2–8 are typically charged a co-pay for care for non-service-related health conditions; co-pay amounts are similar to those charged via employer-sponsored health insurance. Regardless of priority group, all veterans are entitled to free mental health services for MST and issues related to readjusting to civilian life. Any tests and exams needed to assess health status for the purposes of assigning priority group are provided free of charge; X-rays, immunizations, preventative screenings, lab tests, smoking cessation programs, and weight loss programs are also free. Most maternity-related health care is provided at no cost; however, those in priority groups 6, 7, and 8 are charged co-pays for certain specialty consultations and procedures. Pregnancy termination is not covered under VA benefits.

Most veterans are eligible for insurance coverage through TRICARE. This is the same fee-for-service program that provides health insurance to active duty military and their dependents. It includes coverage for preventative care, treatment, prescription medications, vision care, dental care, and certain mental health, reproductive health, and disability-related services. Like most health insurance programs for civilians, TRICARE includes varying levels of coverage, each with a different monthly premium. Some veterans combine TRICARE with other types of health insurance, including private, employer-sponsored, and/or other government-sponsored health insurance. For example, veterans aged 65 or older and who meet the requirements for Medicare parts A and B are also eligible for TRICARE for Life, a program that enables approved individuals to receive care from any health-care provider who accepts Medicare. Those enrolled in TRICARE for Life pay premiums for Medicare part B coverage as well as an annual deductible; once their deductible is met, subscribers are then responsible for 20 percent of costs associated with approved health services. Yet the TRICARE system has been widely criticized. Elective health services, chiropractic care, abortion, many dental procedures, and certain types of contraception are not covered. In addition, while active duty military personal who are diagnosed with gender dysphoria may receive hormonal and counseling options under TRICARE, gender-affirming surgical procedures are not routinely covered for veterans. While some veterans may be able to secure a waiver that provides coverage for gender-affirming surgery, the process of obtaining such a waiver can be time-consuming, discouraging, and constitute a significant barrier to care. In addition, many veterans find it difficult to understand coverage guidelines. Furthermore, it can be difficult to locate a health-care provider that accepts TRICARE and is accepting new patients. Those receiving TRICARE benefits may also have to file their own claims, something that is associated with increased errors and delays in reimbursement.

The VA Health System in Crisis

The VA health-care system is extensive. It is comprised of over 1,300 unique health facilities, including over 170 medical centers and nearly 1,200 outpatient facilities. The vast majority of these facilities are located in urban or suburban areas; thus, veterans in rural areas often face geographic barriers when seeking care at the VA. Those who must travel long distances to receive care at VA facilities may receive reimbursement for certain travel expenses. In addition, veterans who live a great distance from VA facilities may receive approval to obtain care outside of the VA system. However, such approval must be secured prior to receiving nonemergency medical care. Many veterans find the process for securing such approval rather confusing, however, and it is not always clear why some requests are granted while others are denied. Each year, the VA health system provides care to nearly 10 million veterans. However, only about two-thirds of all veterans qualify for services through the VA health system. Those who were dishonorably discharged, did not serve for the full period for which they were called to active duty (typically a minimum of 24 continuous months), or were reservists who participated in military training but never served in active duty are ineligible for VA health care. Of those who qualify, only about half pursue care through the VA system and, instead, opt for care through other providers. Consequently, many argue that the system remains underutilized. The VA health system has been plagued by problems for decades. Problems including waste of resources and inadequate care provided in VA facilities were documented as early as the 1940s; inadequate funding and poor quality of care due to heavy caseloads emerged as significant concerns in the 1970s; and in the 1980s and 1990s, concerns surfaced concerning unethical practices in some VA facilities (e.g., employing physicians with revoked or suspended licenses, noncompliance with legal requirements for research, and performing unnecessary surgical procedures).

In the first decade of the twenty-first century, veterans seeking care through VA facilities commonly experienced lengthy waiting times to receive care, often over two months. In VA facilities in multiple states, veterans were exposed to and, in some cases, contracted potentially deadly infectious diseases (e.g., hepatitis, HIV, and Legionnaires' Disease) because medical equipment had not been properly disinfected or because other sanitation protocols had not been followed. Ongoing problems with inaccurate record-keeping, understaffing, bribes paid to VA officials, and inappropriate use of funds were also documented. In January 2014, widespread problems within the VA health system emerged as a national scandal. Ultimately, and in response to mounting pressure from politicians as well as veterans' groups, Eric K. Shinseki, Secretary for Veterans Affairs, submitted his resignation on May 30, 2014. Ten days later, the VA released an internal audit that presented damning evidence about the state of the VA health system. Chief among its findings was the fact that wait times exceeded 90 days for most new veterans seeking health care; furthermore, over 100,000 veterans who had requested medical care at the VA during the previous decade had never been given an appointment. The VA also admitted that some veterans had died while waiting to receive health care. In the wake of the scandal, there were changes to administration and oversight within the VA system. Similarly, the VA scheduling and appointment system was updated. The Veterans Access Choice and Accountability Act of 2014 (VACAA) was also implemented. It permitted veterans to seek private care outside of the VA system if they could not get a VA appointment within 30 days or if they faced substantial burdens (e.g., related to their unique medical conditions and/or geographic distance) that diminished their access to VA facilities. It also provided increased funding for staffing of VA health facilities and expansion of telemedicine and mobile health clinics. Despite this, long wait times and chronic understaffing remained concerns at many VA facilities. In 2018, the Mission Act was implemented as an additional measure to promote increased access to health care for veterans. Despite this, many veterans continue to struggle to access VA health services; others remain skeptical about the quality of care available at VA facilities and, thus, are discouraged from pursuing treatment. In addition, evidence from the COVID-19 pandemic indicates that the VA health system remains inefficient, lacks adequate training for staff (e.g., recognizing and adequately responding to signs of suicidal ideation), and is underfunded. In recent years, evidence of ongoing bias and discrimination—specifically based on gender identity, race, ethnic identity, sexual orientation, and sex—in VA health facilities has also emerged.

Other Issues

Veterans also encounter other issues with quality of care. For example, although veterans with limb amputations are often provided with prosthetic devices to help restore some measure of function, prosthetic devices in the United States have, until recently, been limited to socket-mounted devices that fit over the residual limb and must be secured with a strap, cuff, or use of suction. Socket-mounted devices work well for some veterans, yet many experience problems with comfort, infection, swelling, circulation, and function. A different category of prostheses—known as osseointegration devices—has been used for more than two decades in countries such as Sweden, Australia, Germany, and France. Such devices are anchored to a biocompatible component that is implanted into the bone of the residual stump. Osseointegration prostheses are stronger, more durable, promote increased strength and flexibility, and minimize some risks associated with socket-mounted prostheses. Despite these benefits, veterans were not offered osseointegration options until fairly recently. In 2020, the US Food and Drug Administration (FDA) approved the Osseoanchored Prostheses for the Rehabilitation of Amputees (OPRA) Implant System. OPRA may only be used for lower limb amputations if the residual limb terminates above the knee. As of June 2022, no other osseointegration devices had received FDA approval. Many veterans and veteran support organizations such as the Wounded Warriors Project continue to draw attention to the lack of options and the need for improved care for veterans with amputations.

There are also ongoing issues with the recognition of and response to the health concerns of veterans who served in specific military campaigns or who were exposed to toxic substances during training or other military activities. Veterans who returned from Vietnam, for example, voiced concerns about various types of cancer and other health issues they believed were caused by exposure to Agent Orange. Although the last US military troops left Vietnam in 1973, it took nearly two decades for the US Congress to pass the Agent Orange Act of 1991. It acknowledged the connection between the herbicide and poor health and also approved benefits for those veterans with health conditions related to exposure. Veterans who had served as part of ground forces in Vietnam were routinely granted such benefits. However, those involved in air or sea operations were typically denied such benefits because, according to the VA, they had never set foot in Vietnam and, thus, there was no way to prove they had been exposed to the herbicide. It was not until more than 40 years after US forces exited Vietnam, and only after the decision in the *Gabriel v. Wilkie (2015)* case, that the VA extended benefits to Naval veterans who had docked at certain ports in Vietnam, specifically ports located near where Agent Orange was used. Following the *Procopio v. Wilkie (2019)* decision, VA benefits were finally extended to Navy veterans who served in open waters off the shores of Vietnam. During that same year, the Blue Water Navy Vietnam Veterans Act was passed. It acknowledged exposure to Agent Orange among naval forces and approved them for VA disability benefits. Unfortunately, some veterans remain unaware of such benefits or encounter significant problems with processing their applications. It is estimated that thousands of veterans afflicted with health maladies related to Agent Orange exposure died before receiving such benefits. Similar patterns of denial regarding certain health conditions related to military experience and corresponding delays in benefits have been noted among Gulf War veterans and those exposed to PFAS.

LIVING ENVIRONMENT AND SOCIAL CONTEXT

Some of the most significant challenges veterans face relate to social dynamics. On an individual level, they may struggle to transition from the more scheduled routine of military life to the relatively less structured norms of civilian life. In addition, relationships can be strained, particularly for veterans who feel socially isolated, have service-related disabilities and/or suffer from mental illness, and encounter anti-military discrimination in their personal or professional lives. Many veterans encounter significant and persistent barriers that diminish their access to basic needs. Support services specifically for veteran populations are also inadequate to meet demand. Additionally, stereotypes of military experiences and veteran populations continue to permeate media and popular culture. This not only contributes to the military-civilian divide but also minimizes attention to the experiences and needs of particular groups of veterans. Thus, such representations can diminish the social well-being and mental health of veterans.

Social Dynamics

Many veterans find it difficult to adjust to post-military civilian life. In many respects, military life is often fast-paced and dictated by a rigid hierarchy and strictly controlled schedules. Civilian life, in contrast, can seem relatively chaotic and unstructured. For example, civilian workplaces and educational institutions are often competitive and lack the camaraderie and sense of collective purpose that is common among military units. Furthermore, there is more free time associated with civilian life. This can leave many veterans feeling restless, bored, frustrated, and anxious. Such feelings are most common among veterans whose military service ended less than a year ago but tend to diminish as time goes by. However, certain groups of veterans are at increased risk of problems related to civilian life. This includes veterans who are unemployed, lack a strong social support system, are geographically isolated, lack meaningful and consistent connections with other veterans and veterans' support organizations, have significant service-related disabilities, and are housing insecure and/or food insecure. Veterans with various mental health disorders are also among those most likely to experience problems adjusting to civilian life. For example, those with depression may find their symptoms increase and become more severe in the period immediately following military discharge. Similarly, the less structured components of civilian life can exacerbate symptoms for veterans with anxiety disorders. Anti-military discrimination can also make it difficult for veterans to adjust to civilian life. Such discrimination has been documented in employment, educational, and other social institutions. It is associated with increased risk of social isolation, low self-esteem, and stress among veterans and can exacerbate other health conditions. Participation in veterans' organizations can help ease the transition to civilian life and connect veterans with various support services. Yet sexism, racism, homophobia, and other forms of discrimination within such groups often discourage individuals from participating and increase feelings of social isolation.

Housing insecurity continues to plague veteran populations. It is most common among veterans with physical disabilities, or PTSD, are unemployed, and/or lack access to adequate financial resources. Yet structural components of American society also diminish veterans' access to adequate shelter. The United States has a chronic shortage of accessible housing for individuals with disabilities. At present, less than 5 percent of all housing meets legal standards of accessibility for individuals with mobility impairments, sensory deprivation, and other significant disabilities, including veterans. Furthermore, many veterans encounter anti-military sentiment when attempting to secure housing. At present, there is no federal law that prohibits housing discrimination related to military or veteran status. Some states, however, have implemented fair housing standards that protect veterans; examples include Massachusetts, Illinois, Washington, and Rhode Island. Yet even in states where such legislation exists, discriminatory attitudes and practices that impede access to housing for veterans persist. Lack of affordable (including subsidized) and safe housing in the United States as well as poor credit scores among some veterans are also factors that contribute to housing insecurity. Veterans may also encounter unique housing-related issues in different geographic locations. For example, veterans who reside in urban areas are more likely to encounter loud noises related to traffic, construction, and other activities; however, much of existing housing does not include architectural features (e.g., open floor plans, soundproofing, and adequate lighting) that promote a sense of calmness and reduce triggers for individuals with PTSD and other mental health conditions. In contrast, those in rural areas often must contend with geographic and transportation-related barriers that diminish their access to housing support services. Food insecurity is also an issue. Structural inequities such as food deserts, inadequate nutritional programs for low-income populations, and insufficient economic support services for veteran populations have been identified as key factors that contribute to food insecurity among this population, especially those who are elderly and/or disabled.

Representations in Mass Media and Popular Culture

Attitudes about military personnel and veterans are heavily influenced by media and various forms of popular culture (e.g., films, television series, and video games). Although there is some degree of diversity in such representations, there tends to be an overreliance on a limited range of rather simplistic stereotypes to depict the identities, experiences, and needs of military personnel. Some of the most prominent themes among such representations include the drug-addicted veteran; the emotionally distant veteran; the traumatized veteran (e.g., having severe and complex PTSD); the heroic veteran; the dangerous/violent veteran; the drug/alcohol-addicted veteran; the weak veteran (often used to depict those who were captured by enemy forces or who were discharged from the military due to physical injury, illness, or mental health issues); and the hyper-masculine veteran. Additionally, veterans continue to be represented primarily as cisgender males; when cisgender female veterans are depicted, they are often shown as victims—especially victims of sexual assault—or as having only a supporting, noncombat role in military operations. Heterosexism and homophobia also continue to influence representations of veterans; depictions of veterans who identify as lesbian, gay, bisexual, transgender, or gender nonbinary are scarce. Veterans who are members of racial and ethnic minority groups also continue to be underrepresented in media and popular culture.

Representations of veterans in mass media and popular culture have been identified as a key factor in perpetuating what is commonly referred to as the military-civilian divide. This refers to the limited—and largely inaccurate—knowledge that civilian populations have of military operations and the experiences of military forces and, by extension, the experiences of veteran populations. Thus, although the US voting public and US political institutions continue to express strong support for troops and veterans, the reality is that dominant representations found in US mass media and popular culture contribute to a lack of understanding of how family members, friends, and even social institutions can best meet the needs of veterans. Furthermore, such representations can also impact the self-concept of veterans, including their understanding of typical and expected behaviors among veteran populations within the unique context of American society. This has been shown to exacerbate the difficulties many veterans experience when making the transition to civilian life. It also contributes to social isolation, depression, anxiety, and stress among veteran populations and impacts their experiences in employment, educational, and social settings.

CHAPTER THIRTEEN

Women and Girls

Cisgender women and girls (those whose gender identity coincides with sex assigned at birth) have some unique health concerns when compared to cisgender men and boys. Many of these concerns are related to chromosomes, anatomy, secondary sex characteristics, and hormones. Consequently, biological determinants of health continue to receive considerable attention in studies that focus on women's and girl's health. Yet due largely to the influence of feminists who campaigned for women's rights and gender equality from the nineteenth century onward, attention to the effects of social determinants of the health of women and girls has steadily expanded over the past century. Such attention is now common among health-care providers and academic researchers; it is also found in the work of multilateral agencies such as the World Health Organization and Pan American Health Organization, and within the US government, public health programs, and nonprofit organizations.

This chapter focuses on social factors that influence the health of cisgender women and girls. Research continues to demonstrate that bias, discrimination, and other manifestations of gender inequality within American culture contribute to the burden of disease among this population. Particular areas of concern include economic inequities, social biases, discrimination within the US health-care system, exposure to certain types of violence, and social roles that continue to disadvantage females in their personal and professional lives. Furthermore, such disadvantage is evident throughout the lifespan, from birth to death. It is especially pronounced for women and girls who identify as Black, Indigenous, and People of Color (BIPOC) as well as elderly women, the poor, immigrants, lesbians, and bisexuals.

CURRENT STATE OF HEALTH

During infancy and childhood, cisgender girls are overall healthier and have lower rates of mortality than cisgender boys. They are less likely to be born prematurely and less prone to respiratory illnesses, health complications, injuries, and certain types of genetic disorders. Research has linked such differences to sex chromosomes and hormones, specifically as these seem to promote increased immune system function and reduce susceptibility to certain diseases among females during infancy, childhood, and throughout the lifespan. Certain types of accidents and injuries are also significant considerations. Rates of drowning are lower for girls. Adolescent girls who drive automobiles are less likely than boys to be involved in accidents. Yet some health problems are more common among girls including chronic conditions such as food allergies, asthma, hypertension, and diabetes. Additionally, girls are more likely than boys to die or suffer serious injury when involved in auto accidents. Violence also impacts girls differently than boys—girls constitute less than 15 percent of children who die from gun violence each year, yet they are nine out of ten homicide victims of teen dating violence. Approximately one in nine girls will experience sexual abuse before age 18. Some genetic diseases (e.g., Turner syndrome and Rett syndrome) occur only in females. Rates of obesity are also a concern. Prevalence of obesity is similar among cisgender girls and boys during the first decade of life, yet adolescent females are more likely to be overweight or obese than their male peers. At present, approximately one in five girls aged 6–17 meets the medical guidelines for obesity. Prevalence is higher among Indigenous (30 percent), Hispanic/Latinx/Chicanx (HLC) (25 percent), and Black (24 percent) populations but lower among non-HLC whites (16 percent) and Asians (9 percent).

Mental health is another pressing health concern for girls. During the first decade of life, rates of diagnosis for most mental health disorders do not vary greatly between girls and boys. However, during adolescence, incidence of anxiety, depression, social anxiety, bipolar disorder, and borderline personality disorder are two to three times higher among girls. In addition, girls are less likely to be diagnosed with autism spectrum disorders, attention-deficit hyperactivity disorders, and conduct disorders but at least twice as likely as boys to develop eating disorders during childhood and adolescence. Although male and female cisgender teens use alcohol and illegal drugs at roughly the same rates, girls more often engage in substance abuse, develop an addiction, and have suicidal thoughts after using such substances. They are also at increased risk of developing PTSD and, consequently, are more likely than boys to engage in non-suicidal self-injury and attempt suicide; however, they are less likely than boys to die by suicide.

Gender disparities in mental health persist in adulthood. Women are twice as likely as men to develop a mental health disorder and more likely to receive mental health services including counseling, medication, and hospitalization. Each year, one-fourth of women experience a mental health problem; two-thirds of women will have a diagnosable mental illness during their lifetime and the most common are anxiety, depression, eating disorders, impulse control disorders, and substance abuse disorders. Rates of diagnosis are highest among non-HLC white, middle-class women, something that reflects ongoing barriers to mental health care that continue to disproportionately disadvantage BIPOC and poor populations. Risks of mental illness increase during pregnancy and the post-partum period.

Physical health considerations are also significant for adult women. Nearly 40 percent of women have a chronic health condition. They are more likely than men to be overweight or obese, and rates are highest among low-income populations. At present, nearly 70 percent of American women are overweight or obese and rates have steadily increased since the 1970s. Reproductive and sexual health issues are also common. Over 70 percent of women will experience a hormonal imbalance in their lifetimes. Such imbalances can cause irregular menstrual cycles, polycystic ovarian syndrome, infertility, aggravated menopause symptoms, mood swings, acne, sleep disturbances, and decreased sex drive. Women are twice as likely as men to contract a sexually transmitted disease (STD). Furthermore, pregnancy and childbirth pose unique health risks including gestational diabetes, certain infections, preeclampsia, and hemorrhage.

Certain autoimmune diseases (e.g., lupus, Graves' disease, rheumatoid arthritis, and Hashimoto's disease) are more common in women. Women also have higher rates of Alzheimer's disease (the fifth leading cause of death among women), lower respiratory tract diseases (the fourth leading cause of death among women), stroke (the third leading cause of death among women), multiple sclerosis, and osteoporosis. Cancers are, collectively, the second leading cause of death among women; cancers of the breast, reproductive tract (e.g., uterine, ovarian, cervical, vaginal, and vulvar), skin, lungs, colon, and rectum are especially common. Although they typically have lower risk of heart disease, women who have a heart attack are more likely than men to experience long-term health problems and to die. Heart disease is the leading cause of death among women.

ECONOMIC FACTORS

Women and girls tend to have fewer economic resources than men and boys. Such disparities are due, in part, to differences in patterns of paid employment. Yet practices that discriminate against women and girls—including those that diminish the value of their work, compensate them less than their male peers, and contribute to various forms of sex and gender discrimination—are equally significant. The economic marginalization of women and girls is so pervasive that it is often referred to as the feminization of poverty. It is associated with diminished physical, mental, and social health throughout the lifespan.

Paid Employment

A strong economy promotes access to paid employment for women and adolescent girls, thereby enhancing their earnings and purchasing power while also decreasing their risk of poverty. Married women who work for wages experience greater autonomy and decision-making power within their households. Among women and adolescent girls, employment is often associated with enhanced self-esteem and a sense of purpose beyond familial roles and academic responsibilities. Employment can also promote social connections, thereby promoting the mental health of women and girls. Those who work for wages are often more physically active than those who do not and, therefore, may enjoy physical health benefits.

Employment can also facilitate access to health insurance, paid sick leave, flexible spending accounts for health and childcare, and paid vacation leave. Such benefits are important for all women, yet they are especially significant for unmarried women who cannot access benefits through a spouse and for those who are heads of households and, therefore, whose benefits also offer advantages for their dependents. A unique benefit that is gaining in popularity is employee wellness programs. Typically offered in the workplace setting or online, these often focus on smoking cessation, stress-reduction techniques, healthy eating, and fitness. Women are more likely than men to participate in such programs.

However, in times of economic recession, the employment of women and girls suffers. During the Great Recession (December 2007–June 2009), approximately 2.7 million women lost their jobs. While this was lower than the rate of job loss among men for the same period, women lost jobs at a higher rate than men in certain industries, including construction, manufacturing, and local government. In the ensuing years, women's return to employment lagged behind that of men, particularly in retail, education, health care, business, and professional services. The COVID-19 pandemic also had a profound impact on women's employment. They lost more jobs than men in all industries and overall job loss was greatest in industries that employed a greater number of women than men (including travel, entertainment, beauty services, childcare, elementary and secondary education, and hospitality). Rates of job loss were especially high among BIPOC women. During some portions of the pandemic, recorded job losses occurred entirely among women while employment rates among men remained unchanged or increased.

The Gender Wage Gap and Earnings

The gender wage gap refers to difference in average earnings between full-time female and male employees. At present, women earn only about 82 cents for every $1 earned by males. The gap persists at all levels of employment, regardless of work experience or education, and becomes greater as women age. It also varies by race and ethnicity. For every $1 earned by white males, Asian women earn about 90 cents; white women earn 79 cents; Black women earn 62 cents; Indigenous women earn 57 cents; and HLC women earn 54 cents. The wage gap can impair women's ability to pay for basic needs, including preventative health care and treatment. Yet it is also associated with diminished self-esteem as well as higher rates of depression and anxiety.

Over the courses of their lives, American women earn less than American men. This is due, in part, to the wage gap. Yet women also have lower overall rates of participation in the labor force than men. Approximately 55 percent of adult women (compared to nearly 70 percent of adult men) work for wages. Single women and women with minor children are currently less likely to participate in paid labor than they were at the start of the twenty-first century. This may be due, in part, to their increased participation in postsecondary education. Yet in recent years, increasing emphasis on traditional family values and gender roles has prompted some married women with children to withdraw from the workforce. Other familial responsibilities—such as caring for aging parents—have also been linked to reduced labor force participation among some middle-aged women.

Women are more likely to work part-time than men. Such work is associated with diminished access to health insurance, paid sick leave, and other benefits. Despite the fact that they often have duties that are similar to full-time employees, part-time workers typically earn wages that are considerably lower. Although some women choose part-time work, many are part of the involuntary part-time workforce—those actively seeking yet unable to find full-time work. In some cases, such individuals will work more than one part-time job in order to increase overall income. Women currently make up more than half of all Americans who work multiple jobs and the practice is especially common among women who are widowed, divorced, or separated as well as those without a college degree. Yet working multiple part-time jobs is associated with increased stress, fatigue, sleep disruption, physical injury, and exposure to hazardous conditions in the workplace. It can also cause strain in family relationships and friendships due to unpredictable scheduling and limited time for leisure and socializing. Those who work multiple part-time jobs are typically ineligible for benefits. However, their total income may render them ineligible for government-sponsored health insurance or community health services for low-income populations.

Employment Sectors and Sex Discrimination

Women and adolescent girls tend to be concentrated in sectors of the workforce with lower average pay. Examples include service industries such as food service; cleaning and custodial services; clerical support; pet services; and beauty-related services. Additionally, just over 75 percent of teachers from preschool through high school and approximately 95 percent of childcare workers are women. Importantly, when women are employed in sectors that are traditionally male dominated, such as construction, firefighting, aviation, architecture, finance, manufacturing, finance, and software technology, they are less likely to occupy higher-paying managerial or supervisory roles. This marginalization of women in leadership roles is known as the glass ceiling and it is especially pronounced for BIPOC women. It has long been recognized as a manifestation of systemic sex and gender discrimination and has been documented among Fortune 500 companies, S&P 500 companies, political bodies, educational institutions, and health-care entities. While there has been a marginal increase in women in leadership positions in recent decades, those who do break through the glass ceiling often experience diminished mental wellness due to marginalization and stigmatization from co-workers.

Furthermore, women employed in male-dominated industries such as construction and manufacturing often find that safety equipment—including hard hats, safety gloves, and harnesses—is designed for the average male body. Women tend to be shorter and differently proportioned than men. Therefore, such equipment often does not fit women properly and, therefore, increases their risk of injuries and exposure to hazardous materials. Yet this problem is not exclusive to construction and manufacturing. During the COVID-19 pandemic, female health-care workers increasingly complained that personal protective equipment (PPE)—such as gowns, gloves, and face masks/face shields—was too large or otherwise ill-fitting and, thus, increased their risk of exposure to potentially fatal pathogens.

There has been increased attention to sex and gender discrimination in the workplace since the mid-twentieth century. This has been prompted by state and federal policies—including the Equal Pay Act of 1963, Title VII of the Civil Rights Act of 1964, the Equal Employment Opportunity Act of 1972, and the Pregnancy Discrimination Act of 1978—as well as high-profile sexual harassment cases, and social change efforts (e.g., the Me Too Movement and the Time's Up Movement). Data indicate that nearly 80 percent of those who report such discrimination are cisgender women; 40 percent of female employees experience some form of sex or gender discrimination during their lifetime. Rates are fairly consistent across age groups and racial and ethnic groups, yet lesbian and bisexual women report higher rates of discrimination than heterosexual/straight women. Workplace discrimination is more common in industries that have been traditionally male dominated and in the entertainment, hospitality, and service industries. Flight attendants, food services workers, and those employed in the sex work industry (e.g., erotic dancing, escort services, pornography, and prostitution) are often targeted. Many workplaces attempt to combat such discrimination through employee training programs, but others do not. Yet even when such programs are mandatory, they are often perfunctory, ineffective, and not adequately enforced.

Sex and gender discrimination in the workplace take a variety of forms. Examples include paying women less than men for the same work, questioning women's leadership abilities or competency just because they are women, passing women over for promotions even though they are qualified, giving women less desirable work assignments, and socially ostracizing women in male-dominated workplaces. Sexual harassment is a unique category of discrimination and is divided into two categories. The first is hostile environment; it occurs when the workplace includes behaviors, comments, or images of a sexual nature that interfere with an individual's ability to do their job and that a reasonable person would find intimidating or offensive. The second type, quid pro quo, occurs when the harasser requests sexual acts in exchange for workplace advancement or with the indication that the victim will be demoted, fired, or penalized if they fail to comply. Stalking and cyberstalking are also forms of sexual harassment.

Over 80 percent of American women experience workplace sexual harassment at some point in their lives. It can impair mental health and increases stress, job dissatisfaction, depression, anxiety, and low self-esteem. Sexual harassment is one of the most commonly cited reasons that women quit their jobs, especially lesbian, bisexual, and BIPOC women. Victims also face physical health risks due to sleep disorders, chest pain, breathing difficulties, and other physical symptoms associated with stress disorders. They are also more likely to abuse alcohol and drugs (including prescriptions and illegal substances), socially isolate from support networks, engage in high-risk sexual behaviors, and experience PTSD. Common health problems among victims of sexual assault and rape include STDs, unintended pregnancy, sexual dysfunction, chronic pelvic pain, and traumatic injuries. Sexual harassment most directly harms the victim but also contributes to decreased job satisfaction; higher rates of job turnover; and increased rates of anxiety, fear, sleep disorders, headaches, and stomach aches among those who witness such abuse.

Victims of sex and gender discrimination in the workplace are legally entitled to damages, including monetary compensation and punitive damages. Additionally, perpetrators may face fines, loss of employment, and/or jail time. Victims may file a grievance through human resources or their employee union or they may pursue legal action either by hiring a private attorney or filing a formal complaint with the Equal Employment Opportunities Commission (EEOC). Yet less than 15 percent of all sex discrimination and only 1 percent of all sexual harassment are reported. Reasons for not reporting vary considerably. Many women fear they will not be believed or will be blamed. Others fear retaliation (such as job loss), despite the fact that all forms of retaliation against those who file complaints are illegal. Some do not file reports due to shame or embarrassment or because they lack faith in workplace reporting mechanisms. The cost of hiring a private attorney can be prohibitive. Investigations by the EEOC may take up to a year but a resolution may be reached more quickly via mediation.

The Feminization of Poverty

Women and girls are overrepresented among America's poor and are more likely than their male counterparts to live in poverty and lack the economic and material resources necessary to meet their basic needs. This is true among all racial and ethnic groups and throughout the lifespan but is more pronounced for BIPOC, elderly, lesbian, and bisexual women. Economic and material scarcity has a variety of negative impacts on mental and physical health. Some infectious diseases are more common among low-income populations. These are collectively referred to as diseases of poverty and include TB, chronic respiratory illnesses, and diarrheal diseases. Rates of HIV infection, obesity, and death from breast cancer are also higher among low-income women.

Poverty is associated with food insecurity and low-quality diet, factors that increase incidence of stunting and malnutrition in young girls and chronic health issues such as hypertension, diabetes, kidney disease, coronary heart disease, obesity, stroke, and various types of cancer among adolescent girls and adult women. Low-income women—especially those with dependent children—face increased risk of housing insecurity, homelessness, and exposure to environmental hazards such as temperature extremes, allergens, and toxic building materials; those without stable housing are more likely to be victims of sexual violence and physical assault. Rates of depression, anxiety, panic disorder, and PTSD are high among low-income women. Poverty also reduces life expectancy—on average, women with the lowest household incomes live a decade less than women with the highest household incomes.

Poverty also impairs health-seeking behaviors among women and girls. Those with incomes less than 200 percent of the Federal Poverty Level (FPL) are twice as likely as more affluent women to postpone preventative care, forgo prescription medication, cut pills in half or dilute liquid medications to make them last longer, skip recommended treatments, and have problems accessing mental health services. They are also more likely to encounter difficulties paying for childcare or transportation or taking time off of work in order to attend medical appointments. Low-income women also have fewer choices among providers, health-care facilities, and types of treatment. Among low-income women, over 60 percent find it difficult to pay for necessities due to health-related expenses and medical debt. Approximately one in four American women reported difficulties paying medical bills during the COVID-19 pandemic.

Furthermore, gender norms may encourage mothers to prioritize the needs of their children or the family unit over their own health and well-being. This can have long-term implications for all low-income women, but especially for those with disabilities and BIPOC women who are more likely to have chronic health conditions and require ongoing medical care and prescription medications. Additionally, women encounter higher average lifetime health expenses than men. Some of these expenses are related to reproductive health care, yet others stem from increased rates of certain diseases and disorders among women and their tendency to utilize health-care services more frequently than men. For economically vulnerable women—especially unmarried heads of household and those with chronic health conditions or disabilities—health expenses can push them into poverty.

Among populations over age 65, women are more likely than men to live in poverty. They are also less likely to have retirement accounts and own property, stock, or other assets. Economic scarcity is especially high among retired and elderly women with disabilities; lesbian and bisexual women; BIPOC women; and those who are divorced, widowed, or never married. In addition, and because women tend to live longer than men, elderly women typically spend more years living in poverty than elderly males. Health-care costs have been identified as a significant barrier to care for elderly women. They encounter higher average health-care costs than elderly males, and such costs consume a larger portion of the average annual income among elderly women.

Women and girls do benefit from various social programs that provide support for low-income Americans. For example, women constituted over half of all unemployment recipients in 2020. Yet unemployment benefits provide only limited income and may make it difficult for women to meet their basic needs. In addition, health insurance is available through programs such as the Children's Health Insurance Program (CHIP), Medicare, and Medicaid. Women are twice as likely as men to rely on Medicaid. During 2019, over 25 million adult women received Medicaid; another 2 million women met federal eligibility guidelines for Medicaid but were not enrolled. Women are also the majority of Medicare recipients (about 57 percent) and nearly 70 percent of women who receive Medicare have two or more chronic health conditions. Despite expanded access to health insurance prompted by the Patient Protection and Affordable Care Act (ACA) of 2010, over 10 percent of American adult women under the age of 65 were uninsured in 2019. Community health clinics that offer low-cost or free health services can help meet their health-care needs. Yet such services are limited, particularly in rural areas, and often do not include advanced diagnostic procedures, surgical options, or certain medications.

Government-sponsored food and nutrition programs are available to those who meet income guidelines. These include the Supplemental Nutrition Assistance Program (SNAP) and the Special Supplemental Nutrition Program for Women, Infants, and Children (commonly referred to as WIC). Women represent over 60 percent of nonelderly SNAP recipients; over one-third of all SNAP recipients in 2019 were BIPOC women. Of those households that receive SNAP benefits and have minor children, nearly 90 percent are headed by single mothers. The WIC program provides nutritional support to 6–8 million people annually, including over 1.5 million pregnant and breastfeeding women. Yet such programs are underfunded and not able to meet demand. Community food banks may also help meet the nutritional needs of low-income populations. National data indicates that low-income women, particularly those who have limited education, are unmarried, and are raising children are the most common users of food banks. However, such programs often face obstacles in getting food to those most in need (especially in rural areas), maintaining a consistent supply of food, and offering food that meets dietary restrictions or food preferences. Furthermore, many women report that the stigma associated with reliance on government and community support programs discourages them from participating.

EDUCATION ACCESS AND QUALITY

Since the 1980s, women and girls have outperformed their male peers in scholastic pursuits, something that is evident in degree completion rates and performance on certain standardized tests. It is clear that education and health are interconnected for women and girls—access to high-quality education improves their health, while good health improves their access to education. However, there are significant disparities in education access and quality among different demographic groups and, consequently, the health-related benefits of education are not equally available to all women and girls. Furthermore, and although it is clear that educational settings can promote positive social connections and psychological well-being, educational settings can also contribute to poor health outcomes for some women and girls, particularly for BIPOC, LGBTQIA, low-income, and disabled populations.

Educational Enrollment and Achievement

Historically, females in the United States were discouraged from pursuing education, particularly as such pursuits were deemed counter to their social roles as daughters, wives, and mothers. Yet during the twentieth century, their participation in higher education increased dramatically. By 1980, over half of college students were women and during the 1980–1 academic year, women earned more than half of all bachelor's degrees. They have done so every year since and, at present, earn approximately 57 percent of undergraduate degrees, 60 percent of master's degrees, and 53 percent of doctoral degrees. Many have linked this drastic increase in women's postsecondary degree completion to feminist social change efforts and changing gender norms. Others have pointed to the influence of Title IX of the Education Amendments Act of 1972 (commonly referred to as Title IX) which prohibits sex discrimination in public education. Interestingly, however, and despite the fact that over half of all currently enrolled college students are women, they remain underrepresented in traditionally male-dominated academic fields including mathematics, engineering, computer science, architecture, and physical/earth sciences.

Indigenous, Black, and HLC women are less likely to pursue postsecondary education than white and Asian women; those who do enroll are more likely to pursue a two-year degree rather than a four-year degree and less likely to complete their education. Among those with disabilities, women are more likely than men to earn their degree, yet they are less likely to graduate than women without disabilities. Women who are raising children also have lower rates of degree completion than their non-parenting peers. Within the context of preschool, primary, and secondary educational settings, the enrollment of girls is on par with that of boys. However, whereas males constituted the majority of those who earned high school diplomas in the United States in the mid-twentieth century, rates began to shift in the 1970s and by the 1980s, more girls than boys successfully completed high school. Despite more than three decades of efforts to rectify the gender gap in standardized test performance, boys still earn higher scores than girls on the math portion of standardized tests (such as the SAT and ACT) while girls perform better on the verbal reasoning and writing portions of such exams. Girls are about half as likely to drop out of school as boy. Thus, girls of all racial and ethnic groups and all income levels are more likely than their male peers to complete high school. Yet dropout rates remain disproportionately high among low-income, HLC, Black, lesbian, and bisexual girls as well as those with disabilities.

Benefits of Educating Women and Girls—Health and Beyond

There is a two-way, multifaceted connection between education and health for girls and women. This means that access to high-quality education contributes to improved health while good health promotes improved academic achievement and completion rates. Furthermore, education not only benefits females throughout their lifetimes but also benefits their families, communities, and broader society in a variety of ways. Enhanced educational attainment promotes health literacy among women and girls. Those who complete a college degree have higher rates of health literacy than women who do not attend college. They typically have a more accurate understanding of medical diagnoses, health insurance coverage, and treatments. They are also more likely to engage in behaviors that promote their health, particularly as related to diet, exercise, and preventative health screenings. They are also less likely to smoke, use illegal drugs, and abuse alcohol. They also demonstrate increased ability to advocate for themselves in health-care settings by asking questions, requesting second opinions, and filing complaints if mistreated.

Many continue to promote the education of women and girls as a public health imperative. Advanced education is linked with increased life expectancy, decreased incidence of certain types of diseases and disabilities, improved sexual and reproductive health, and reduced strain on the US health-care system. Women who earn a bachelor's degree live, on average, 10 years longer than those who do not complete high school and 5 years longer than those with a high school diploma; for women with graduate or professional degrees, life expectancy is 12 years longer when compared to those with high school diplomas. Rates of certain communicable diseases and chronic diseases are lower among women who have earned a bachelor's degree. Adolescent girls who regularly attend school are less likely to get married before they reach adulthood, contract a STD, or experience an unintended pregnancy; they are also more likely to adhere to safe-sex practices. Similarly, rates of unintended pregnancy and STDs are lower among adult women with a college degree. They also tend to have healthier pregnancy outcomes; give birth to fewer children; and promote good health for their children, other family members, friends, and within their communities. College-educated women generally have higher average lifetime earnings and, therefore, are more able to afford preventative care as well as treatment. Consequently, they are less likely to require support from government health programs for low-income populations.

School settings can also help foster friendships and mentoring relationships that promote mental health, social connections, and academic achievement. Friendships can help girls develop social skills, improve emotional stability, and foster an increased sense of belonging. Healthy friendships with academic peers also reduce stress levels and are associated with decreased incidence and severity of anxiety, depression, and suicidal ideation. Friendships often provide essential support to help adolescent girls cope effectively with the physical, emotional, and social changes common during puberty. For girls with strained family relationships, friends often validate feelings, assist with problem-solving, discourage deviant and aggressive behaviors, and promote academic achievement. Teachers, counselors, and school volunteers can also serve as mentors, thereby helping girls navigate academic and social challenges.

Furthermore, clubs, teams, mentoring programs, and extracurricular activities offered through educational institutions have been shown to have a positive influence on girls' health. Sports and recreational clubs (such as scouting) promote improved cardiovascular health, healthy lifestyles choices, and decrease risk of obesity. Extracurricular activities can promote leadership skills and improved confidence for girls as well as expand their social network. Such activities often facilitate access to enhanced educational, social, and work-related opportunities, including mentoring. Participation in clubs and extracurriculars is associated with higher rates of academic completion, decreased incidence of absenteeism, and lower rates of unintended pregnancy, drug use, and alcohol use among adolescent girls.

Ongoing Challenges

Despite the many health benefits associated with education, there are ongoing challenges. Various federal policies such as the Civil Rights Act of 1964 (CRA), Title IX, and the Americans with Disabilities Act of 1990 (ADA) prohibit discrimination in public education. However, gender inequality in schools persists. Women and girls remain underrepresented in educational curriculum at all levels and in diverse subjects including science, history, art, and literature. Lack of representation of diverse women and girls in the curriculum has been shown to diminish their self-esteem and confidence, reduce their interest in subject matter, and hinder their academic performance. Furthermore, in K-12 and postsecondary institutions, female students continue to be tracked away from science, technology, engineering, and math (STEM) courses. When this occurs, it decreases their confidence in their ability to use STEM skills in all aspects of their lives. It is also associated with increased stress among females who do enroll in such courses.

Representation also remains a problem in educational leadership. Women are overrepresented among K-12 teachers yet underrepresented as administrators in primary, secondary, and postsecondary institutions. In addition, while just over 53 percent of part-time and non-tenure track postsecondary faculty members are women, they constitute only around 42 percent of tenure track faculty overall and only about one-third of full professors. Such disparities are even more pronounced for BIPOC women and those with disabilities. While this diminishes women's earning potential and minimizes their opportunities to influence institutional practices and policies, it also restricts availability of female role models and mentors.

American educational standards regarding sexual and reproductive health have also been widely criticized. Federal law does not require comprehensive sex education in public K-12 schools. Thus, decisions about sex education are left to individual states or school districts. As a result, sex education programs vary widely. Despite the fact that data consistently demonstrate that abstinence-only sex education programs are largely ineffective in delaying sexual activity among teens and preventing rates of unintended pregnancy and STDs, only twenty states require that sex education include information about contraception and only seventeen require that sex education curriculum be medically accurate. Another twenty-one states do not require any type of sex education. Although lack of medically sound, comprehensive sex education that includes attention to diverse gender and sexual identities and preferences is detrimental to the health of all students, it is especially harmful to girls and young women as they are more vulnerable to STDs and given the risks pregnancy poses to their physical and mental health.

Although education can promote positive self-esteem and social connections for girls, it can also be a significant source of stress and contribute to poor mental health. Such outcomes are especially pronounced among BIPOC populations. For example, Black, HLC, and Indigenous girls routinely receive harsher punishment in schools (including physical punishment and arrest) and are expelled more frequently for both academic and behavioral infractions than Asian and white students, even for similar offenses. They are also more likely to be punished for dress code violations. Similar outcomes have been noted for lesbian and bisexual students. These differences have been critiqued as part of the undue policing of girls of color and sexual minorities and are regarded by many as key components of the school-to-prison pipeline for such students.

Furthermore, in those educational settings where students and staff are predominantly white, BIPOC girls are more likely to feel lonely and stigmatized and to be victims of bullying. Overall, boys are more likely to be victims and perpetrators of bullying. Yet girls are more likely to engage in relational aggression that includes name-calling, exclusion, and spreading rumors; such aggression is linked to poor mental health outcomes and social isolation. Girls are also more likely to be the victims of sexual bullying including both in-person and via social media. Girls and women with disabilities are also more likely than nondisabled students to experience stress and social marginalization in educational settings. In recent years, and although the ADA requires accommodations for students with disabilities, there has been increasing evidence that American schools are doing a poor job meeting the needs of such students, especially those with mental illnesses. At the postsecondary level, nontraditional female students—including older women and single mothers—are also more likely to report feeling stigmatized and unwelcomed at school, something that can impair their academic achievement and diminish their desire to complete their degree.

Low English literacy (LEL) and limited English proficiency (LEP) remain ongoing concerns in educational settings. At present, women and girls aged 16 and over represent half of the nearly 44 million individuals with LEL and LEP in the United States. Such populations are less likely to meet grade-level academic standards, more likely to miss school, and less likely to graduate than their peers. They are also more likely to be socially marginalized within educational settings and, thus, to struggle with low self-esteem, anxiety, and depression. Girls with LEP are also less likely to pursue postsecondary education and vocational training. Preliminary data suggests that during the COVID-19 pandemic, the challenges faced by girls and women with LEP were compounded by the gendered digital divide. This refers to the limited access to and understanding of the various types of digital technologies required for online learning that disproportionately impacts females, particularly low-income populations. The digital divide is associated with diminished academic achievement, heightened anxiety about school, and increased social isolation.

Low-income girls and women also face some unique challenges within the context of educational settings. In K-12 settings, they are more likely to participate in free or reduced lunch programs; while such programs can promote nutritional health, they can also be a source of embarrassment, particularly when recipients do not receive the same food choices as other students or are otherwise identified to their peers or teachers. Low-income women and girls are also more likely to experience what is known as period poverty—the inability to afford menstrual products—and, consequently, to miss school during their menstrual periods. In addition, they are more likely to be employed than their more affluent peers and are often tasked with caring for younger siblings or aging relatives when the family cannot afford hired caretakers. Such responsibilities can increase stress and contribute to sleep deprivation. In addition, low-income girls and women often face difficulties accessing educational opportunities beyond the classroom such as field trips, experiential learning, and internships, something that diminishes their education and can leave them feeling ostracized and marginalized among their peers. Additionally, girls in low-income families are more likely to be unsupervised during time periods when they are not in school (e.g., after school, during holidays or summer break). Unsupervised girls are more likely to use drugs, tobacco products, and alcohol, to feel lonely, and to become sexually active before high school.

HEALTH-CARE ACCESS AND QUALITY

Women are more likely than men to seek out health-care services and to receive preventative, diagnostic, pharmaceutical, and other services for both physical and mental health. Despite this, significant barriers can and do diminish their access to health care. Additionally, biases related to sex and gender remain ongoing problems in the US health-care system. Such biases have been documented in medical research, medical education, health-care employment, and clinical care. Consequently, women and girls are more likely than men and boys to be misdiagnosed, have their symptoms dismissed, receive inferior quality of care, and face various types of medical abuse.

Access to Health Care

Geographic considerations are significant to understanding access to health care for women and girls. Rural women and girls tend to be in worse overall health than those in more urban areas and have higher rates of unintentional injury, automobile accidents, high blood pressure, high cholesterol, cardiac disease, cigarette smoking, alcohol consumption, cervical cancer, stroke, obesity, suicide, diabetes, and use of illegal drugs. They also tend to marry younger, have more children, and experience higher rates of social isolation and interpersonal violence than women and girls in urban areas. Yet limited availability of health-care services in rural areas diminishes their access to care. Lack of family planning, abortion services, emergency care, prenatal care, mental health, and substance abuse treatment are especially common in rural areas. Some rural residents must travel hours to reach health-care services. Geographic barriers have been linked to undertreatment for acute and chronic health conditions among rural women and girls. Such barriers also delay diagnosis of serious diseases such as cancer and HIV, thereby increasing risk of poor health outcomes and death. Yet those in urban and suburban areas may also experience geographic barriers to care, especially those who do not own a vehicle or do not live near public transportation.

Physical access is also diminished by the lack of accessible health-care facilities for those with disabilities. Women are more likely than men to have a disability; at present, one in five adult women has a disability. Because women typically live longer than men, they are more likely to experience aging-related decline in mobility, dexterity, or sensory functions. Yet many health-care facilities lack structural components—including elevators, access ramps, and adjustable exam tables—that promote access for disabled populations. This is most common in rural areas but has also been noted at urban health facilities that are located in older buildings.

Economic barriers to health care remain significant for women, particularly elderly, disabled, and BIPOC populations who are disproportionately represented among the poor. While women are as likely to have health insurance as men, women generally have higher health expenses but fewer economic resources. Some do qualify for government-sponsored insurance or health services for low-income populations, yet such programs are limited in scope and may not cover all necessary health treatments. Furthermore, and because they typically do not qualify for assistance through government programs, many immigrant women find health care in the United States unaffordable.

Informational access also warrants attention. Those with LEL and LEP often have difficulties understanding information from health-care providers, including diagnoses and treatment instructions. The use of language access services and telehealth options has improved in recent years. Yet some women and girls are hesitant to use such services because they fear loss of privacy. This is especially true for those seeking care for certain mental health disorders, reproductive and sexual health care, or gender-based violence. In addition, and although computing technology can help facilitate increased access to health care for some populations, elderly women are among those most likely to lack access to computing technology and to have limited understanding of how to use such technology for telehealth visits. Such concerns are even more pronounced for those with cognitive decline and memory loss.

Another type of access relates to culturally competent care. Such care respects a patient's cultural identity, beliefs, and values and incorporates such components into their treatment plan. Promoting culturally competent care has been shown to improve health outcomes for women and girls. Yet barriers to such care remain ongoing problems and disproportionately impact poor, BIPOC, immigrant, and sexual minority women and girls, thereby diminishing their health and reducing health-care-seeking behaviors among these populations. Lack of culturally competent care is especially pronounced in the areas of sexual and reproductive health, mental health, and certain cultural health practices (sometimes referred to as complementary and alternative treatments).

Bias in the US Health-Care System

Sex and gender bias in health care have been documented in medical research, employment, education, and practice. Such bias reflects broader societal gender norms and perpetuates gender inequalities; thus, it violates federal and state laws regarding fair and equal treatment in health care. Such bias also runs counter to ethics as defined by professional health organizations including the American Medical Association, American College of Obstetricians and Gynecologists, and American Nurses Association. Various organizations and advocacy groups (e.g., the Women's Health Movement, American Medical Women's Association, Black Women's Health Imperative, Asian Women for Health, and Gay and Lesbian Medical Association) continue to challenge such bias as part of ongoing efforts to advocate for sex and gender equity in the US health-care system.

Historically, women have been excluded and underrepresented as participants in clinical trials. Thus, the physical body and health needs of men and their responses to various surgical, dietary, behavioral, and pharmaceutical treatments have largely been regarded as "the norm" in medical research. Some well-known examples include the Physicians' Health Study and the Multiple Risk Factor Intervention Trial; both focused on heart disease and then applied their findings to all populations, despite the fact that women have different risk factors for and symptoms of heart disease than men. Similarly, the Baltimore Longitudinal Study of Aging excluded women for the first 20 years. Even when research has focused specifically on women's health issues—such as uterine cancer, breast cancer, and menopause—women have sometimes been excluded. Such exclusion minimizes and denies the very real and important differences in anatomy, hormones, chromosomes, and other biological factors between cisgender women and cisgender men. Although women's inclusion in clinical trials has increased over the past 50 years, it is still not on par with men. This is especially true for BIPOC and elderly women. Furthermore, the digital divide exacerbates such disparities, particularly as studies that rely on electronic recruitment methods have markedly lower rates of BIPOC women as participants than studies that use more traditional recruitment methods. Consequently, evidence-based understanding of the health needs and efficacy of various types of treatment for diverse groups of women remains inadequate.

Gender bias has also been documented in medical education and employment. Women constitute over half of those admitted to and who graduate from medical schools. Yet they hold less than 25 percent of all faculty and leadership positions in such institutions. Gender disparities are also evident among the health-care workforce. Ninety percent of all nurses are women, yet women represent only about one-third of all physicians. Female physicians tend to be concentrated in obstetrics and gynecology, pediatrics, palliative care, and dermatology but underrepresented in higher-paying specialties such as neurology, thoracic surgery, orthopedics, oncology, cardiology, and vascular surgery. The gender wage gap persists in health-care professions and women are less likely than men to receive promotions but more likely to report difficulty maintaining an effective work-life balance. Sexual harassment remains an ongoing problem in health care, and BIPOC women are disproportionately the targets of such harassment. Estimates indicate that half of all female health-care workers and nearly 80 percent of female nurses experience sexual harassment from co-workers, patients, or family members of patients.

Yet gender bias is also pervasive in health-care practice. Such bias diminishes quality of care and health outcomes; it disproportionately impacts BIPOC, poor, elderly, lesbian, and bisexual women and those with disabilities. When women and girls seek care, their symptoms are often dismissed or minimized by health-care providers; this is well documented in relation to anxiety, depression, chest pain, and suicidal ideation. They are more likely than men to be given sedatives than analgesics for pain and face longer wait times when they do receive pain medication. Women also encounter longer wait times for emergency care, surgical procedures, and organ transplantation. Among patients with heart disease, women are more often advised to modify their diet and increase physical activity, but men are more often given medication. In addition, abuse of women in the realm of sexual and reproductive health persists. Such abuse has been recognized as a violation of basic human rights and medical ethics, yet it takes a variety of forms including obstetric violence, coercive contraceptive practices (including forced sterilization), and lack of informed consent for various medical procedures used during childbirth.

LIVING ENVIRONMENT AND SOCIAL CONTEXT

Environmental and social factors bear considerably on the health and well-being of women and girls. They are more likely than men and boys to live in unhealthy built environments and to be exposed to certain harmful components of natural environments. This is especially true for low-income populations and those who lack secure housing. Gendered social norms and related gender roles remain a salient feature of American society. Research consistently links such norms and roles to health, demonstrating that more traditional ideas about gender are linked to diminished well-being for women and girls.

Neighborhoods and Housing

Health problems that stem from living environment—including both natural environment and built spaces—are more common in women and girls. Some of these differences have been linked to biological and physiological factors such as sex hormones, women's lower average body weight, and women's higher average percentage of body fat (a key consideration in relation to fat soluble toxins). Yet others reflect economic disparities. Because they are more likely to live in poverty, women and girls face increased risk of exposure to contaminated air and water, extreme weather conditions, natural disasters (such as hurricanes, tornadoes, monsoons, wildfires, and droughts), and vector-borne diseases (such as those transmitted by insects, animals, viruses, rodents, and other species). Low-income women and girls also are more likely to live and work in areas with toxic building materials such as asbestos, phthalates, insecticides, and volatile organic compounds.

Socioeconomic status is also a key consideration when examining the health-related aspects of built environments, including in urban, suburban, and rural areas. Examinations of community health demonstrate a clear link between health and average household income. Those who reside in communities where incomes meet or exceed national averages are generally healthier and have longer average life expectancy than those in poorer communities. Some of this is due to the lifestyle choices available to those with higher incomes. However, the overall economy and related tax base within a community also confers what are known as place-based health benefits. This means that residents of middle-income and high-income communities generally enjoy health benefits as a result of their access to higher-quality infrastructure related to education, health care, employment, housing, social opportunities, commerce, and recreational activities. Those living in more affluent communities have better access to nutritious food, parks and green spaces, reliable transportation, and safety services (e.g., fire departments and police services). Such communities are also generally more accessible for those with disabilities.

In contrast, low-income communities continue to be plagued by persistent segregation, low-quality and inadequate housing, overcrowding, weak infrastructure, pollution, and disinvestment. Such factors undermine economic opportunities for residents, thereby perpetuating the cycle of poverty and impairing health. Nutritional health is a significant concern in poor communities particularly due to limited access to healthy food options and overconcentration of fast-food restaurants and convenience stores. Targeted advertising for tobacco products, soft drinks, fast food, and alcohol has also been shown to have a negative impact on health of residents in low-income communities. Given their overrepresentation among America's poor, BIPOC, disabled, elderly, lesbian, and bisexual women and girls are especially vulnerable to the place-based health risks. Furthermore, women and girls who cannot afford stable housing are especially vulnerable to health risks due to physical and sexual violence.

Gendered Social Roles and Health Impacts

Gendered social roles continue to influence the experiences and opportunities available to women and girls. In 2021, the United States ranked lower than Canada, most high-income European nations, and several middle- and low-income nations in Central America, Africa, and eastern Europe in regard to gender equality. Discriminatory attitudes that diminish women's opportunities and their achievements have been documented in all American social institutions, including employment, education, families, government, legislation, and religion. Additionally, women's political empowerment and safety remain ongoing concerns. This is not to suggest that all women and girls have the same experiences with sex and gender discrimination. Indeed, such discrimination manifests differently for different subpopulations depending on social identities and access to resources.

The community in which an individual is born and raised has a significant influence on their attitudes about gender equality as adults. Those who grow up in areas where gender norms are more rigid and reflect the belief that women's interests and skills are fundamentally different from and inferior to men's are more likely to espouse such ideas in adulthood. This is true not only for men but also for women and has been shown to influence women's decisions about employment, marriage, and childbearing. Attitudes about the importance of combatting sexism in American society are sharply divided along political lines as well as by age and educational attainment. Those with a bachelor's degree, who are Democrats, and under age 35 are more likely to identify gender inequity as an ongoing problem in American society than less educated, Republican, and older populations. There are also significant variations by geographic region. Women's rights and opportunities are strongest in the northeast, upper Midwest, and on the west coast while attitudes that regard women as subordinate to men and that reinforce rigid gender roles remain more prominent in southern states and non-coastal western states. Women are twice as likely as men to indicate that more needs to be done to combat existing gender inequalities.

Gendered social roles are evident in caretaking work. Within the context of heterosexual, married, cisgender relationships, women continue to be tasked with majority of unpaid work associated with caring for children, elderly, or ill family members. Additionally, and because women continue to be tasked with the majority of household cleaning tasks, they are more frequently exposed to cleaning products and solvents. Many of these substances contain neurotoxins, carcinogens, endocrine disruptors, and caustic ingredients. They can irritate the eyes, skin, and respiratory tract and have been linked to respiratory ailments, headaches, chemical burns, allergic reactions, and certain types of cancer.

Women also continue to be tasked with the majority of emotional labor and practical tasks involved in maintaining social relationships on behalf of the family unit. This includes planning and communicating with extended family about holidays and celebrations. It also includes managing the family calendar and planning recreational and leisure pursuits for families. Women who do not have children or who do not participate in caretaking work are often deemed unfeminine and selfish; they are frequently socially marginalized within their families and broader communities. The gendering of emotional labor has also been noted among adolescents in relation to social events and celebrations. It has also been documented in workplace settings as women are more often expected to provide emotional support, solve interpersonal conflicts among co-workers, and arrange social activities even when such tasks are not part of their formal work responsibilities. Yet women's emotional work also involves modifying their affect in order to appease others and present themselves as more feminine. This is evident, for example, among political candidates and elected officials. BIPOC women often feel increased pressure to engage in such emotional modification due to stereotypes about their supposed inherent emotionality.

Gender roles and related discrimination have been shown to contribute to chronic stress among women and girls. Such stress is associated with higher incidence and severity of depression, anxiety, and PTSD. Furthermore, it contributes to lowered self-confidence and self-esteem, factors that have been linked to increased risk of eating disorders and self-harming behaviors as well as decreased performance in education and employment. Stress also contributes to many chronic physical health conditions among women and girls including chronic pain, musculoskeletal disorders, high blood pressure, digestive issues, diabetes, and sleep disturbances. It is also associated with higher rates of tobacco, drug, and alcohol use and abuse as well as higher incidence of unintended pregnancy and STDs. Chronic stress related to gender norms has been linked to interpersonal conflict: women and girls who experience sex and gender discrimination are more likely to have unhealthy relationships with family, friends, and co-workers. Chronic stress can also lead to burnout, a condition characterized by exhaustion, reduced ability to manage responsibilities, social disengagement, and increased feelings of pessimism, distrust, and low self-worth.

Gender-Based Violence

Gender-based violence (GBV) refers to harmful acts that target individuals because of their gender identity or sex. Common forms include intimate partner violence (IPV), sexual harassment, and sexual violence (including rape and sexual assault). However, other forms of GBV such as forced sterilization, obstetric violence, and stalking have received increasing attention in recent years. Although GBV can and does impact men and boys, women and girls are most often the victims of such violence, both in the United States and globally. The US Department of State and the US Department of Justice have recognized GBV as an ongoing threat to national security and a significant public health problem. Despite efforts from federal, state, and local governments, including the Violence against Women Act of 1994, such violence persists and has been documented among all demographic groups. However, data demonstrates that BIPOC women, women with disabilities, lesbian, bisexual, and incarcerated women are disproportionately impacted by such violence.

IPV (sometimes referred to as domestic violence, dating violence, or family violence) refers to violence between individuals involved in a marital, dating, or familial relationship. It can include physical acts, threats, coercion, verbal abuse, economic abuse, social isolation, blaming, and intimidation in an effort to control or exercise power over an individual. While IPV most often occurs between spouses or dating partners, it has been documented in other relationships as well including abuse of parents by minor children, abuse between siblings, and abuse between in-laws. IPV that occurs in marriage or between dating partners can occur during the relationship or after it has ended. Approximately one in four adult women will be the victim of IPV that involves physical acts of violence during her lifetime. However, IPV remains underreported. Even prior to puberty, many girls have been socialized to accept IPV as a normal part of interpersonal and romantic relationships. By the time they reach adulthood, 40 percent of young women will have experienced some form of abuse in a dating relationship. Such abuse among younger generations increasingly involves use of digital formats (such as texting) and social media.

Common mental health disorders among IPV survivors include anxiety, depression, suicidal ideation, and PTSD. Due to the shame and embarrassment common among survivors of IPV, they often self-isolate and disconnect from their support networks, something that leaves them more vulnerable to the influence of their abuser. The physical abuse associated with IPV often causes bruises, sprains, broken bones, concussions, missing teeth, cuts, and burns. IPV also increases risk of miscarriage, stillbirth, pregnancy complications, and risk of death. When IPV occurs in a household or other setting where a gun is present, a woman is five times more likely to be killed by her abuser. Although IPV most directly harms the physical and psychological health of the victim, there are also risks to others who witness such abuse. PTSD, behavioral disorders, substance abuse, anxiety disorders, emotional detachment, interpersonal conflict, and depression are common among children and teenagers who grow up in households where IPV occurs. There have been increased efforts to train law enforcement officers and health-care providers to recognize and respond to signs of IPV. Yet such training is limited, and many continue to criticize the dismissive attitudes demonstrated by some professionals in relation to IPV.

Some groups of women and girls are particularly vulnerable to GBV. Nearly four-fifths of Indigenous women will be victims of IPV during their lifetimes and they are murdered at a rate 10 times the national average. Furthermore, and despite the fact that thousands of Indigenous individuals are missing in the United States, law enforcement investigations into their disappearances are often mishandled and done in a cursory manner. Such disappearances are also underreported by news media, something that inhibits efforts to locate missing individuals. In November 2021, President Biden issued an executive order to address the crisis of murdered and missing Indigenous Americans. Yet critics argue that such an order does little to change dominant attitudes that continue to marginalize Indigenous women and girls, both in the United States more broadly and in their own communities. Undocumented immigrant women and girls are also especially vulnerable to gender-based violence. Although some enter the United States seeking work, others are trafficked into the country. National data indicate that half of all trafficking victims are adult women while another one-fourth are minor girls. GBV is often used by employers and traffickers to intimidate, punish, or otherwise control undocumented women and girls. Many of these women and girls encounter language barriers that diminish their ability to seek legal or medical support when such violence occurs. Yet others are fearful that if they report such violence, they will be prosecuted for not entering the country through legal channels.

Sexual violence is another type of GBV. It sometimes occurs within the context of IPV. However, it is perpetrated in a wide variety of contexts including in the workplace as well as military, correctional, health care, educational, and religious institutions. Sexual violence takes various forms including sexual assault (unwanted sexual touching or forcing someone to perform sex acts), rape (forced or coerced sexual activity that involves penetration), incest (between immediate family members), child sexual abuse (perpetrated against a minor), drug-facilitated abuse (when alcohol or controlled substances are used to impair the victim's ability to provide consent), and sexual harassment (unwanted touching, sexual advances, statements, or related activities that occur in work or educational settings). Sexual violence costs the United States just over $125 billion each year due to medical care, legal and judicial services, social support, and lost productivity. At present, less than 2 percent of perpetrators of sexual violence are convicted.

Legal definitions of sexual violence vary from state to state. Although such violence remains underreported, it is estimated that over 1,200 individuals are victims of sexual assault every day in the United States. Ninety percent of victims of rape are women and nearly one-fifth of American women will be victims of rape or attempted rape during their lifetimes. In most cases of sexual violence, the perpetrator is known to the victim; the majority of sexual assaults occur in or near the victims' home or another location frequented by the victim (such as their workplace, school, or the home of a friend or relative). Victims of sexual violence experience some of the same health risks as victims of other forms of GBV but are at greater risk for STDs, unintended pregnancy, and trauma to the genital region.

Representation in Community Leadership

Gender norms also contribute to the ongoing marginalization of women and girls in political leadership. Although ambition, assertiveness, and decisiveness are often regarded as advantageous—and even essential—for male politicians, voters are more likely to deem such traits undesirable for female politicians. Despite the increase in the number of women elected to US Congress in 2019, gender parity in politics remains elusive and, consequently, women's perspectives and needs remain marginalized. At present, only 27 percent of US Congressional seats, one-third of elected statewide positions, and one-fourth of mayorships for cities with populations over 30,000 are held by women. Only one woman, Kamala Devi Harris, has ever been elected to serve as vice president of the United States and no woman has ever been elected president. Disparities by race are even more pronounced: BIPOC women represent only one-fifth of all women in the US Congress, one-fourth of women governors, and one-third of women in state legislatures. In addition, young women and poor women are underrepresented among elected officials. Women who are Republicans are less likely to be elected than Democrats.

Women continue to be underrepresented in other leadership positions as well, including in religious institutions. Orthodox Jews, Latter-Day Saints, Southern Baptists, and Roman Catholics do not permit women to be ordained. Among major religions that do allow women clerics, over half have never had a female in the top leadership position. Moreover, the total number of women who have ever been appointed to a top leadership position among all major religious groups in the United States remains in the single digits. Girls who grow up with female clergy as role models benefit both psychologically and with regard to educational achievement. However, many Americans remain opposed to women as religious leaders. Such attitudes are more pronounced among men than women and among Evangelicals.

Influence of Popular Culture

Studies of television, movies, advertisements, magazines, video games, and other genres of popular culture demonstrate that traditional gender norms and related stereotypes are pervasive. Even preschool-aged children internalize such representations in ways that impact their neurological functioning and, thus, influence how they make sense of the world and interact with others. Women and girls continue to be demeaned and objectified in popular culture. Females are more often presented as supporting characters rather than in leading roles, something that has been shown to diminish girls' self-esteem and their perception of opportunities available to females. Common stereotypes portray women as overly emotional, primarily interested in the domestic sphere, naive, and obsessed with relationships, appearance, and shopping. BIPOC and immigrant women remain underrepresented in popular culture. When included, they are often portrayed as less feminine and less attractive than white women born in the United States, particularly via caricatures that represent them as bossy, angry, criminal, or scheming to take advantage of men or government support systems. Other times, they are exoticized, hyper-sexualized, de-humanized, and presented as sexual deviants, something evident in stereotypes of the Black Jezebel, the Asian temptress, and the spicy Latina. Indigenous women remain largely absent in American popular culture; when they are represented, they are often cast as a love interest of a white man, the target of sexual violence, or played by white actors (a practice commonly referred to as "whitewashing"). Women over 50 and those with disabilities continue to be underrepresented in popular culture and are typically portrayed as asexual and in poor health. Heterosexual, young, white, attractive, thin, and able-bodied females continue to be overrepresented.

Gender stereotypes in popular culture have been linked to various types of violence against women and girls, including IPV, rape, sexual assault, and sexual harassment. In addition, the internalization of such stereotypes decreases satisfaction with appearance and body image among women and girls, thereby increasing their risk for eating disorders. In recent years, social media platforms have been particularly scrutinized and criticized for reinforcing unrealistic standards of beauty and contributing to eating disorders, especially among teens and young adults. Gender norms in popular culture also encourage women and girls to alter their appearance and appeal through body modification and beautification. Thus, it is common for them to use perfume, hair dyes, and cosmetics as well as salon procedures such as artificial nails, eyelash extensions, or modification of the hair (including extensions, perms, chemical straightening, and bleaching). Such substances and procedures expose users to a variety of hazardous chemicals and have been linked to increased risk of respiratory problems, chemical burns, vision problems, skin irritation, headaches, and damage to organs including the lungs, kidneys, and liver. For those employed in salons—who are disproportionately BIPOC women—the risks are even more pronounced due to regular exposure to toxins as part of their work responsibilities. Although some cosmetic brands and salons offer nontoxic and organic options, these are typically considerably more expensive than standard options and, therefore, not affordable to most women and girls.

Yet popular culture increasingly serves as a way to contest and disrupt traditional gender norms and related roles. Some films, television programs, video games, and even children's books have been noted for creating more dynamic and authentic portrayals of women and girls and presenting them in more active roles. Thus, and given the ways it influences people both emotionally and cognitively, popular culture can also serve as an avenue to challenge biases and foster social change that promotes more egalitarian and equitable gender norms in American culture.

BIBLIOGRAPHY AND FURTHER READING

Chapter 1: Asian, Pacific Islander, and Desi American (APIDA) Populations

Acoba, Jared, Susie A. Chen, Charles F. Miller, and Ian Okazaki. *Understanding and Improving Lung Cancer Treatment in Asian Americans and Pacific Islanders in the Community Setting.* Rockville, MD: Hawaii Society for Clinical Oncology (accessed July 5, 2022). https://www.accc-cancer.org/docs/projects/resources/pdf/LungCancerTools/aapi-whitepaper.

Act to Change. *2021 Asian American Bullying Survey Report.* Walnut, California: Act to Change, 2021. https://acttochange.org/wp-content/uploads/2021/05/Asian-American-Bullying-Report_FINAL.pdf.

Balingit, Mirah, Hannah Natanson, and Yutao Chen. "As Schools Reopen, Asian American Students Are Missing from Classrooms." *The Washington Post.* March 4, 2021. https://www.washingtonpost.com/education/asian-american-students-home-school-in-person-pandemic/2021/03/02/eb7056bc-7786-11eb-8115-9ad5e9c02117_story.html.

Casabianca, Sandra Silva. "Asian-American Racism Takes Devastating Toll on Community." *PsychCentral.* March 24, 2021. https://psychcentral.com/news/anti-asian-racism-mental-health-impact.

Chau, Victoria, and Perry Chan. "One Size Does Not Fit All: Appreciating the Diversity of Asian Americans, Native Hawaiians, and Pacific Islanders (AANHPI) and the Implications for Mental Health." *Substance Abuse and Mental Health Services Administration, U.S. Department of Health and Human Services* (blog). May 25, 2021. https://www.samhsa.gov/blog/one-size-does-not-fit-all-appreciating-diversity-asian-americans-native-hawaiians-pacific.

Chen, Moon S., Jr., and Julie Dang. "Hepatitis B among Asian Americans: Prevalence, Progress, and Prospects for Control." *World Journal of Gastroenterology* 21, 42 (November 14, 2015): 11924–30. https://www.ncbi.nlm.nih.gov/pmc/articles/PMC4641114/.

Chu, Rose C., and Benjamin D. Sommers. *Health Insurance Coverage Changes since Implementation of the Affordable Care Act: Asian Americans and Pacific Islanders.* Issue Brief No. HP-2021-11. Washington, DC: Office of the Assistant Secretary for Planning and Evaluation, U.S. Department of Health and Human Services, 2021.

Cumming, Carmen Sanchez, and Kathryn Zickuhr. "Jobs Report: Amid Continued Job Gains, Asian American, Native Hawaiian, and Pacific Islander Workers Experience the U.S. Labor Market in Different and Often Hidden Ways." *Washington Center for Equitable Growth.* May 6, 2022. https://equitablegrowth.org/jobs-report-amid-continued-job-gains-asian-american-native-hawaiian-and-pacific-islander-workers-experience-the-u-s-labor-market-in-different-and-often-hidden-ways/.

DeQuattro, Kimberly, Laura Trupin, Louse B. Murphy, Stephanie Rush, Lindsey A. Criswell, Cristina M. Lanata, Maria Dall-Era, Patricia Katz, and Jinoos Yazdany. "High Disease Severity among Asian Patients in a US Multiethnic Cohort of Individuals with Systemic Lupus Erythematosus." *Arthritis Care and Research* 74, 6 (June 2022): 896–903.

Do, Quyen A., Joyce P. Yang, Karie A. Gaska, Kayla Knopp, and Shelby B. Scott. "Centering Asian American Women's Health: Prevalence of Health Care Discrimination and Associated Health Outcomes." *Journal of Racial and Ethnic Health Disparities* (February 23, 2022). https://link.springer.com/article/10.1007/s40615-022-01267-w.

Holland, Ariel T., and Latha P. Palaniappan. "Problems with the Collection and Interpretation of Asian-American Health Data: Omission, Aggregation, and Extrapolation." *Annals of Epidemiology* 22, 6 (2012): 397–405.

Hollister, Sarah. "Placenta Burial Rituals." *Placenta Risks: Sonoma County Breastfeeding Coalition.* August 16, 2018. https://placentarisks.org/wp-content/uploads/2018/09/Placenta-burial-rituals-from-around-the-world-handout.pdf.

Hu, Cathy. "Fighting the Stigma: Mental Health among Asian Americans and Pacific Islanders." *Urban Institute*. May 20, 2019. https://www.urban.org/urban-wire/fighting-stigma-mental-health-among-asian-americans-and-pacific-islanders.

Jang, Yuri, and Miyong T. Kim. "Limited English Proficiency and the Health Service Use in Asian Americans." *Journal of Immigrant and Minority Health* 21, 2 (April 2019): 264–70. https://www.ncbi.nlm.nih.gov/pmc/articles/PMC6252148/.

Kawakami, Keilyn Leina'ala, Shelley Muneoka, Rachel L. Burrage, Leslie Tanoue, Kilohana Haitsuka, and Kathryn L. Braun. "The Lives of Native Hawaiian Elders and Their Experiences with Health Care." *Frontiers in Public Health* 2022, 10 (February 22, 2022). https://www.ncbi.nlm.nih.gov/pmc/articles/PMC8902069/ #:~:text=Colonization%20led%20to%20militarization%2C%20widespread,Hawaiians%20(27%E2%80%9329.

Lim, Sungwoo, Stella S. Yi, Nneka Lundy de la Cruz, and Chau Trinh-Shervin. "Defining Ethnic Enclave and Its Association with Self-Reported Health Outcomes among Asian Americans in New York City." *Journal of Immigrant and Minority Health* 19, 1 (2017): 138–46. https://stacks.cdc.gov/view/cdc/40039.

Liou, Wayne, Eugene Tian, and Joseph Roos. *Hawaii's Labor Market Impact during COVID-19.* Honolulu, Hawaii: State of Hawaii Department of Business, Economic Development, and Tourism, 2021.

Liu, Ruyu. "Not Your Model Minority: Asian Americans Face Food Insecurity." *Nutribites: Nutrition Research, One Bite at a Time.* May 5, 2021. https://nutribites.blog/2021/05/05/not-your-model-minority-asian-americans-face-food-insecurity/.

McTaggart, Ninochka, Michele Meyer, Meredith Conroy, Romeo Perez, Cameron Espinoza, Sarah Trinh, Pamela Campos, Emma Burrows, Jenna Virgo, Camryn Brennan, Isabel Dolan, Cris Ackel, and Sofie Christensen. *I Am Not a Fetish or Model Minority: Redefining What It Means to Be API in the Entertainment Industry*. Los Angeles, CA: Geena Davis Institute on Gender in Media, 2021.

Menath, Anisha. "Let's Talk about APIDA Mental Health and the Impact of COVID-19." *Pactie-Cal Matters*. November 10, 2021. https://pacificties.org/lets-talk-about-apida-mental-health-and-the-impact-of-covid-19/.

Min, Lucy Y., Rehnuma B. Islam, Nikhila Gandrakota, and Megha K. Shah. "The Social Determinants of Health Associated with Cardiometabolic Diseases among Asian American Subgroups: A Systematic Review." *BMC Health Services Research* 22, 257 (February 25, 2022). https://bmchealthservres.biomedcentral.com/articles/10.1186/s12913-022-07646-7.

Morey, Brittney N., Gilbert C. Gee, Salma Shariff-Marco, Juan Yang, Laura Allen, and Scarlett Lin Gomez. "Ethnic Enclaves, Discrimination, and Stress among Asian American Women: Differences by Nativity and Time in the United States." *Cultural Diversity and Ethnic Minority Psychology* 26, 4 (2020): 460–71.

Namkung, Victoria. "Why Asian American Kids Are Under-Diagnosed When It Comes to Learning Disabilities." *NBCnews.com*. October 1, 2021. https://www.nbcnews.com/news/asian-america/asian-american-kids-are-diagnosed-comes-learning-disabilities-rcna2425.

Nguyen, Bach Mai Dolly, Pedro Noguera, Nathan Adkins, and Robert T. Teranishi. "Ethnic Discipline Gap: Unseen Dimensions of Racial Disproportionality in School Discipline." *American Educational Research Journal* 56, 5 (2019): 1973–2003.

Pang, Daniel, and Jung Hun Choi. "Why Does Homeownership Vary So Widely within the AAPI Community?" *Urban Institute*. December 15, 2021. https://www.urban.org/urban-wire/why-does-homeownership-vary-so-widely-within-aapi-community.

Pillai, Drishti, Aggie J. Yellow Horse, and Russell Jeung. *The Rising Tide of Violence and Discrimination against Asian American and Pacific Islander Women and Girls*. stopaapihate.org. 2021. https://stopaapihate.org/aapi-women-and-girls-report/.

Pillai, Drishti, Nambi Ndugga, and Samantha Artiga. "Health Care Disparities among Asian, Native Hawaiian, and Other Pacific Islander (NHOPI) People." *KFF: Kaiser Family Foundation*. May 27, 2022. https://www.kff.org/racial-equity-and-health-policy/issue-brief/health-care-disparities-among-asian-native-hawaiian-and-other-pacific-islander-nhopi-people/.

Rubin-Miller, Lily, Christopher Alban, Samantha Artiga, and Sean Sullivan. "COVID-19 Racial Disparities in Testing, Infection, Hospitalization, and Death: Analysis of Patient Epic Data." *KFF: Kaiser Family Foundation*. September 16, 2020. https://www.kff.org/report-section/covid-19-racial-disparities-in-testing-infection-hospitalization-and-death-analysis-of-epic-patient-data-issue-brief/.

Sabato, Todd M. "Deconstructing the Model Minority Myth: Exploring Health Risk Behaviors of American Asian and Pacific Islander Young Adults." *Journal of Health Disparities Research and Practice* 10, 3 (Fall 2017): 136–52.

Westfall, Chris. "Battling Discrimination and the Bamboo Ceiling." *Forbes*. September 14, 2021. https://www.forbes.com/sites/chriswestfall/2021/09/14/discrimination-and-bamboo-ceiling-the-unconscious-bias-facing-asian-american-managers/?sh=69e01d1023dc.

Williams, Andrew D., Lynne C. Messer, Jenna Kanner, Sandie Ha, Katherine L. Gantz, and Pauline Mendola. "Ethnic Enclaves and Pregnancy and Behavior Outcomes among Asian/Pacific Islanders in the USA." *Journal of Racial and Ethnic Health Disparities* 7, 2 (2020): 224–33. https://www.ncbi.nlm.nih.gov/pmc/articles/PMC7104626/.

Yi, Stella S., Simona C. Kwon, Rachel Suss, Lan N. Đoàn, Iyanrick John, Nadia S. Islam, and Chau Trinh-Shevrin. "The Mutually Reinforcing Cycle of Poor Quality Data and Racialized Stereotypes That Shapes Asian American Health." *Health Affairs* 41, 2 (February 2022). https://www.healthaffairs.org/doi/10.1377/hlthaff.2021.01417.

Yuen, Nancy Wang, Stacy L. Smith, Katherine Pieper, Marc Choueiti, Kevin Yao, and Dana Dinh. *The Prevalence and Portrayal of Asian and Pacific Islanders across 1,300 Popular Films*. Los Angeles, California: USC Annenberg Inclusion Initiative, May 2021. https://www.nytimes.com/2021/05/18/movies/asian-pacific-islanders-film.html.

Chapter 2: Black Populations

Amuchie, Nnennaya. "'The Forgotten Victims' How Racialized Gender Stereotypes Lead to Police Violence against Black Women and Girls: Incorporating an Analysis of Police Violence into Feminist Jurisprudence and Community Activism." *Seattle Journal for Social Justice* 14, 3 (2018): 627–68.

Asare, Janice Gassam. "3 Ways Intergenerational Trauma Still Impacts the Black Community Today." *Forbes*. February 14, 2022. www.forbes.com/sites/janicegassam/2022/02/14/3-ways-intergenerational-trauma-still-impacts-the-black-community-today/?sh=766850e93cf6.

"Black and African American Communities and Mental Health." *Mental Health America*. www.mhanational.org/issues/black-and-african-american-communities-and-mental-health (accessed March 18, 2023).

Carbado, Devon W. *Unreasonable: Black Lives, Police Power, and the Fourth Amendment*. New York: The New Press, 2022.

Chavis, Kami. "The Dangerous Expansion of Stand-Your-Ground Laws and Its Racial Implications." *Duke Center for Firearms Law*. January 18, 2022. https://firearmslaw.duke.edu/2022/01/the-dangerous-expansion-of-stand-your-ground-laws-and-its-racial-implications/.

Choi, Soon Kyu, Bianca D.M. Wilson, and Christy Mallory. "Black LGBT Adults in the US: LGBT Well-Being at the Intersection of Race." *The Williams Institute*. January 2021. https://williamsinstitute.law.ucla.edu/publications/black-lgbt-adults-in-the-us/.

Correll, Joshua, Sean M. Hudson, Steffanie Guillermo, and Debbie S. Ma. "The Police Officer's Dilemma: A Decade of Racial Bias on the Decision to Shoot." *Social and Personality Psychology Compass* 8, 5 (2014): 201–13.

Dennard, Elizabeth, Elizabeth Kristjansson, Nedelina Tchangalova, Sarah Totton, Donna Windham, and Annette O'Connor. "Food Insecurity among African Americans in the United States: A Scoping Review." *PLOS ONE* 17, 9 (2022). https://journals.plos.org/plosone/article?id=10.1371/journal.pone.0274434.

Ellis, Katrina, Hillary K. Hecht, Tiffany L. Young, Seyoung Oh, Shikira Thomas, Lori S. Hoggard, Zaire Ali, Ronke Olawale, Dana Carthron, Giselle Corbie-Smith, and Eugenia Eng. "Chronic Disease among African American Families: A Systematic Scoping Review." *Preventing Chronic Disease: Public Health Research, Practice, and Policy* 17 (December 31, 2020). www.cdc.gov/pcd/issues/2020/19_0431.htm.

Fleming, Kristine M. "Observing from a Lens of Equity: Recognizing the Impact of Segregated Recreation." *Parks & Recreation Magazine*. August 19, 2021. www.nrpa.org/partks-recreation-magazine/2021/september/observing-from-a-lens-of-equity/.

Forde, Allana T., Danielle M. Crookes, Shakira F. Suglia, and Ryan T. Demmer. "The Weathering Hypothesis as an Explanation for Racial Disparities in Health: A Systematic Review." *Annals of Epidemiology* 33 (May 2019): 1–18. www.sciencedirect.com/science/article/pii/S1047279718300802.

Goldhill, Olivia. "Shuttered Hospitals, Soaring COVID-19 Deaths: Rural Black Communities Lose a Lifeline in the Century's Worst Health Crisis." *STAT News*. May 26, 2021. www.statnews.com/2021/05/26/shuttered-hospitals-soaring-covid19-deaths-rural-black-communities-lose-lifeline-in-pandemic/.

Hankerson, Sidney H., Nathalie Moise, Diane Wilson, Bernadine Y. Waller, Kimberly T. Arnold, Cristiane Duarte, Claudio Lugo-Candelas, Myrna M. Weissman, Milton Wainberg, Rachel Yehuda, and Ruth Shim. "The Intergenerational Impact of Structural Racism and Cumulative Trauma of Depression." *The American Journal of Psychiatry* 179, 6 (June 2022). Available: https://ajp.psychiatryonline.org/doi/10.1176/appi.ajp.21101000.

Hasan, Tashfia, Katherine Lucas Mckay, and Joanna Smith-Ramani. *Disparities in Debt: Why Debt Is a Driver in the Racial Wealth Gap*. Washington, DC: The Aspen Institute Financial Security Program, 2022. Available: www.aspeninstitute.org/wp-content/uploads/2022/02/FINAL-ASP-FSW_Disparities-in-Debt_020722-3.pdf.

Heitzig, Nancy A. *The School-to-Prison Pipeline: Education, Discipline, and Racialized Double Standards*. Santa Barbara, CA: Praeger, 2016.

Isong, Inyang A., Sowmya R. Rao, Marie-Abèle Bind, Mauricio Avendaño, Ichiro Kawachi, and Tracy K. Richmond. "Racial and Ethnic Disparities in Early Childhood Obesity." *Pediatrics* 141, 1 (2018): e20170865. Available: www.ncbi.nlm.nih.gov/pmc/articles/PMC5744272/.

Johnson, David Kyle. "Confirmation Bias and Police Brutality." *Psychology Today*. June 1, 2020. www.psychologytoday.com/us/blog/logical-take/202006/confirmation-bias-and-police-brutality.

Loh, Tracy Hadden, Christopher Coes, and Becca Buthe. "The Great Real Estate Reset—Separate and Unequal: Persistent Residential Segregation Is Sustaining Racial and Economic Injustice in the U.S." *Brookings*. December 16, 2020. www.brookings.edu/essay/trend-1-separate-and-unequal-neighborhoods-are-sustaining-racial-and-economic-injustice-in-the-us/.

Mahowald, Lindsay. "Black LGTBQ Individuals Experience Heightened Levels of Discrimination." *Center for American Progress*. July 13, 2021. www.americanprogress.org/article/black-lgbtq-individuals-experience-heightened-levels-discrimination/.

Martin, David. "The Birth of Jim Crow in Alabama, 1865-1896." *National Black Law Journal* 13, 1 (1993): 184–97.

Martin, Kimberly J., Annette L. Stanton, and Kerri L. Johnson. "Current Health Care Experiences, Medical Trust, and COVID-19 Vaccination Intention and Uptake in Black and White Americans." *Health Psychology*, October 13, 2022. https://psycnet.apa.org/fulltext/2023-08280-001.html.

Masters, N. Tatiana, Taryn P. Lindhort, and Marcia K. Meyers. "Jezebel at the Welfare Office: How Racialized Stereotypes of Poor Women's Reproductive Decisions and Relationships Shape Policy Implementation." *Journal of Poverty* 18, 2 (2014): 109–29.

Muvuka, Baraka, Ryan M. Combs, Suur D. Ayangeakaa, Nida M. Ali, Monica L. Wendel, and Trinidad Jackson. "Health Literacy in African-American Communities: Barriers and Strategies." *Health Literacy Research and Practice* 4, 3 (July 2020): e138–e143. www.ncbi.nlm.nih.gov/pmc/articles/PMC7365659/.

Nichols, Andrew Howard. *'Segregation Forever'?: The Continued Underrepresentation of Black and Latino Undergraduates in the Nation's 101 Most Selective Public Colleges and Universities*. Washington, DC: The Education Trust, 2020. https://edtrust.org/wp-content/uploads/2014/09/Segregation-Forever-The-Continued-Underrepresentation-of-Black-and-Latino-Undergraduates-at-the-Nations-101-Most-Selective-Public-Colleges-and-Universities-July-21-2020.pdf.

Omenka, Ogbannaya I., Dennis P. Watson, and Hugh C. Hendrie. "Understanding the Healthcare Experiences and Needs of African Immigrants in the United States: A Scoping Review." *BMC Public Health* 20, 27 (2020). https://bmcpublichealth.biomedcentral.com/articles/10.1186/s12889-019-8127-9.

Parker, Kim, Juliana Horowitz, and Brian Mahl. "On Views of Race and Inequality, Blacks and Whites Are Worlds Apart." *Pew Research Center*. June 27, 2016. www.pewresearch.org/social-trends/2016/06/27/on-views-of-race-and-inequality-blacks-and-whites-are-worlds-apart/.

Parks, Gregory S., and Danielle C. Heard. "'Assassinate the Nigger Ape': Obama, Implicit Imagery, and the Dire Consequences of Racist Jokes." *Cornell Law Faculty Working Papers*. Paper 61. August 14, 2009. http://scholarship.law.cornell.edu/clsops_papers/61.

Pennsylvania Coalition against Rape. *Racism and Sexual Violence: What's the Connection?* Enola, PA: Pennsylvania Coalition against Rape, 2017. https://pcar.org/sites/default/files/resource-pdfs/tab_2017_racismsexual_violence_connections-508d.pdf.

Pittman, Cassi. "'Shopping While Black: Black Consumers' Management of Racial Stigma and Racial Profiling in Retail Settings." *Journal of Consumer Culture* 20, 1 (2020): 3–22.

Profit, Jochen, Jeffrey B. Gould, Mihoko Bennett, Benjamin A. Goldstein, David Draper, Ciaran S. Phibbs, and Henry C. Lee. "Racial/Ethnic Disparity in NICU Quality of Care Delivery." *Pediatrics* 140, 3 (2017). www.ncbi.nlm.nih.gov/pmc/articles/PMC5574732/.

Ramirez, Stephen A. "The Racist Roots of the War on Drugs and the Myth of Equal Protection for People of Color." *University of Arkansas at Little Rock Law Review* 44, 4 (2022). https://lawrepository.ualr.edu/cgi/viewcontent.cgi?article=2106&context=lawreview.

Reyes, Maritza Vasquez. "The Disproportional Impact of COVID-19 on African-Americans." *Health and Human Rights* 22, 2 (December 2020): 299–307. www.ncbi.nlm.nih.gov/pmc/articles/PMC7762908/#:~:text=Approximately%2097.9%20out%20of%20every,Asians%20(40.4%20per%20100%2C000.

Riley, Emmitt Y., and Clarissa Peterson. "I Can't Breathe: Assessing the Role of Racial Resentment and Racial Prejudice in Whites' Feelings Toward Black Lives Matter." *National Review of Black Politics* 1, 4 (2020): 496–515.

Roberts, Dorothy. *Killing the Black Body: Race, Reproduction, and the Meaning of Liberty*. New York: Vintage Books, 1997.

Rothstein, Richard. *The Color of Law: A Forgotten History of How Our Government Segregated America*. New York: W.W. Norton & Company, Inc., 2017.

Sawyer, Wendy. "Visualizing Disparities in Mass Incarceration." *Prison Policy Initiative*. July 27, 2020. www.prisonpolicy.org/blog/2020/07/27/disparities/?gclid=EAIaIQobChMI_oHg2oGt_gIVFO3jBx3gPg2jEAAYASAAEgIoffD_BwE.

Serafini, Kelly, Caitlin Coyer, Joedrecka Brown Speights, Dennis Donovan, Jessica Guh, Judy Washington, and Carla Ainsworth. "Racism as Experienced by Physicians of Color in the Health Care Setting." *Family Medicine* 52, 4 (2020): 282–7.

Tamir, Christine, and Monica Anderson. "One-in-Ten Black People Living in the U.S. Are Immigrants." *Pew Research Center*. January 20, 2022. www.pewresearch.org/race-ethnicity/2022/01/20/one-in-ten-black-people-living-in-the-u-s-are-immigrants/.

Taylor, Jamila. "Racism, Inequality, and Health Care for African Americans." *The Century Foundation*. December 19, 2012. https://tcf.org/content/report/racism-inequality-health-care-african-americans/.

Tormala, Teceta Thomas. "Social Representations of Blackness in America: Stereotypes about Black Immigrants and Black Americans." In *Conceptual and Methodological Approaches to Navigating Immigrant Ecologies*, edited by Hui Chu and Barbara Thelamour, 89–106. New York, NY: Springer Publishing, 2021.

Weller, Christian E. "African Americans Face Systemic Obstacles to Getting Good Jobs." *Center for American Progress*. December 5, 2019. www.americanprogress.org/article/african-americans-face-systematic-obstacles-getting-good-jobs/.

Willis, Henry A., Effua A. Sosoo, Donte L. Bernard, Aaron Neal, and Enrique W. Neblett. "The Associations between Internalized Racism, Racial Identity, and Psychological Distress." *Emerging Adulthood* 9, 4 (2021): 384–400.

Yearby, Ruqaiijah, Brietta Clark, and José F. Figueroa. "Structural Racism in Historical and Modern US Health Care Policy." *Health Affairs* 41, 2 (February 2022). www.healthaffairs.org/doi/10.1377/hlthaff.2021.01466.

Chapter 3: Disabled Populations

Altiraifi, Azza. "Advancing Economic Security for People with Disabilities." *CAP: Center for American Progress*. July 26, 2019. www.americanprogress.org/article/advancing-economic-security-people-disabilities/.

American College of Rheumatology. *Rheumatic Diseases in America: Confronting the Challenge*. simpletasks.org. May 2021. https://simpletasks.org/wp-content/uploads/2021/05/Rheumatic-Diseases-in-America-White-Paper.pdf.

Bureau of Labor Statistics. *Persons with a Disability: Labor Force Characteristics–2022*. USDL-23-0351. Washington, DC: U.S. Department of Labor, 2023. www.bls.gov/news.release/pdf/disabl.pdf.

Centers for Disease Control and Prevention. "Vision Health Initiative." www.cdc.gov/visionhealth/index.htm (accessed May 4, 2023).

Coleman-Jensen, Alisha. "Thirty Years after Enactment of the Americans with Disabilities Act, Disabilities Remain a Risk Factor in Food Insecurity." *Amber Waves Magazine*. December 7, 2020. www.ers.usda.gov/amber-waves/2020/december/thirty-years-after-enactment-of-the-americans-with-disabilities-act-disabilities-remain-a-risk-factor-for-food-insecurity.

Cooks-Campbell, Allaya. "Disability Inclusion in the Workplace: The What, Why, and How." *BetterUp*. September 16, 2021. www.betterup.com/blog/disability-inclusion.

Crossley, Mary. "Disability Cultural Competence in the Medical Profession." *Saint Louis University Journal of Health Law & Policy* 9, 1 (2015): 89–110.

Deighton, Katie. "Disabled Shoppers Struggle with Inaccessible Self-Checkouts." *The Wall Street Journal*. November 21, 2022. www.wsj.com/articles/disabled-shoppers-struggle-with-inaccessible-self-checkouts-11668808226.

Diversability. “Invisible Disabilities 101: What You Need to Know.” January 30, 2021. https://mydiversability.com/blog/invisible-disabilities.

Garland-Thomson, Rosemarie. *Extraordinary Bodies: Figuring Physical Disability in American Culture and Literature*. 20th Anniversary Ed. New York, NY: Columbia University Press, 2017.

Gilmour, Allison F., Douglas Fuchs, and Joseph H. Wehby. “Are Students with Disabilities Accessing the Curriculum? A Meta-Analysis of the Reading Achievement Gap between Students with and without Disabilities.” *Exceptional Child* 85, 3 (2018): 329–46.

Goodman, Nanette, Bonnie O’Day, and Michael Morris. *Financial Capability of Adults with Disabilities*. Washington, DC: National Disability Institute, 2019. www.nationaldisabilityinstitute.org/wp-content/uploads/2019/01/ndi-finra-report-2017.pdf.

Grigorovich, Alisa. “Governing ‘Risky’ Sexualities: Representations of Dementia and Sexuality in the New Media.” *Disability Studies Quarterly* 40, 3 (2020). https://dsq-sds.org/article/view/6877/5704.

Harrell, Erika. “Crime against People with Disabilities, 2009-2019: Statistical Tables.” NCJ 301367. *Bureau of Justice Statistics*. November 2021. https://bjs.ojp.gov/content/pub/pdf/capd0919st.pdf.

Houchins, David E., Wendy Peia Oakes, and Zachary G. Johnson. “Bullying and Students with Disabilities: A Systematic Literature Review of Intervention Studies.” *Remedial and Special Education* 37, 5 (2016): 259–73.

Iezzoni, Lisa I., Sowmya R. Rao, Julia Ressalam, Dragana Bolcic-Jankovic, Nicole D. Agaraonnik, Karen Donelan, Tara Lagu, and Eric G. Campbell. “Physicians’ Perceptions of People with Disabilities and Their Health Care.” *Health Affairs* 40, 2 (2021). www.healthaffairs.org/doi/10.1377/hlthaff.2020.01452?url_ver=Z39.88-2003&rfr_id=ori%3Arid%3Acrossref.org&rfr_dat=cr_pub±±0pubmed.

Johnson, Richard W. *Later-Life Household Wealth before and after Disability Onset*. Washington, DC: The Urban Institute, 2017. www.urban.org/sites/default/files/publication/90531/later-life_household-wealth-before-and-after-disability-onset.pdf.

Jones, Angela. “‘I Can’t Really Work Any “Normal” Job’: Disability, Sexual Ableism, and Sex Work.” *Disability Studies Quarterly*. Special Issue on Sex Work and Disability. 42, 2 (2022). https://dsq-sds.org/index.php/dsq/article/view/9094/7750.

Kaye, H. Stephen. “Disability-Related Disparities in Access to Health Care before (2009-2010) and after (2015-2017) The Affordable Care Act.” *AJPH: American Journal of Public Health* 109, 7 (July 2019): 1015–2021. https://ajph.aphapublications.org/doi/pdf/10.2105/AJPH.2019.305056?role=tab.

Kennedy, Jae, and Elizabeth G. Wood. *Disability-Based Disparities in Social Determinants of Health among Working-Age Adults: Evidence from the 2018 National Health Interviews Survey*. Spokane, WA: Collaborative on Health Reform and Independent Living, 2020.

Kenyon, Mara. “What Is SPD? Sensory Processing Disorder 101.” *NAPA*. May 18, 2020. https://napacenter.org/what-is-a-sensory-processing-disorder/.

Lagu, Tara, Carol Haywood, Kimberly Reimold, Christene DeJong, Robin Walker Sterling, and Lisa I. Iezonni. “‘I Am Not the Doctor for You’: Physicians’ Attitudes about Caring for People with Disabilities.” *Health Affairs* 41, 10 (2022). www.healthaffairs.org/doi/full/10.1377/hlthaff.2022.00475.

Lake, Jaboa, Valeria Novack, and Mia Ives-Rublee. “Recognizing and Addressing Housing Insecurity for Disabled Renters.” *CAP: Center for American Progress*. May 27, 2021. www.americanprogress.org/article/recognizing-addressing-housing-insecurity-disabled-renters/.

Longmore, Paul K. *Why I Burned My Book and Other Essays on Disability*. Philadelphia, PA: Temple University Press, 2003.

Mader, Jackie. “How Teacher Training Hinders Special Needs Students.” *The Atlantic*. March 1, 2017. www.theatlantic.com/education/archive/2017/03/how-teacher-training-hinders-special-needs-students/518286/.

Marini, Irmo, Noreen M. Graf, and Michael J. Millington. *Psychosocial Aspects of Disability: Insider Perspectives and Strategies for Counselors*. New York, NY: Springer Publishing Company, 2018.

Minnesota Governor's Council on Developmental Disabilities. *Parallels in Time: A History of Developmental Disabilities*. https://mn.gov/mnddc/parallels/index.html (accessed May 12, 2023).

National Center for College Students with Disabilities. https://nccsd.ici.umn.edu (accessed May 12, 2023).

National Center for Education Statistics. "Table 1: Public high school 4-year adjusted cohort graduation rate (ACGR), by race/ethnicity and selected demographic characteristics for the United States, the 50 states, the District of Columbia, and Puerto Rico: School year 2019–20." *Common Core of Data: America's Public Schools* (accessed May 3, 2023). https://nces.ed.gov/ccd/tables/ACGR_RE_and_characteristics_2019-20.asp.

National Council on Disability. *The Current State of Health Care for People with Disabilities*. www.ncd.gov/publications/2009/Sept302009#Gaps (accessed May 12, 2023).

Ouellette, Alicia. "People with Disabilities in Human Subjects Research: A History of Exploitation, a Problem of Exclusion." Albany Law School Research Paper. November 22, 2019. Available: https://papers.ssrn.com/sol3/papers.cfm?abstract_id=3492078.

Perry, David M., and Lawrence Carter-Long. *The Ruderman White Paper on Media Coverage of Law Enforcement Use of Force and Disability: A Media Study (2013-2015) and Overview*. Boston, MA: Ruderman Family Foundation, March 2016. https://rudermanfoundation.org/wp-content/uploads/2017/08/MediaStudy-PoliceDisability_final-final.pdf.

Pham, Bach. "The Challenges of Eating and Grocery Shopping for People with Disabilities." *Free Times*. September 25, 2019. www.postandcourier.com/free-times/food/the-challenges-of-eating-and-grocery-shopping-for-people-with-disabilities/article_8d129a08-def3-11e9-a89c-03c56ff37a80.html.

Rembis, Michael, Catherine J. Kudlick, and Kim E. Nielsen, eds. *The Oxford Handbook of Disability History*. New York, NY: Oxford University Press, 2018.

Richards, Stephen B., Michael P. Brady, and Ronald L. Taylor. *Cognitive and Intellectual Disabilities: Historical Perspectives, Current Practices, and Future Directions*. New York: Routledge, 2015.

Saleh, Naveed. "How the Stigma of Mental Health Is Spread by the Media." *Verywell Mind*. January 16, 2023. www.verywellmind.com/mental-health-stigmas-in-mass-media-4153888.

Scheckler, Samara, Jennifer Molinsky, and Whitney Airgood-Obrycki. "How Well Does Housing Stock Meet Accessibility Needs? An Analysis of the 2019 American Housing Survey." *Joint Center for Housing Studies, Harvard University*. March 2022. www.jchs.harvard.edu/sites/default/files/research/files/harvard_jchs_housing_stock_accessibility_scheckler_2022_0.pdf.

Schifter, Laura A., Todd Grindal, Gabriel Schwartz, and Thomas Hehir. "Students from Low-Income Families and Special Education." *The Century Foundation*. January 17, 2019. https://tcf.org/content/report/students-low-income-families-special-education/.

Thomas, Katie. "The Story of Thalidomide in the U.S., Told Through Documents." *The New York Times*. March 23, 2020. www.nytimes.com/2020/03/23/health/thalidomide-fda-documents.html.

United Nations Office at Geneva. "Disability Inclusive Language Guidelines." www.ungeneva.org/sites/default/files/2021-01/Disability-Inclusive-Language-Guidelines.pdf (accessed April 25, 2023).

U.S. Department of Health and Human Services. "National CLAS Standards." *Think Cultural Health*. https://thinkculturalhealth.hhs.gov/clas (accessed May 15, 2023).

VanPuymbrouck, Laura, Carli Friedman, and Heather Feldner. "Explicit and Implicit Disability Attitudes of Healthcare Providers." *Rehabilitation Psychology*, 65, 2 (2020): 101–12.

Villegas, Tim. "A History of Educating Children with Disabilities in America." *Think Inclusive*. June 22, 2021. www.thinkinclusive.us/post/young-man-with-an-autistic-twin-brother-makes-documentary-about-the-history-of-special-education.

Wang, Ziru, Xiaoli Xu, Qiong Han, Jiayao Jiang, Guo-Xin Ni. "Factors Associated with Public Attitudes towards Persons with Disabilities: A Systematic Review." *BMC Public Health* 21, 1058 (2021). https://bmcpublichealth.biomedcentral.com/articles/10.1186/s12889-021-11139-3.

Welding, Lyss. "Students with Disabilities in Higher Education: Facts and Statistics." *Best Colleges*. March 29, 2023. www.bestcolleges.com/research/students-with-disabilities-higher-education-statistics/#:~:text=College%20Graduation&text=Nearly%2020%25%20of%20 25-34,doubled%20between%202008%20and%202021.

Woodgate, Roberta L., Miriam Gonzalez, Lisa Demczuk, Wanda M. Snow, Sarah Barriage, and Susan Kirk. "How Do Peers Promote Social Inclusion of Children with Disabilities? A Mixed-Methods Systematic Review." *Disability and Rehabilitation* 42, 18 (2020): 2553–79.

Chapter 4: Elderly Populations

Administration on Aging. *2020 Profile of Older Americans*. Washington, DC: U.S. Department of Health and Human Services, Administration on Community Living, 2021. https://acl.gov/sites/default/files/Aging%20and%20Disability%20in%20America/2020ProfileOlderAmericans.Final_.pdf.

Administration on Aging. *Profile of American Indians and Alaskan Natives Age 65 and Over*. Washington, DC: U.S. Department of Health and Human Services, Administration on Community Living, 2017. https://acl.gov/sites/default/files/Aging%20and%20Disability%20 in%20America/2017OAProfileAIAN508.pdf.

Axelrod, Josh, Samantha Balaban, and Scott Simon. "Isolated and Struggling, Many Seniors Are Turning to Suicide." *NPR: National Public Radio*. July 27, 2019. https://www.npr.org/2019/07/27/745017374/isolated-and-struggling-many-seniors-are-turning-to-suicide.

Bellport, Lori. "How Understanding the 5 Stages of Aging Can Help with Aging in Place." *Live in Place Designs*. https://liveinplacedesigns.com/the-5-stages-of-aging-at-home/ (accessed June 9, 2022).

Borelli, Cara M., Dara Grennan, and Christopher C. Muth. "Causes of Memory Loss in Elderly Persons." *Journal of the American Medical Association* 323, 5 (2020): 486. https://jamanetwork.com/journals/jama/fullarticle/2760393.

Bowsher, Karla. "Here's How Much Retiree Households Spend in a Year." *Money Talks News*. September 27, 2021. https://www.moneytalksnews.com/4-genius-ways-to-protect-your-retirement-savings/.

Christ, Amber, and Tracey Gronniger. *Older Women and Poverty*. Washington, DC: Justice in Aging, 2020. https://justiceinaging.org/wp-content/uploads/2020/08/Older-Women-and-Poverty.pdf.

Cohen, Robin A., Amy E. Cha, Emily P. Terlizzi, and Michael E. Martinez. "Demographic Variation in Health Insurance Coverage: United States, 2019." *National Health Statistics Reports*. No. 159 (June 29, 2021). https://www.cdc.gov/nchs/data/nhsr/nhsr159-508.pdf.

Cromartie, John. "Rural Aging Occurs in Different Places for Very Different Reasons." *U.S. Department of Agriculture*. July 30, 2021. https://www.usda.gov/media/blog/2018/12/20/rural-aging-occurs-different-places-very-different-reasons#:~:text=As%20the%20United%20 States%20population,in%20urban%20(metro)%20areas.

Cubanski, Juliette, Wyatt Koma, Anthony Damico, and Tricia Neuman. "How Many Seniors Live in Poverty?" *KFF: Kaiser Family Foundation*. November 19, 2018. https://www.kff.org/report-section/how-many-seniors-live-in-poverty-issue-brief/#:~:text=There%20are%20some%20 notable%20gender,14.1%25%20of%20older%20Hispanic%20men.

Dionigi, Rylee A. "Stereotypes of Aging: Their Effects on the Health of Older Adults." *Journal of Geriatrics* 2015 (November 12, 2015). https://www.hindawi.com/journals/jger/2015/954027/.

Doyle, Latasha. "4 Cultural Differences to Be Mindful of When Caring for Seniors." *Care.com*. February 18, 2021. https://www.care.com/c/cultural-differences-caring-for-seniors/.

"Elder Abuse." *National Institute on Aging*. July 29, 2020. https://www.nia.nih.gov/health/elder-abuse.

Estes, Clary. "Historic High Rates of STIs among Older Americans." *Forbes*. February 26, 2020. https://www.forbes.com/sites/claryestes/2020/02/26/historic-high-rates-of-stis-among-older-americans/?sh=71ee87f64c39.

Ford-Martin, Paula. "Types of Dementia." *WebMD*. September 29, 2020. https://www.webmd.com/alzheimers/guide/alzheimers-dementia#091e9c5e8001055b-2-7.

Gaugler, Joseph, Tricia Johnson, Allison Marin, and Jennifer Weuve. "2020 Alzheimer's Disease Facts and Figures." *Alzheimer's & Dementia* 16 (2020): 391–460. https://alz-journals.onlinelibrary.wiley.com/doi/epdf/10.1002/alz.12068.

"Get the Facts on Falls Prevention." *NCOA: National Council on Aging*. June 14, 2021. https://www.ncoa.org/article/get-the-facts-on-falls-prevention.

Ghosh, Palash. "A Third of Seniors Seek to Work Well Past Retirement Age, Or Won't Retire at All, Poll Finds." *Forbes*. May 6, 2021. https://www.forbes.com/sites/palashghosh/2021/05/06/a-third-of-seniors-seek-to-work-well-past-retirement-age-or-wont-retire-at-all-poll-finds/?sh=514c02726b95.

Graham, Judith. "'They Treat Me Like I'm Old and Stupid': Seniors Decry Health Providers' Bias." *KHN: Kaiser Health News*. October 20, 2021. https://khn.org/news/article/ageism-health-care-seniors-decry-bias-inappropriate-treatment/.

Hartline-Grafton, Heather. "Hunger Is a Health Issue for Older Adults: Food Insecurity, Health, and Federal Nutrition Programs." *Food Research & Action Center*. December 2019. https://frac.org/wp-content/uploads/hunger-is-a-health-issue-for-older-adults-1.pdf.

"Hearing Loss: A Common Problem for Older Adults." *National Institute on Aging*. https://www.nia.nih.gov/health/hearing-loss-common-problem-older-adults (accessed June 13, 2022).

"Higher Ed, Lower Risk." *ALZ Magazine* (Summer 2021). https://www.alz.org/news/2021/higher-ed-lower-risk.

Jacobson, Gretchen, Aimee Cicchiello, Arnav Shah, Michelle M. Doty, and Reginald D. Williams. "When Costs Are a Barrier to Getting Health Care: Reports from Older Adults in the United States and Other High-Income Countries." *The Commonwealth Fund*. October 1, 2021. https://www.commonwealthfund.org/publications/surveys/2021/oct/when-costs-are-barrier-getting-health-care-older-adults-survey#:~:text=Key%20Findings%3A%20One%2Dfifth%20of,%2Dof%2Dpocket%20health%20costs.

Jaffe, Ina. "Older Americans Are Increasingly Unwilling—or Unable—to Retire." *NPR: National Public Radio*. October 2, 2019. https://www.npr.org/2019/10/02/751797229/the-new-realities-of-work-and-retirement.

Kernisan, Leslie, and Paula Spencer Scott. *When Your Aging Parent Needs Help: A Geriatrician's Step-By-Step Guide to Memory Loss, Resistance, Safety Worries, and More*. San Francisco: Better Health While Aging, 2021.

Kushel, Margot. "Homelessness among Older Adults: An Emerging Crisis." *Generations Journal* (Summer 2020). https://generations.asaging.org/homelessness-older-adults-poverty-health.

Lamb, Sandra. "When Thinner Isn't Better: Extra Pounds May Keep Some People Healthier after a Certain Age." *AARP*. June 13, 2019. https://www.aarp.org/health/healthy-living/info-2019/weight-concerns-after-80.html.

Lem, Ellyn A. *Gray Matters: Finding Meaning in the Stories of Later Life*. New Brunswick, NJ: Rutgers University Press, 2020.

Morrow-Howell, Nancy, Natalie Galucia, Emma Swinford, and Tanner Meyer. "Challenges and Opportunities of Age Diverse Universities: Perspectives from Admissions and Career Services." *Gerontology & Geriatrics Education* (December 17, 2020). https://cpb-us-w2.wpmucdn.com/sites.wustl.edu/dist/1/2391/files/2021/02/Challenges-and-opportunities-of-age-diverse-universities_-Perspectives_FINAL_PUBLISHED.pdf.

Mullen, Nadia, Arne Stinchcombe, Charles Seguin, Shawn Marshall, Gary Naglie, Mark J. Rapoport, Holly Tuokko, and Michel Bédard. "Perceived Community Age-Friendliness Is Associated with Quality of Life among Older Adults." *Journal of Applied Gerontology* 41, 5 (2022): 1274–82.

Newman, Michelle G., and Nur Hani Zainal. "The Value of Maintaining Social Connections for Mental Health in Older People." *Lancet Public Health* 5, 1 (January 2020): e12–e13. https://www.ncbi.nlm.nih.gov/pmc/articles/PMC7261393/.

Pacific ADA Center, ADA National Network. *Health Care and the Americans with Disabilities Act*. 2020. https://adata.org/sites/adata.org/files/files/Health%20Care%20and%20the%20ADA%20FINAL%202-11-2020.pdf.

Papke, David Ray. "Ageism in American Culture." *Hedgehogs and Foxes: The Law and Humanities Blog*. August 7, 2018. https://hedgehogsandfoxes.org/index.php/2018/08/07/ageism-in-american-culture/.

Peters, Matthew E., and Raquel C. Gardner. "Traumatic Brain Injury in Older Adults: Do We Need a Different Approach?" *Concussion* 3, 3 (September 20, 2018). https://www.futuremedicine.com/doi/10.2217/cnc-2018-0001.

Prunhuber, Patti, and Vivian Kwok. *Issue Brief: Low-Income Older Adults Face Unaffordable Rents, Driving Housing Instability and Homelessness*. Washington, DC: Justice in Aging, February 2021. https://justiceinaging.org/wp-content/uploads/2021/02/Older-Adults-Rental-Housing-Burdens.pdf.

Remillard, Elena T., Margaret L. Campbell, Lyndsie M. Koon, and Wendy A. Rogers. "Transportation Challenges for Persons Aging with Mobility Disability: Qualitative Insights and Policy Implications." *Disability and Health Journal* 15, 1 Supplement (January 2022). https://www.sciencedirect.com/science/article/pii/S1936657421001825.

Rosenfeld, Jordan. "Seniors Need Sexual Healthcare Too." Medical Economics. May 1, 2019. https://www.medicaleconomics.com/view/seniors-need-sexual-healthcare-too.

Sadighi Akha, Amir A. "Aging and the Immune System: An Overview." *Journal of Immunological Methods* 463 (December 2018): 21–6.

Schanzenbach, Diane Whitmore, Ryan Nunn, and Lauren Bauer. *The Changing Landscape of American Life Expectancy*. Washington, DC: The Hamilton Project, June 2016. https://www.hamiltonproject.org/assets/files/changing_landscape_american_life_expectancy.pdf.

Seegert, Liz. "Doctors Are Ageist—and It's Harming Older Patients." *NBCnews.com*. June 26, 2019. https://www.nbcnews.com/think/opinion/doctors-are-ageist-it-s-harming-older-patients-ncna1022286.

Selassie, Gelila. "Health Disparities Facing Older Adults of Color amid COVID-19: Guest Blog by Justice in Aging." *National Health Law Program*. August 24, 2020. https://healthlaw.org/health-disparities-facing-older-adults-of-color-amid-covid-19-guest-blog-by-justice-in-aging/.

"Senior Consumer Debt Report, 2020: Credit Cards, Auto Loans, Mortgages for Ages 65+ and COVID-19." *SeniorLiving.org*. October 6, 2020. https://www.seniorliving.org/senior-debt-annual-report/.

Shirey, Lee, and Laura Summer. "Obesity among Older Americans." *Health Policy Institute, Georgetown University*. https://hpi.georgetown.edu/obesity2/ (accessed June 15, 2022).

Smith, Stacy L., Katherine Pieper, Marc Choueiti, Artur Tofan, Anne-Marie Depauw, and Ariana Case. *Seniors on the Small Screen: Aging in Popular Television Content*. Los Angeles, CA: USC Annenberg School for Journalism and Communication, 2017. https://assets.uscannenberg.org/docs/Seniors_on_the_Small_Screen-Dr_Stacy_L_Smith_9-12-17.pdf.

Span, Paula. "Exploring the Health Effects of Ageism." *The New York Times*. April 23, 2022. https://www.nytimes.com/2022/04/23/health/ageism-levy-elderly.html

Tepper, Taylor. "America's Seniors in Debt: A Growing Problem." *Forbes*. March 29, 2021. https://www.forbes.com/advisor/retirement/seniors-debt-statistics/.

Terry, Sabrina. "Poor Older People: The Graying of Racial and Gender Wealth Inequality." *National Community Reinvestment Coalition*. November 20, 2019. https://ncrc.org/poor-old-people-the-graying-of-racial-and-gender-wealth-inequality/.

"The U.S. Population Is Aging." *The Urban Institute*. https://www.urban.org/policy-centers/cross-center-initiatives/program-retirement-policy/projects/data-warehouse/what-future-holds/us-population-aging#:~:text=The%20US%20Population%20Is%20Aging%20%7C%20Urban%20Institute&text=The%20number%20of%20Americans%20ages,quadruple%20between%202000%20and%202040 (accessed June 9, 2022).

"Tips for Improving Communication with Older Patients." *National Institute for Aging*. https://www.nia.nih.gov/health/tips-improving-communication-older-patients (accessed June 15, 2022).

Torborg, Lisa. "Mayo Clinic Q and A: Weight Loss in Older Adults Can Signal Underlying Issues." *Mayo Clinic News Network*. August 11, 2015. https://newsnetwork.mayoclinic.org/discussion/mayo-clinic-q-and-a-weight-loss-in-older-adults-can-signal-underlying-health-issue/.

Tran, Victoria. "Asian American Seniors Are Often Left out of the National Conversation on Poverty." *The Urban Institute*. May 31, 2017. https://www.urban.org/urban-wire/asian-american-seniors-are-often-left-out-national-conversation-poverty.

Waggoner, John. "Student Loan Debt Is an Unheralded Burden for Older Borrowers." *AARP*. October 30, 2021. https://www.aarp.org/money/credit-loans-debt/info-2021/student-debt-crisis-for-older-americans.html#:~:text=Of%20the%20%241.6%20trillion%20in,five%2Dfold%20increase%20from%202004.

Weiss, Barry D. "Elder Care Provider Professional Sheets: Health Literacy." *Arizona Center on Aging, University of Arizona College of Medicine, Tucson*. August 2019. https://www.uofazcenteronaging.com/care-sheet/providers/health-literacy.

Wisniewski, Molly. "Understanding Terms of Endearment: The 'Do's' and 'Don'ts' of Calling the Older Adults in Our Care 'Sweetie' and 'Honey'." *The Upside of Aging* (blog). January 30, 2018. https://theupsidetoaging.com/2018/01/30/%E2%80%8Bunderstanding-terms-of-endearment-the-dos-and-donts-of-calling-the-older-adults-in-our-care-sweetie-or-honey-%E2%80%8B/.

Woody, Imani. "Suicide and LGBTQ+/SGL Older Adults." *SAGE Advocacy & Services for LGBTQ+ Elders*. March 21, 2016. https://www.sageusa.org/suicide-and-lgbtqsgl-older-adults/.

Chapter 5: Hispanic, Latinx, Chicanx (HLC) Populations

Arciniega, G. Miguel, and Terence J. G. Tracey. "Toward a Fuller Concept of Machismo: Development of a Traditional Machismo and Caballerismo Scale." *Journal of Counseling Psychology* 55, 1 (2008): 19–33. http://www.ncdsv.org/images/JCP_TowardFullerConceptionMachismo_2008.pdf.

Asante-Muhammad, Dedrick, and Diego Hernandez. "Latinos, the Racial Wealth Divide and Rebuilding the American Middle Class." *National Community Reinvestment Coalition*. October 15, 2019. https://ncrc.org/latinos-the-racial-wealth-divide-and-rebuilding-the-american-middle-class/.

Barna, Mike. "Life Expectancy for US Hispanics Drops Drastically during Pandemic." *The Nation's Health* 51, 7 (2021): 9. https://www.thenationshealth.org/content/51/7/9.1.

Blossom, Priscilla. "We Need to Talk about Marianismo." *HipLATINA*. March 13, 2018. https://hiplatina.com/marianismo/.

Brown, Sarah, and Katherine Mangan. "Everyone Wants to Be a Hispanic Serving Institution." *Chronicle of Higher Education*. December 1, 2021. https://www.chronicle.com/article/everyone-wants-to-be-a-hispanic-serving-institution.

Carrazana, Chabeli. "On LGBTQ+ Equal Pay Day, the U.S. Still Doesn't Know the Size of the Wage Gap." *PBS.org*. June 16, 2021. https://www.pbs.org/newshour/economy/on-lgbtq-equal-pay-day-the-u-s-still-doesnt-know-the-size-of-the-wage-gap.

Case, Ariana, Zoily Mercado, and Karla Hernandez. *Hispanic and Latino Representation in Film: Erasure on Screen and behind the Camera across 1,300 Popular Movies*. Los Angeles, CA: USC Annenberg Inclusion Initiative, September 2021. https://assets.uscannenberg.org/docs/aii-hispanic-latino-rep-2021-09-13.pdf.

Chabram-Dernersesian, Angie, and Adela de la Torre. *Speaking from the Body: Latinas on Health and Culture*. Tucson, AZ: University of Arizona Press, 2008.

Chong, Nilda. *The Latino Patient: A Cultural Guide for Health Care Providers*. Boston, MA: Intercultural Press, 2002.

Esperanza United. *Latinas and Intimate Partner Violence: Evidence-Based Facts.* St. Paul, MN: Esperanza United, 2021. https://esperanzaunited.org/wp-content/uploads/2021/09/3.11.73-Factsheet_GeneralIPV2021-1.pdf.

Espinoza, Omar. "Social and Economic Factors Leading to Health Disparities in the Latino Populations Living in the United States." *Grace Peterson Nursing Research Colloquium* 4 (2019). https://via.library.depaul.edu/cgi/viewcontent.cgi?article=1367&context=nursing-colloquium.

Frey, William H. "Neighborhood Segregation Persists for Black, Latino or Hispanic, and Asian Americans." *Brookings*. April 6, 2021. https://www.brookings.edu/research/neighborhood-segregation-persists-for-black-latino-or-hispanic-and-asian-americans/.

Gándara, Patricia. "The Potential and Promise of Latino Students." *American Educator*. Spring 2017. https://www.aft.org/ae/spring2017/gandara.

Gast, Julie, Terry Peak, and Anne Hunt. "Latino Health Behavior: An Exploratory Analysis of Health Risk and Health Protective Factors in a Community Sample." *American Journal of Lifestyle Medicine* 14, 1 (2017): 97–106.

Grace, Karen Trister, Kamila A. Alexander, Noelene K. Jeffers, Elizabeth Miller, Michele R. Decker, Jacquelyn Campbell, and Nancy Glass. "Experiences of Reproductive Coercion among Latina Women and Strategies for Minimizing Harms: 'The Path Makes Us Strong.'" *Journal of Midwifery and Women's Health* 65, 2 (March 2020): 248–56.

Gramlich, John. "Hispanic Dropout Rate Hits New Low, College Enrollment at New High." *Pew Research Center*. September 29, 2017. https://www.pewresearch.org/fact-tank/2017/09/29/hispanic-dropout-rate-hits-new-low-college-enrollment-at-new-high/.

Green Latinos. "Fact Sheet: Latino Communities and the Climate Crisis." *Environmental Defense Fund*. October 2020. https://www.edf.org/sites/default/files/documents/LatinosandtheClimateCrisis_Factsheet_Oct2020_Final3.pdf.

Grover, Michael. "What a $400 Emergency Expense Tells Us about the Economy." *Federal Reserve Bank of Minneapolis*. June 11, 2021. https://www.minneapolisfed.org/article/2021/what-a-400-dollar-emergency-expense-tells-us-about-the-economy.

Guerrero, Erick, Dennis Kao, and Brian E. Perron. "Travel Distance to Outpatient Substance Use Disorder Treatment Facilities for Spanish-Speaking Clients." *International Journal of Drug Policy* 24, 1 (2013): 38–45.

Guzman, Joseph. "Hate Crimes against Latinos Rose in 2019 Pushing Overall Figure to Highest in a Decade." *The Hill*. November 17, 2020. https://thehill.com/changing-america/respect/equality/526364-hate-crimes-against-latinos-rose-in-2019-pushing-overall.

Haro, Alein Y., Randall Kuhn, Michael A. Rodriguez, Nik Theodore, Edwin Melendez, and Abel Valenzuela, Jr. "Beyond Occupational Hazards: Abuse of Day Laborers and Health." *Journal of Immigrant and Minority Health* 22 (2020): 1172–83.

Klerman, Jacob Alex, and Michelle Blocklin. "Tailoring Job Training Programs for Hispanics." *National Research Center on Hispanic Children and Families*. April 17, 2019. https://www.hispanicresearchcenter.org/research-resources/tailoring-job-training-programs-for-hispanics/.

Krogstad, Jens Manuel, and Mark Hugo Lopez. "Coronavirus Economic Downtown Has Hit Latinos Especially Hard." *Pew Research Center*. August 4, 2020. https://www.pewresearch.org/hispanic/2020/08/04/coronavirus-economic-downturn-has-hit-latinos-especially-hard/.

"Latinx/Hispanic Communities and Mental Health." *Mental Health America* (accessed February 22, 2022). https://www.mhanational.org/issues/latinxhispanic-communities-and-mental-health#:~:text=Serious%20mental%20illness%20(SMI)%20rose,range%20between%20 2008%20and%202018.

Machado, Amanda. "Why Many Latinos Dread Going to the Doctor: How Cultural Barriers Can Be More Important Than Income." *The Atlantic*. May 7, 2014. https://www.theatlantic.com/health/archive/2014/05/why-many-latinos-dread-going-to-the-doctor/361547/.

Mahowold, Lindsay. "Hispanic LGBTQ Individuals Encounter Heightened Discrimination." *Center for American Progress*. July 29, 2021 https://www.americanprogress.org/article/hispanic-lgbtq-individuals-encounter-heightened-discrimination/.

Mays, Mackenzie. "Why Are Birth Rates Higher for Latina Teens Than Others? It's Complicated, Experts Say." *USC Center for Health Journalism*. July 23, 2017. https://centerforhealthjournalism.org/fellowships/projects/why-are-birth-rates-higher-latina-teens-others-it%E2%80%99s-complicated-experts-say.

Medina, Yolanda. "Low Literacy Hispanics: A Case Study." Presented at Literacy Texas Conference, February 2017. Available: https://present5.com/low-literacy-hispanics-a-case-study-mrs-yolanda/.

Mireles-Rios, Rebeca, Victor M. Rios, and Augustina Reyes. "Pushed out for Missing School: The Role of Social Disparities and School Truancy in Dropping Out." *Education Sciences* 14, 4 (2020): 108–22. https://www.mdpi.com/2227-7102/10/4/108/htm.

Mora, G. Cristina. *Making Hispanics: How Activists, Bureaucrats, and the Media Constructed a New American*. Chicago, IL: University of Chicago Press, 2014.

Mora, Marie T., and Alberto Dávila. "The Hispanic-White Wage Gap Has Remained Wide and Relatively Steady." *Economic Policy Institute*. July 2, 2018. https://www.epi.org/publication/the-hispanic-white-wage-gap-has-remained-wide-and-relatively-steady-examining-hispanic-white-gaps-in-wages-unemployment-labor-force-participation-and-education-by-gender-immigrant/.

National Partnership for Women and Families. *Beyond Wages: Effects of the Latina Wage Gap*. Washington, DC: National Partnership for Women and Families, March 2021. https://www.nationalpartnership.org/our-work/resources/economic-justice/fair-pay/latinas-wage-gap.pdf.

Office of the Assistant Secretary for Planning and Evaluation, U.S. Department of Health and Human Services. *Health Insurance Coverage and Access to Care among Latinos: Recent Trends and Key Challenges*. Issue Brief No. HP-2021-2. Washington, DC: U.S. Department of Health and Human Services. October 2021. https://aspe.hhs.gov/sites/default/files/documents/68c78e2f b15209dd191cf9b0b1380fb8/ASPE_Latino_Health_Coverage_IB.pdf.

"*Promotores y Promotoras de Salud*." MHP Salud. https://mhpsalud.org/our-chw-initiatives/promotoras-de-salud/ (accessed March 9, 2022).

Rivera, David B., John P. Brady, and Aaron J. Blashill. "Traditional Machismo, Caballerismo, and the Pre-Exposure Prophylaxis (PrEP) Cascade among a Sample of Latino Sexual Minority Men." *Journal of Sexual Research* 58, 1 (2021): 21–8.

Rivera, Gustavo. *Television Viewing and Latino Stereotypes*. University of the Pacific, Thesis. 2021. https://scholarlycommons.pacific.edu/uop_etds/3756.

Rundle, Anne, Maria Carvalho, and Mary Robinson, eds. *Cultural Competence in Health Care: A Practical Guide*. San Francisco, CA: Jossey-Bass, 2002.

Sanchez, Claudio. "English Language Learners: How Your State Is Doing?" *NPR.org*. February 23, 2017. https://www.npr.org/sections/ed/2017/02/23/512451228/5-million-english-language-learners-a-vast-pool-of-talent-at-risk.

Shapiro, Doug, Afet Dundar, Faye Huie, Phoebe Khasiala Wakhungu, Xin Yuan, Angel Nathan, and Youngsik Hwang. *Completing College: A National View of Student Attainment Rates by Race and Ethnicity – Fall 2010 Cohort* (Signature Report No. 12b). Herndon, VA: National Student Clearinghouse Research Center, 2017. https://nscresearchcenter.org/wp-content/uploads/Signature12-RaceEthnicity.pdf.

Simón, Yara. "Latino, Hispanic, Latinx, Chicano: The History behind the Terms." *History.com*. September 16, 2020. https://www.history.com/news/hispanic-latino-latinx-chicano-background.

U.S. Bureau of Labor Statistics. "Household Data Annual Averages, Employed Persons by Detailed Industry, Sex, Race, and Hispanic or Latino Identity." *U.S. Bureau of Labor Statistics*. January 20, 2022. https://www.bls.gov/cps/cpsaat18.htm.

Vázquez, Karina Elizabeth, Sadie Wenger, and Danny Frascella. "Vulnerable Bodies: Domestic Violence in the Hispanic/Latinx Community during a Pandemic." *Latinx Talk*. October 15, 2020. https://latinxtalk.org/2020/10/15/vulnerable-bodies-domestic-violence-in-the-hispanic-latinx-community-during-a-pandemic/.

Wilson, Biana D.M., Christy Mallory, Lauren Bouton, and Soon Kyu Choi. *Latinx LGBT Adults in the US: Well-Being at the Intersection of Race*. Los Angeles, CA: UCLA School of Law Williams Institute, 2021. https://williamsinstitute.law.ucla.edu/wp-content/uploads/LGBT-Latinx-SES-Sep-2021.pdf.

Zamarripa, Ryan, and Lorena Roque. "Latinos Face Disproportionate Health and Economic Impacts from COVID-19." *Center for American Progress*. March 5, 2021. https://www.americanprogress.org/article/latinos-face-disproportionate-health-economic-impacts-covid-19/#:~:text=Effects%20of%20COVID%2D19%20on%20Latino%20employment&text=The%20initial%20employment%20shock%20from,a%2014.2%20percentage%2Dpoint%20jump.

Chapter 6: Homeless and Housing Insecure Populations

ACOG Committee on Health Care for Underserved Women. *Health Care for Homeless Women*. Committee Opinion No. 576. Washington, DC: American College of Obstetricians and Gynecologists, 2013. https://www.acog.org/-/media/project/acog/acogorg/clinical/files/committee-opinion/articles/2013/10/health-care-for-homeless-women.pdf.

Andrews, Jeff. "Zumper National Rent Report." *Zumper.com*. January 27, 2022. https://www.zumper.com/blog/rental-price-data/.

Balasuriya, Lilanthi, Eliza Buelt, and Jack Tsai. "The Never-Ending Loop: Homeless, Psychiatric Disorder, and Mortality." *Psychiatric Times* 37, 5 (May 29, 2020). https://www.psychiatrictimes.com/view/never-ending-loop-homelessness-psychiatric-disorder-and-mortality.

Bersin, Josh. "Why Aren't Wages Keeping Up? It's Not the Economy, It's Management." *Forbes*. October 31, 2018. https://www.forbes.com/sites/joshbersin/2018/10/31/why-arent-wages-keeping-up-its-not-the-economy-its-management/?sh=310ca3f2397e.

Boone, Alistair. "Why Can't We Get an Accurate Count of the Homeless Population?" *Pacific Standard*. March 7, 2019. https://psmag.com/social-justice/why-cant-we-count-the-homeless-population.

Capps, Kristin. "The High Cost of Clearing Tent Cities." *Bloomberg*. April 12, 2021. https://www.bloomberg.com/news/articles/2021-04-12/the-high-cost-of-clearing-homeless-encampments.

Centers for Disease Control and Prevention. "Homelessness as a Public Health Law Issue: Selected Resources." March 2, 2017. https://www.cdc.gov/phlp/publications/topic/resources/resources-homelessness.html.

Centers for Disease Control and Prevention. "Interim Guidance on People Experiencing Unsheltered Homelessness." February 10, 2022. https://www.cdc.gov/coronavirus/2019-ncov/community/homeless-shelters/unsheltered-homelessness.html.

Cooper, David, Elise Gould, and Ben Zipperer. "Low Wage Workers Are Suffering from a Decline in the Real Value of the Federal Minimum Wage." *Economic Policy Institute*. August 27, 2019. https://www.epi.org/publication/labor-day-2019-minimum-wage/.

DiPietro, Barbara. "Five Ways Medicaid Expansion Is Helping Homeless Populations Ten Years after The ACA Became Law." *Health Affairs Forefront*. February 27, 2020. https://www.healthaffairs.org/do/10.1377/forefront.20200225.434660/full/.

Flach, Yuri, and Timothy S. Razza. "Suicidality in Homeless Children and Adolescents: A Systematic Review." *Aggression and Violent Behavior* 64 (2022): 1–9.

Gilens, Martin. *Why Americans Hate Welfare: Race, Media, and the Politics of Antipoverty Policy*. Chicago, IL: University of Chicago Press, 1999.

Gilmer, Cyndi, and Kristy Buccieri. "Homeless Patients Associate Clinician Bias with Suboptimal Care for Mental Illness, Addictions, and Chronic Pain." *Journal of Primary Care and Community Health* 11 (2020): 1–7. https://www.ncbi.nlm.nih.gov/pmc/articles/PMC7059226/pdf/10.1177_2150132720910289.pdf.

Golabek-Goldman, Sarah. "Ban the Address: Combating Employment Discrimination against the Homeless." *The Yale Law Journal* 126, 6 (2017): 1788–868. https://www.yalelawjournal.org/pdf/h.1788.Golabek-Goldman.1868_9wo15f6u.pdf.

Grajo, Lenin C., Sharon A. Gutman, Hannah Gelb, Katie Langan, Karen Marx, Devon Paciello, Christie Santana, Ashley Sgandurra, and Krysti Teng. "Effectiveness of a Functional Literacy Program for Sheltered Homeless Adults." OTJR: Occupation, Participation, and Health 40, 1 (2019): 17–26. https://journals.sagepub.com/doi/pdf/10.1177/1539449219850126.

Grumet, Julie Goldstein. *Improving Care for Homeless Patients at Risk for Suicide*. Washington, DC: Zero Suicide Institute. January 30, 2018. https://zerosuicide.edc.org/sites/default/files/Zero%20Suicide%20Improving%20Care%20for%20Homeless%20Patients%20at%20Risk%20for%20Suicide%201.30.18.PPT_.Transcript.pdf.

Holtzman, Ben. "When the Homeless Took Over." *Shelterforce: The Original Voice of Community Development*. October 11, 2019. https://shelterforce.org/2019/10/11/when-the-homeless-took-over/.

Howard, Miles. "Tiny Houses—Not a Big Enough Solution." *Shelterforce*. January 10, 2020. https://shelterforce.org/2020/01/10/tiny-houses-not-a-big-enough-solution/.

HUD Exchange. "Homelessness Assistance Programs." U.S. Department of Housing and Urban Development. https://www.hudexchange.info/homelessness-assistance/ (accessed February 8, 2022).

Hu, Winnie. "'Hostile Architecture': How Public Spaces Keep the Public Out." *The New York Times*. November 8, 2019. https://www.nytimes.com/2019/11/08/nyregion/hostile-architecture-nyc.html.

Ingram, Erin S., John M. Bridgeland, Bruce Reed, and Matthew Atwell. *Hidden in Plain Sight: Homeless Students in America's Public Schools*. Washington, DC: Civic Enterprises and Hart Research Associates, 2017. https://www.americaspromise.org/sites/default/files/d8/2016-12/HiddeninPlainSightFullReportFINAL_0.pdf.

Kaste, Martin. "Homeless Camps Are Often Blamed for Crime but Experts Say It's Not So Simple." *NPR*. January 24, 2022. https://www.npr.org/2022/01/24/1074577305/homeless-crime-experts.

Kelly-Blake, Karen. "Patient Dumping: Why Are Patients Disposable?" *MSU Bioethics*. July 26, 2018. https://msubioethics.com/2018/07/26/patient-dumping-why-are-patients-disposable/.

Kritz, Fran. "Expired, Lost, and Stolen: Cell Phones, Critical for Homeless People, Can Be Tough to Get and Keep." *California Health Report*. January 11, 2019. https://www.calhealthreport.org/2019/01/11/expired-lost-stolen-cell-phones-critical-homeless-people-can-tough-get-keep/.

Kusmer, Kenneth. *Down and Out on the Road: The Homeless in American History*. New York: Oxford University Press, 2002.

Lee, Alexandria. "Disparities in Health Care for the Homeless." *Loma Linda University Health, Institute for Health Policy and Leadership*. January 22, 2021. https://ihpl.llu.edu/blog/disparities-health-care-homeless.

"Median Sales Price of Houses Sold for the United States." *Fred Economic Data, St. Louis Fed*. January 26, 2022. https://fred.stlouisfed.org/series/MSPUS.

Meehan, Mary. "Unsheltered and Uncounted: Rural America's Hidden Homeless." *NPR*. July 4, 2019. https://www.npr.org/sections/health-shots/2019/07/04/736240349/in-rural-areas-homeless-people-are-harder-to-find-and-to-help.

Meinbresse, Molly, Lauren Brinkley Rubenstein, Amy Grassette, Joseph Benson, Carol Hall, Reginald Hamilton, Marianne Malott, and Darlene Jenkins. "Exploring the Experiences of Violence among Individuals Who Are Homeless Using a Consumer-Led Approach." *Violence and Victims* 29, 1 (2014): 122–36. https://nhchc.org/wp-content/uploads/2019/08/vv-29-1_ptr_a8_122-136.pdf.

Muniz, Hannah, ed. "Student Homelessness and Basic Needs Insecurity." *Best Colleges*. September 29, 2021. https://www.bestcolleges.com/resources/homeless-student-guide/#:~:text=Others%20may%20live%20in%20shelters,same%20in%202020%20at%2014%25.

Musumeci, MaryBeth. "Medicaid Work Requirements at the U.S. Supreme Court." *KFF: Kaiser Family Foundation*. February 11, 2021. https://www.kff.org/policy-watch/medicaid-work-requirements-at-u-s-supreme-court/.

Nagourney, Adam. "Old and on the Streets: The Greying of America's Homeless." *The New York Times*. May 31, 2016. https://www.nytimes.com/2016/05/31/us/americas-aging-homeless-old-and-on-the-street.html.

National Low Income Housing Coalition. *Out of Reach: The High Cost of Housing*. Washington, DC: National Low Income Housing Coalition, 2021. https://nlihc.org/sites/default/files/oor/2021/Out-of-Reach_2021.pdf.

Odoh, Chisom, Jennifer I. Vidrine, Michael S. Businelle, Darla E. Kendzor, Pooja Agrawal, and Lorraine R. Reitzel. "Health Literacy and Self-Rated Health among Homeless Adults." Health Behavior Research 2, 4 (2019): 1–13. https://www.ncbi.nlm.nih.gov/pmc/articles/PMC8218643/pdf/nihms-1601682.pdf.

Omeed, Memar, James R. Bell, and Benjamin Caughlin. "Review of Dermatological Problems among the Homeless." *ARC Journal of Dermatology* 3, 3 (2018): 1–6.

Oshin, Olafimihan. "California College Allowing Homeless Students to Sleep in Parked Cars." *The Hill*. November 3, 2021. https://thehill.com/homenews/state-watch/579936-california-college-allowing-homeless-students-to-sleep-in-cars-in.

Park, Alice. "Study Tracks Changing Perception of Homelessness." *Yale News*. October 24, 2017. https://yaledailynews.com/blog/2017/10/24/study-tracks-changing-perception-of-homelessness/.

Parker, Njeri. "The Many Forms of Homelessness." JOIN PDX (blog). January 25, 2019. https://joinpdx.org/the-many-forms-of-homelessness/.

Pavlakis, Alexandra E. "COVID-19 Pandemic Poses Unique Challenges for Students Who Are Homeless." *The Conversation*. February 23, 2022. https://theconversation.com/covid-19-pandemic-poses-unique-challenges-for-students-who-are-homeless-174860.

Rainey, Rebecca, and Chris Marr. "Minimum Wage Levels Will Rise in Half of American States in 2022." *Bloomberg Law*. December 30, 2021. https://news.bloomberglaw.com/daily-labor-report/minimum-wage-levels-will-rise-in-half-of-american-states-in-2022.

Ross, Martha, and Nicole Bateman. "Low Unemployment Isn't Worth Much If Jobs Barely Pay." *Brookings*. January 8, 2020. https://www.brookings.edu/blog/the-avenue/2020/01/08/low-unemployment-isnt-worth-much-if-the-jobs-barely-pay/.

Silfee, Denise. "There's a Lack of Access to Clean Water for Many Homeless People in Eugene." *KLCC: NPR for Oregonians*. January 11, 2019. https://www.klcc.org/health-medicine/2019-01-11/theres-a-lack-of-access-to-clean-water-for-many-homeless-people-in-eugene.

Smith, Doug, and Benjamin Oreskes. "Are Many Homeless People in L.A. Mentally Ill? New Findings Back the Public's Perception." *Los Angeles Times*. October 7, 2019. https://www.latimes.com/california/story/2019-10-07/homeless-population-mental-illness-disability.

Spencer, Kyle. "In College and Homeless." *The New York Times*. February 20, 2022. https://www.nytimes.com/2020/02/20/education/learning/college-homeless-students.html.

Stasha, Smiljanic. "The State of Homelessness in the US—2021." *Policy Advice*. April 22, 2021. https://policyadvice.net/insurance/insights/homelessness-statistics/.

Sutherland, Harper, Mir M. Ali, and Emily Rosenoff. *Health Conditions among Individuals with a History of Homelessness: ASPE Research Brief*. Washington, DC: U.S. Department of Health and Human Services, February 8, 2021. https://aspe.hhs.gov/reports/health-conditions-among-individuals-history-homelessness-research-brief-0.

"Taking Away Medicaid for Not Meeting Work Requirements Harms People Experiencing Homelessness." *Center on Budget and Policy Priorities*. March 10, 2020. https://www.cbpp.org/sites/default/files/atoms/files/4-18-18health.pdf.

The Homeless Period Project. https://www.homelessperiodproject.org/ (accessed February 14, 2022).

U.S. Department of Veterans Affairs. "Heightened Risk of Suicide among Veterans Who Have Experienced Homelessness." *From Science to Practice* (accessed February 14, 2022). https://www.mentalhealth.va.gov/suicide_prevention/docs/Literature_Review_FSTP_Homelessness_508_FINAL_07-11-2019.pdf.

Watson, Juliet. "'Just a Piece of Meat': How Homeless Women Have Little Choice but to Use Sex for Survival." *The Conversation*. August 12, 2018. https://theconversation.com/just-a-piece-of-meat-how-homeless-women-have-little-choice-but-to-use-sex-for-survival-101113.

Wells, Megan. "Rates of Violence against the Homeless Are Worse Than You Think." *Lexipol*. April 20, 2020. https://www.gov1.com/public-safety/articles/rates-of-violence-against-the-homeless-are-worse-than-you-think-PZ7QgDNA4F2MXDwf/.

Wiltz, Teresa. "'A Pile Up of Inequities': Why People of Color Are Hit Hardest by Homelessness." *The Pew Charitable Trusts*. March 29, 2019. https://www.pewtrusts.org/en/research-and-analysis/blogs/stateline/2019/03/29/a-pileup-of-inequities-why-people-of-color-are-hit-hardest-by-homelessness.

Chapter 7: Incarcerated Populations

Administration for Native Americas, Administration for Children and Families, U.S. Department of Health and Human Services. *Improving Outcomes for American Indian/Alaskan Native People Returning to the Community from Incarceration: A Resource Guide for Service Providers*. Washington, DC: U.S. Department of Health and Human Services, 2021. https://aspe.hhs.gov/sites/default/files/documents/87b6927ebbd6583df77f31ef4648cbac/improving-aian-reentry-toolkit.pdf.

Benns, Whitney. "American Slavery, Reinvented." *The Atlantic*. September 21, 2015. https://www.theatlantic.com/business/archive/2015/09/prison-labor-in-america/406177/.

Bernd, Candace, Zoe Loftus-Farren, and Maureen Nandini Mitra. *America's Toxic Prisons: The Environmental Injustices of Mass Incarceration*. Berkeley, CA: Earth Island Institute, 2017. https://www.earthisland.org/journal/americas-toxic-prisons/.

Bowman, Scott Wm., ed. *Color behind Bars: Racism in the U.S. Prison System*. Santa Barbara, CA: Praeger, 2014.

"Correctional Education: Adult Education and Literacy." U.S. Department of Education, Office of Career, Technical, and Adult Education. https://www2.ed.gov/about/offices/list/ovae/pi/AdultEd/correctional-education.html (accessed January 25, 2022).

Eisen, Lauren-Brooke. "Charging Inmates Fees behind Bars May Violate the Excessive Fines Clause." *The Brennan Center for Justice*. July 31, 2014. https://www.brennancenter.org/our-work/research-reports/paying-your-time-how-charging-inmates-fees-behind-bars-may-violate.

Eisler, Peter, Linda So, Jason Szep, Grant Smith, and Ned Parker. *A Hidden Crisis in America's Jails: Dying Inside, A Reuters Investigation*. https://www.reuters.com/investigates/section/usa-jails/ (accessed January 20, 2022).

"Ending Mass Incarceration." *Vera Institute of Social Justice*. https://www.vera.org/ending-mass-incarceration (accessed January 11, 2022).

Fassler, Joe, and Claire Brown. "Prison Food Is Making Inmates Disproportionately Sick." *The Atlantic*, December 27, 2017. https://www.theatlantic.com/health/archive/2017/12/prison-food-sickness-america/549179/.

Feldman, Amanda, "Incarcerated Women: Reproductive Healthcare Concerns Silenced by the Prison Litigation Reform Act" (2020). *Upper Level Writing Requirement Research Papers*. 38. https://digitalcommons.wcl.american.edu/stu_upperlevel_papers/38.

Ford, Matt. "America's Largest Mental Health Hospital Is a Jail." *The Atlantic*. June 8, 2015. https://www.theatlantic.com/politics/archive/2015/06/americas-largest-mental-hospital-is-a-jail/395012/.

Ghandnoosh, Nazgol. *Race and Punishment: Racial Perceptions of Crime and Support for Punitive Policies*. Washington, DC: The Sentencing Project, 2014. https://www.sentencingproject.org/publications/race-and-punishment-racial-perceptions-of-crime-and-support-for-punitive-policies/.

Gibbons, Alexandra, and Rashawn Ray. "The Societal Benefits of Postsecondary Prison Education." *The Brookings Institute*. August 20, 2021. https://www.brookings.edu/blog/how-we-rise/2021/08/20/the-societal-benefits-of-postsecondary-prison-education/.

Hawks, Laura, Steffie Woolhandler, and Danny McCormick. "COVID-19 in Prisons and Jails in the United States." *JAMA Internal Medicine*, April 28, 2020. https://jamanetwork.com/journals/jamainternalmedicine/fullarticle/2765271.

Jain, Nishi. "Risk of Death among Recently Released Inmates." *International Collegiate Journal of Science*. January 13, 2021. https://ncjs.us/risk-of-death-among-recently-released-inmates/.

Jenkins, Jimmy. "Medical Debt from In-Prison Injuries Is Chasing Inmates after Release." *NPR: National Public Radio*. May 27, 2019. https://www.npr.org/2019/05/27/727373494/medical-debt-from-in-prison-injuries-is-chasing-inmates-after-release.

Landgrave, Michelangelo, and Alex Nowrasteh. "Incarcerated Immigrants in 2016: The Numbers, Demographics, and Countries of Origin." *The CATO Institute: Immigration Research and Policy Brief*. June 4, 2018. https://www.cato.org/sites/cato.org/files/pubs/pdf/irpb7.pdf.

Lockwood, Beatrix, and Nicole Lewis. "The Hidden Cost of Incarceration." *The Marshall Project*. December 17, 2019. https://www.themarshallproject.org/2019/12/17/the-hidden-cost-of-incarceration.

Looney, Adam, and Nicholas Turner. *Work and Opportunity before and after Incarceration*. Washington, DC: The Brookings Institution, 2018. https://www.brookings.edu/wp-content/uploads/2018/03/es_20180314_looneyincarceration_final.pdf.

Markshamer, Jody, and Harper Jean Tobin. *Standing with LGBT Prisoners: An Advocate's Guide to Ending Abuse and Combating Imprisonment*. Washington, DC: National Center for Transgender Equality, 2014. https://transequality.org/sites/default/files/docs/resources/JailPrisons_Resource_FINAL.pdf.

Medina, Eduardo. "Detainees Sue Arkansas Jail That Gave Them Ivermectin to Treat COVID." *The New York Times*. January 17, 2022. https://www.nytimes.com/2022/01/17/us/ivermectin-covid-arkansas-jail.html.

Michaels, Samantha. "Jail Is a Terrible Place to Have a Period. One Woman Is on a Crusade to Make It Better." *Mother Jones*. February 21, 2019. https://www.motherjones.com/crime-justice/2019/02/jail-california-tampons-menstruation-paula-canny-sanitary-pads/.

Morris, Robert E. "Health Care for Incarcerated Adolescents: Significant Needs with Considerable Obstacles." *AMA Journal of Ethics* 7, 3 (2005): 244–8. https://journalofethics.ama-assn.org/article/health-care-incarcerated-adolescents-significant-needs-considerable-obstacles/2005-03.

National Prison Rape Elimination Commission. *Standards for the Prevention, Detection, Response, and Monitoring of Sexual Abuse in Adult Prisons and Jails*. Washington, DC: National Crime Justice and Reference Service, 2009.

Ositelu, Monique O. *Equipping Individuals for Life Beyond Bars: The Promise of Higher Education and Job Training in Closing the Gap in Skills for Incarcerated Populations*. Washington,

DC: New America, 2019. https://s3.amazonaws.com/newamericadotorg/documents/Interior_Text_-_Life_Beyond_Bars_v3_VLiTdnh.pdf.
Peiffer, Emily, Sarah Gillespie, Samantha Batko, Zach VeShancey, and Ben Cartoff. "Five Charts that Explain the Homeless-Jail Cycle and How to Break It." *The Urban Institute*. September 16, 2020. https://www.urban.org/features/five-charts-explain-homelessness-jail-cycle-and-how-break-it.
Primus, Eve Brensike. "Defense Counsel and Public Defence." In *Reforming Criminal Justice: Pretrial and Trial Processes*, edited by Erik Luna, 3, 121–45. Phoenix, AZ: Academy for Justice, 2017. https://repository.law.umich.edu/cgi/viewcontent.cgi?article=1113&context=book_chapters.
"Prison Conditions." *Equal Justice Initiative*. https://eji.org/issues/prison-conditions/ (accessed January 17, 2022).
Saar, Malika Saada, Brittany Bisnott, and Faiza Mathon-Mathieu. *Mothers behind Bars: A State-By-State Report Card and Analysis of Federal Policies on Conditions of Confinement for Pregnant and Parenting Women and the Effect on Their Children*. Washington, DC: National Women's Law Center and the Rebecca Project for Human Rights, 2010.
Sarrett, Jennifer. "US Prisons Hold More Than 550,000 People with Intellectual Disabilities—They Face Exploitation and Harsh Treatment." *The Conversation*. May 7, 2021. https://theconversation.com/us-prisons-hold-more-than-550-000-people-with-intellectual-disabilities-they-face-exploitation-harsh-treatment-158407.
Schwartzapfel, Beth, and Jimmy Jenkins. "Inside the Nation's Overdose Crisis in Prisons and Jails." *The Marshall Project*. July 15, 2021. https://www.themarshallproject.org/2021/07/15/inside-the-nation-s-overdose-crisis-in-prisons-and-jails.
Shulein, Orli, Risa Klemme, Kurt Johnson, and Mark Harniss. "Traumatic Brain Injury in Corrections." *Brain Injury Association of America*. https://www.biausa.org/public-affairs/media/traumatic-brain-injury-in-corrections#:~:text=Researchers%20estimate%20that %20up%20to,(TBI)%20in%20our%20prisons.&text=One%20study%20suggests%20that%20people,individuals%20to%20have%20multiple%20TBIs (accessed January 19, 2022).
Stabley, Justin. "People Leaving Prison Have a Hard Time Getting Jobs. The Pandemic Has Made Things Worse." *PBS News Hour*. March 31, 2021. https://www.pbs.org/newshour/economy/people-leaving-prison-have-a-hard-time-getting-jobs-the-pandemic-has-made-things-worse.
Trimble, Patricia Elane. "Ignored LGBTQ Prisoners: Discrimination in Education, Rehabilitation, and Mental Health Services during Incarceration." *LGBTQ Policy Journal*. May 22, 2019. https://lgbtq.hkspublications.org/2019/05/22/ignored-lgbtq-prisoners-discrimination-in-education-rehabilitative-and-mental-health-services-during-incarceration/#_edn1.
Widra, Emily, and Tiana Herring. "States of Incarceration: The Global Context 2021." *Prison Policy Initiative*. September 2021. https://www.prisonpolicy.org/global/2021.html.
Zezima, Carolyn. "Incarcerated with Mental Illness: How to Reduce the Number of People with Mental Health Issues in Prisons." *PSYCOM*. https://www.psycom.net/how-to-reduce-mental-illness-in-prisons (accessed January 17, 2022).

Chapter 8: Indigenous Populations

Akee, Randall, and Sarah Reber. "American Indians and Alaska Natives Are Dying of COVID-19 at Shocking Rates." *The Brookings Institution*. February 18, 2021. https://www.brookings.edu/research/american-indians-and-alaska-natives-are-dying-of-covid-19-at-shocking-rates/.
Allard, Mary Dorinda, and Vernon Brundage, Jr. "American Indians and Alaska Natives in the U.S. Labor Force." *Monthly Labor Review*, November 2019. https://www.bls.gov/opub/mlr/2019/article/pdf/american-indians-and-alaska-natives-in-the-u-s-labor-force.htm.
American Association of Medical Colleges. *Diversity in Medicine: Facts and Figures 2019*. www.aamc.org/data-reports/workforce/report/diversity-medicine-facts-and-figures-2019 (accessed October 17, 2022).

"American Indian and Alaska Native Women's Maternal Health: Addressing the Crisis." *National Partnership for Women and Families*. October 2019. https://www.nationalpartnership.org/our-work/resources/health-care/maternity/american-indian-and-alaska.pdf.

Asante-Muhammad, Dedrick, Esha Kamra, Connor Sanchez, Kathy Ramirez, and Rogelio Tec. "Racial Wealth Snapshot: Native Americans." *National Community Reinvestment Coalition*. February 14, 2022. https://ncrc.org/racial-wealth-snapshot-native-americans/.

Bell, Shaquita, Jason F. Deen, Molly Fuentes, and Kelly Moore. "Policy Statement: Caring for American Indian and Alaska Native Children and Adolescents." *Pediatrics* 147, 4 (2021). https://publications.aap.org/pediatrics/article/147/4/e2021050498/180860/Caring-for-American-Indian-and-Alaska-Native.

Biess, Jennifer. "Homelessness in Indian Country Is a Hidden, but Critical, Problem." *The Urban Institute*. April 11, 2017. https://www.urban.org/urban-wire/homelessness-indian-country-hidden-critical-problem.

Buch, Jason. "How Can Police Minimize Racial Profiling of Native Americans, and Others?" *InvestigateWest*. December 20, 2019. www.invw.org/2019/12/20/how-can-police-minimize-racial-profiling-of-native-americans-others.

Center for Behavioral Health Statistics and Quality. *Racial/Ethnic Differences in Substance Use, Substance Abuse Disorders, and Substance Use Treatment Utilization among People Aged 12 and Older (2015-2019)*. Rockville, MD: Substance Abuse and Mental Health Services Administration, 2021. www.samhsa.gov/data/sites/default/files/reports/rpt35326/2021NSDUHSUChartbook102221B.pdf.

Clarren, Rebecca. "Native American Students Face Punitive Discipline, Substandard Curricula." *Investigate West*. July 24, 2017. https://www.invw.org/2017/07/24/native-american-students-in-crisis-from-punitive-discipline-substandard-curricula-declining-federal-funds/.

Dewees, Sarah, and Benjamin Marks. *Twice Invisible: Understanding Rural Native America*. Longmont, CO: First Nations Development Institute, 2017. www.niwrc.org/sites/default/files/files/reports/2017%20Twice%20Invisible%20-%20Research%20Note_0.pdf.

Diamond, Anna. "Inside a New Effort to Change What Schools Teach about Native American History." *Smithsonian Magazine*. September 18, 2019. https://www.smithsonianmag.com/smithsonian-institution/inside-new-effort-change-what-schools-teach-about-native-american-history-180973166/.

Faheid, Dalia. "Indigenous Tribes Facing Displacement in Alaska and Louisiana Say the U.S. Is Ignoring Climate Threats." *Inside Climate News*. September 13, 2021. www.insideclimatenews.org/news/13092021/indigenous-tribes-alaska-louisiana.

Foxworth, Raymond, and Carew Boulding. "Discrimination and Resentment: Examining American Attitudes about Native Americans." *Journal of Race, Ethnicity, and Politics* 7, 1 (2022): 9–36.

Freeman, Miranda, and Alice Ammerman. "Adverse Childhood Experiences and Resilience in Native American Families and Communities." *North Carolina Medical Journal* 82, 6 (2021): 408–13. https://www.ncmedicaljournal.com/content/ncm/82/6/408.full.pdf.

Friedman, Misha. "For Native Americans, Health Care Is a Long, Hard Road Away." *NPR: National Public Radio*. April 13, 2016. www.npr.org/sections/health-shots/2016/4/13/473848341/health-care-s-hard-realities-on-the-reservation-a-photo-essay.

Green, Erica L., and Annie Waldman. "'I Feel Invisible': Native Students Languish in Public Schools." *The New York Times*. December 28, 2018. https://www.nytimes.com/2018/12/28/us/native-american-education.html.

Hall, Emma. "Colleges Are Making Tuition Free for Native Students. Will More Students Graduate?" *NPR*. August 19, 2022. https://www.npr.org/2022/08/19/1117951085/colleges-are-making-tuition-free-for-native-students-will-more-students-graduate.

Hirschfelder, Arlene, and Paulette F. Molin. "I Is for Ignoble: Stereotyping Native Americans." *Jim Crow Museum, Ferris State University*. February 22, 2018. www.ferris.edu/HTMLS/news/jimcrow/native/homepage.htm.

Huggins, Katherine, and Julia Mueller. "Tribal Pharmacy Dispenses Free Meds and Fills Gaps for Native Americans in the City." *Kaiser Health News*. May 24, 2022. www.khn.org/news/article/tribal-pharmacy-native-americans-minneapolis.

"Indigenous Peoples and Violence." *Association of American Indian Affairs* (accessed August 12, 2022). https://www.indian-affairs.org/indigenous-peoples-and-violence.html.

Johnson, Michelle Tyrene. "For Native Americans, Tribal Casinos Help and Hurt." *St. Louis Public Radio*. February 4, 2019. https://www.stlpublicradio.org/projects/fixed-odds/for-native-americans-tribal-casinos-help-and-hurt/.

Manjeshwar, Sanjana. "The Lasting Harms of Toxic Exposure in Native American Communities." *Berkeley Political Review*. July 10, 2021. https://bpr.berkeley.edu/2021/07/10/the-lasting-harms-of-toxic-exposure-in-native-american-communities/.

Maxim, Robert, Randall Akee, and Gabriel R. Sanchez. "For the First Time, the Government Published Monthly Unemployment Data on Native Americans, and the Picture Is Stark." *The Brookings Institution*. February 9, 2022. https://www.borgenmagazine.com/native-american-reservations/.

Melkonian, Stephanie C., Hannah K. Weir, Melissa A. Jim, Bailey Preikschat, Donald Havercamp, and Mary C. White. "Incidence of and Trends in the Leading Cancers with Elevated Incidence among American Indian and Alaska Native Populations, 2012-2016." *American Journal of Epidemiology* 190, 4 (April 2021): 528–38. https://academic.oup.com/aje/article/190/4/528/5922784.

National Indigenous Women's Resource Center. *Expert Panel on Homelessness among American Indians, Alaska Natives, and Native Hawaiians. niwrc.org*. July 21, 2022. Available: www.niwrc.org/resources/report/expert-panel-homelessness-among-american-indians-alaska-natives-and-native.

Petrosky, Emiko, Laura M. Mercer Kollar, Megan C. Kearns, Sharon G. Smith, Carter J. Betz, Katherine A. Fowler, and Delight E. Satter. "Homicides of American Indians/Alaska Natives—National Violent Death Reporting System, 2003-2018." *Surveillance Summaries* 70, 8 (November 19, 2021): 1–19. https://www.cdc.gov/mmwr/volumes/70/ss/ss7008a1.htm.

Poon, Linda. "How 'Indian Relocation' Created a Public Health Crisis." *Bloomberg*. December 2, 2019. https://www.bloomberg.com/news/articles/2019-12-02/what-s-behind-native-american-health-disparities.

Redwood, Diana, Mary C. Schumacher, Elizabeth D. Ferucci, Elvin Asay, Laurie J. Helzer, Lillian Tom-Orme, Sandra L. Edwards, et al. "Physical Activity Patterns of American Indian and Alaska Native People Living in Alaska and the Southwestern United States." *American Journal of Health Promotion* 23, 6 (2019): 388–95.

Riser, Quentin H. , Heather L. Rouse, Cassandra J. Dorius, and Ji Young Choi. "Native American Children and School Readiness: A Nationally Representative Study of Individual and Cumulative Risks." *Children and Youth Services Review* 106 (2019). https://doi.org/10.1016/j.childyouth.2019.104496.

Sherman, Sean. *The Sioux Chef's Indigenous Kitchen*. Minneapolis, Minnesota: University of Minnesota Press, 2017.

Simon, Rachel, Jennifer Giroux, and Julie Chor. "Effects of Substance Use Disorder Criminalization on American Indian Pregnant Individuals." *AMA Journal of Ethics* 22, 10 (2020): E862–867. https://journalofethics.ama-assn.org/article/effects-substance-use-disorder-criminalization-american-indian-pregnant-individuals/2020-10.

Smith, Andrea. *Conquest: Sexual Violence and American Indian Genocide*. Boston, MA: South End Press, 2005.

Solomon, Teshia G. Arambula, Felina M. Cordova, and Fracisco Garcia. "What's Killing Our Children? Child and Infant Mortality among American Indians and Alaska Natives." *National Academy of Medicine*. March 7, 2017. https://nam.edu/whats-killing-our-children-child-and-infant-mortality-among-american-indians-and-alaska-natives/.

Stewart, Ada. "Minorities Are Underrepresented in Clinical Trials." Leader Voice Blog: A Forum for AAFP Leaders and Members. December 4, 2018. https://www.aafp.org/news/blogs/leadervoices/entry/20181204lv-clinicaltrials.html.

Thomas, Morgan, Tara McCoy, Itai Jeffries, Richard Haverkate, Elton Naswood, Jessica Leston, and Laura Platero. "Native American Two Spirit and LGBTQ Health: A Systemic Review of the Literature." *Journal of Gay and Lesbian Mental Health* (2021): 1–36. https://www.tandfonline.com/doi/full/10.1080/19359705.2021.1913462.

Truschel, Lucy, and Cristina Novoa. "American Indian and Alaska Native Maternal and Infant Mortality: Challenges and Opportunities." *Center for American Progress*. July 9, 2018. https://www.americanprogress.org/article/american-indian-alaska-native-maternal-infant-mortality-challenges-opportunities/.

Wang, Leah. "The U.S. Criminal Justice System Disproportionately Hurts Native People: The Data, Visualized." *Prison Policy Initiative*. October 8, 2021. www.prisonpolicy.org/blog/2021/10/08/indigenouspeoplesday/.

Warne, Donald, and Linda Bane Frizzell. "American Indian Health Policy: Historical Trends and Contemporary Issues." *American Journal of Public Health* 104, Suppl. 3 (June 2014): S263–S267.

Whitney, Eric. "Native Americans Feel Invisible in the U.S. Health Care System." NPR: National Public Radio. December 12, 2017. www.npr.org/sections/health-shots/2017/12/12/569910574/native-americans-feel-invisible-in-u-s-health-care-system.

Woodard, Stephanie. "The Police Killings No One Is Talking About." *In These Times*. October 17, 2016. https://inthesetimes.com/features/native_american_police_killings_native_lives_matter.html.

Yeagley, Rebekah May. "Reservations Are the Most Poverty-Stricken Lands in America." *FEE: Foundation for Economic Education*. November 9, 2020. https://fee.org/articles/why-native-american-reservations-are-the-most-poverty-stricken-lands-in-america/?gclid=-EAIaIQobChMIoaSJzdbI-QIVPWpvBB2NMgVjEAAYASAAEgKPC_D_BwE.

Chapter 9: Low-Income Populations

Allyn, Bobby. "College Board Drops Its 'Adversity Score' for Each Student after Backlash." *NPR: National Public Radio*. August 27, 2019. https://www.npr.org/2019/08/27/754799550/college-board-drops-its-adversity-score-for-each-student-after-backlash#:~:text=Announced%20in%20May%2C%20the%20%22adversity,The%20pushback%20was%20swift.

Aurand, Andrew, Dan Emmanuel, Ikra Rafi, Dan Threet, and Diane Yentel. *Out of Reach: The High Cost of Housing*. Washington, DC: National Low Income Housing Coalition, 2021.

Beech, Bettina M., Chandra Ford, Roland J. Thorpe, Jr., Marino A. Bruce, and Keith C. Norris. "Poverty, Racism, and the Public Health Crisis in America." *Frontiers in Public Health* 9 (2021). https://www.frontiersin.org/articles/10.3389/fpubh.2021.699049/full.

Boghani, Priyanka. "What Happened to Poverty in America in 2021." *PBS Frontline*. December 22, 2021. https://www.pbs.org/wgbh/frontline/article/poverty-america-2021-covid-pandemic/#:~:text=The%20Columbia%20team%20estimated%20that,tax%20and%20child%20tax%20credits.

Booker, Karene. "Study: Negative Stereotypes about the Poor Hurt Their Health." *Cornell Chronicle*. July 25, 2012. https://news.cornell.edu/stories/2012/07/negative-stereotypes-about-poor-hurt-their-health.

Center on Budget and Policy Priorities. *Tracking the COVID-19 Economy's Effects on Food, Housing, and Employment Hardships*. August 13, 2020. https://www.cbpp.org/sites/default/files/8-13-20pov.pdf.

Child Care Aware of America. "The US and the High Price of Child Care: An Examination of a Broken System." *childcareaware.org*. Arlington, VA, 2020. https://www.childcareaware.org/our-issues/research/the-us-and-the-high-price-of-child-care-2019/.

Cooper, David. "One in Nine U.S. Workers Are Paid Wages That Can Leave Them in Poverty, Even When Working Full Time." *Economic Policy Institute*. June 15, 2018. https://www.epi.org/publication/one-in-nine-u-s-workers-are-paid-wages-that-can-leave-them-in-poverty-even-when-working-full-time/.

Cunningham, Peter J. "Why Even Healthy Low-Income People Have Greater Health Risks Than Higher- Income People." *The Commonwealth Fund*. September 27, 2018. https://www.commonwealthfund.org/blog/2018/healthy-low-income-people-greater-health-risks.

Dalessandro, Cristen. "'My Family and Friends Thought It Was a Horrible Idea:' The Classed, Gendered Project of Young, Adult Women's Intimacy Choices." *Journal of Youth Studies* 24, 1 (2021): 126–41.

Diallo, Amadou. "After-School Programs Have Either Been Abandoned or Overworked." *Hechinger Report*. April 19, 2021. https://hechingerreport.org/after-school-programs-have-either-been-abandoned-or-overworked/.

Discipline Revolution Project. http://disciplinerevolutionproject.org/ (accessed March 28, 2022).

Duke, Chris C., and Christine Stanik. "Overcoming Low-Income Patients' Concerns about Trust and Respect from Providers." *Health Affairs*. August 11, 2016. https://www.healthaffairs.org/do/10.1377/forefront.20160811.056138/full/.

Duquaine-Watson, Jillian M. *Mothering By Degrees: Single Mothers and the Pursuit of Postsecondary Education*. New Brunswick, NJ: Rutgers University Press, 2017.

Fernald, Marcia, ed. *The State of the Nation's Housing 2020*. Cambridge, MA: Joint Center for Housing Studies of Harvard University, 2020. https://www.jchs.harvard.edu/sites/default/files/reports/files/Harvard_JCHS_The_State_of_the_Nations_Housing_2020_Report_Revised_120720.pdf.

Fry, Richard, and Anthony Cilluffo. "A Rising Share of Undergraduates Are from Poor Families, Especially at Less Selective Colleges." *Pew Research Center*. May 22, 2019. https://www.pewresearch.org/social-trends/2019/05/22/a-rising-share-of-undergraduates-are-from-poor-families-especially-at-less-selective-colleges/.

Garbee, Julia. "A Study of Low-Income Communities and School-to-Prison Pipelines." *The Lowe Down*. December 14, 2021. https://www.lowe-down.org/low-income-communities-breed-school-to-prison-pipelines/.

García, Emma, and Elaine Weiss. *Education Inequalities at the School Starting Gate: Gaps, Trends, and Strategies to Address Them*. Washington, DC: Economic Policy Institute, 2017. https://files.epi.org/pdf/132500.pdf.

Greenfield, Beth. "Harvard Research: Impact of Poverty Begins in the Womb, but It Doesn't Have To." *EMPath: Economic Mobility Pathways*. December 10, 2019. https://www.empathways.org/news/article/harvard-research-impact-of-poverty-begins-in-the-womb-but-it-doesnt-have-to.

Hayes, Tara O'Neill, and Josee Farmer. "Insulin Cost and Pricing Trends." *American Action Forum*. April 2, 2020. https://www.americanactionforum.org/research/insulin-cost-and-pricing-trends/.

Holmes, Seth M. *Fresh Fruit, Broken Bodies: Migrant Farmworkers in the United States*. Berkeley, CA: University of California Press, 2013.

Hughes, Michelle, and Whitney Tucker. "Poverty as an Adverse Childhood Experience." *North Carolina Medical Journal* 79, 2 (2018): 124–6. https://www.ncmedicaljournal.com/content/79/2/124.

Hussar, Bill, Jijun Zhang, Sarah Hein, and Et. Al. *The Condition of Education 2020*. Washington, DC: National Center for Education Statistics, Institute of Education Sciences, 2020. https://nces.ed.gov/pubs2020/2020144.pdf.

Isaacs, Katelin P., Zhe Li, Sharmila Choudhury, and Isaac A. Nicchitta. *The Growing Gap in Life Expectancy by Income: Recent Evidence and Implications for the Social Security Retirement Age*. Washington, DC: Congressional Research Service. Updated July 6, 2021. https://news.harvard.edu/gazette/story/2016/04/for-life-expectancy-money-matters/.

Kang, Esther Yoon-Ji. "Sexually Transmitted Infections Reach Peak Levels; Poor Most at Risk." *NPR.org*. April 23, 2019. https://www.npr.org/local/309/2019/04/23/716545592/sexually-transmitted-infections-reach-peak-levels-poor-most-at-risk.

Kearney, Audrey, Liz Hamel, Mellisha Stokes, and Mollyann Brodie. "Americans' Challenges with Health Care." *KFF: Kaiser Family Foundation*. December 14, 2021. https://www.kff.org/health-costs/issue-brief/americans-challenges-with-health-care-costs/.O.

Lee, De-Chih, Hailun Liang, and Leiyu Shi. "The Convergence of Racial and Income Disparities in Health Insurance Coverage in the United States." *International Journal for Equity in Health* 20 (2021). https://equityhealthj.biomedcentral.com/track/pdf/10.1186/s12939-021-01436-z.pdf.

Leomporra, Annie, and Megan Hustings, eds. *Vulnerable to Hate: A Survey of Bias-Motivated Violence against People Experiencing Homelessness in 2016-2017*. Washington, DC: National Coalition for the Homeless, 2018. https://nationalhomeless.org/wp-content/uploads/2018/12/hate-crimes-2016-17-final_for-web.pdf.

Lewis, Corinne, Laurie Zephyrin, Melinda K. Abrams, and Shanoor Seervai. "Listening to Low-Income Patients and Their Physicians: Solutions for Improving Access and Quality in Primary Care." *The Commonwealth Fund*. May 15, 2019. https://www.commonwealthfund.org/blog/2019/listening-low-income-patients-and-their-physicians–improving-access-and-quality.

Massachusetts Institute of Technology. "Living Wage Calculator." https://livingwage.mit.edu/ (accessed March 23, 2022).

McCorkell, Lisa, and Sara Hinkley. "The Great Recession, Families, and the Safety Net." *Institute for Research on Labor and Employment*. December 19, 2018. https://irle.berkeley.edu/the-great-recession-families-and-the-safety-net/.

McDermott, Nathan. "The Myth of Gay Affluence." *The Atlantic*. March 21, 2014. https://www.theatlantic.com/business/archive/2014/03/the-myth-of-gay-affluence/284570/.

McQueen, Hannah. "The 20 Most Expensive Prescription Drugs in the US." *GoodRx Health*. September 7, 2021. https://www.goodrx.com/healthcare-access/drug-cost-and-savings/20-most-expensive-drugs-in-the-usa.

Moffitt, Robert A., and Stephanie Garlow. "Did Welfare Reform Increase Employment and Reduce Poverty?" *Pathways: A Magazine on Poverty, Inequality, and Social Policy* (Winter 2018): 17–21. https://inequality.stanford.edu/sites/default/files/Pathways_Winter2018_WelfareReform.pdf.

Mueller, Michael, and Emily Hewlett. "Better Ways to Pay for Health Care." *OECD: Better Policies for Better Lives*. June 2016. https://www.oecd.org/els/health-systems/Better-ways-to-pay-for-health-care-FOCUS.pdf.

National Center for Learning Disabilities. *Significant Disproportionality in Special Education: The Role of Income*. Washington, DC: National Center for Learning Disabilities, 2020. https://www.ncld.org/wp-content/uploads/2020/10/2020-NCLD-Disproportionality_-Low-Income-Students_FINAL.pdf.

Parker, Kim, Juliana Menasce Horowitz, and Anna Brown. "About Half of Low-Income Americans Report Household Job Or Wage Loss Due to COVID-19." *Pew Research Center*. April 21, 2020. https://www.pewresearch.org/social-trends/2020/04/21/about-half-of-lower-income-americans-report-household-job-or-wage-loss-due-to-covid-19/.

Rabin, Roni Caryn. "15-Minute Visits Take a Toll on the Doctor-Patient Relationship." *Kaiser Family Foundation*. April 21, 2014. https://khn.org/news/15-minute-doctor-visits/.

The Hope Center for College, Community, and Justice. *#REALCOLLEGE 2021: Basic Needs Insecurity during the Ongoing Pandemic*. Philadelphia, PA: The Hope Center, 2021. https://hope4college.com/wp-content/uploads/2021/03/RCReport2021.pdf.

Tierney, Aaron A., Martin J. Kyalwazi, and Anna Lockhart. "Tackling the Digital Divide by Improving Internet and Telehealth Access for Low-Income Populations." *California Initiative for Health Equity & Action*. Berkeley, CA July 2020. https://healthequity.berkeley.edu/sites/default/files/tacklingthedigitaldivide.pdf.

Vallas, Rebecca, and Shawn Fremstad. "Disability Is a Cause and Consequence of Poverty." *Talk Poverty*. September 19, 2014. https://talkpoverty.org/2014/09/19/disability-cause-consequence-poverty/.

Weinstein, Dana, Kristin (Eun Jung) Jung, Veronica Jauriqui, and Erica L. Rosenthal. *Rags-to-Riches, Welfare Queens, and Broken Families: Media Representations of Poverty and Their Impact on Audiences*. Los Angeles, CA: The Norman Lear Center, 2020. https://learcenter.org/wp-content/uploads/2021/03/povertynarratives_landscapeanalysis.pdf.

Woolf, Steven H., Laudan Aron, Lisa Dubay, Sarah M. Simon, Emily Zimmerman, and Kim X. Luk. *How Are Income and Wealth Linked to Health and Longevity?* Washington, DC: The Urban Institute, 2015. https://www.urban.org/sites/default/files/publication/49116/2000178-How-are-Income-and-Wealth-Linked-to-Health-and-Longevity.pdf.

Chapter 10: Rural Populations

American College of Obstetricians and Gynecologists. "Committee Opinion Number 586: Health Disparities in Rural Women." *ACOG*. February 2014. https://www.acog.org/clinical/clinical-guidance/committee-opinion/articles/2014/02/health-disparities-in-rural-women.

Bauer, Hope H., Carter B. Anderson, Kelly Hirko, and Andrea Wendling. "Barriers to College and Health Care Careers among US Students from a Rural Community." *PRiMER: Peer-Review Reports in Medical Education Research*. March 25, 2019. https://journals.stfm.org/primer/2019/wendling-2018-0053.

Burrows, Elizabeth, Ryung Suh, and Danielle Hamann. *National Rural Health Association Policy Brief: Health Care Workforce Distribution and Shortages in Rural America*. Washington, DC: National Rural Health Association, 2012.

Center on Budget and Policy Priorities. "How Medicaid Work Requirements Will Harm Rural Residents—and Communities." March 1, 2020. https://www.cbpp.org/sites/default/files/atoms/files/8-22-18health.pdf.

Cherry, Debra C., Barbara Huggins, and Karen Gilmore. "Children's Health in the Rural Environment." *Pediatric Clinics of North America*, 54, 1 (2007): 121–33.

Ellison, Ayla. "Why Rural Hospital Closures Hit a Record High in 2020." *Becker's Hospital CFO Report*. March 16, 2021. https://www.beckershospitalreview.com/finance/why-rural-hospital-closures-hit-a-record-high-in-2020.html.

Farragin, Tracey. "Rural Poverty and Well-Being." *Economic Research Service, U.S. Department of Agriculture*. December 2, 2021. https://www.ers.usda.gov/topics/rural-economy-population/rural-poverty-well-being/.

Flowers, Catherine Coleman. *Waste: One Woman's Fight against America's Dirty Little Secret*. New York: The New Press, 2020.

Franz, Berkeley, Lindsay Y. Dhanani, and William C. Miller. "Rural-Urban Differences in Physician Bias Toward Patients with Opioid Use Disorder." *Psychiatric Services* (August 2021): 874–9.

Friedlander, Blaine, and Devon Ryan. "Seven Years of Agricultural Growth Productivity Lost Due to Climate Change." *Stanford University Woods Institute for the Environment*. April 1, 2021. https://woods.stanford.edu/news/seven-years-agricultural-productivity-growth-lost-due-climate-change.

Harris, Adam. "The Education Deserts of Rural America: The College Completion Gap between Rural and Urban Residents Is Widening." *The Atlantic*, July 1, 2019. https://www.theatlantic.com/education/archive/2019/07/education-deserts-across-rural-america/593071/.

Herfort, Noah. "The Impacts of Climate Change on the Rural American Health Care System." *The Climate Institute*. December 5, 2020. https://climate.org/the-impacts-of-climate-change-on-the-american-rural-health-care-system/.

Khazan, Olga. "Rural America's False Sense of Security." *The Atlantic*. November 18, 2021. https://www.theatlantic.com/politics/archive/2021/11/pandemic-covid-urban-rural-divide/620730/.

Lavalley, Megan. *Out of the Loop: Rural Schools Are Largely Left out of Research and Policy Discussions, Exacerbating Poverty, Inequity, and Isolation*. Alexandria, VA: National School Boards Association, Center for Public Education, 2018. https://education.wsu.edu/documents/2018/12/center-public-education-rural-schools-report.pdf/.

Levin, Dan. "In Rural 'Dead Zones,' School Comes on a Flash Drive." *The New York Times*. November 13, 2020. https://www.nytimes.com/2020/11/13/us/wifi-dead-zones-schools.html.

McGraw, George, and Radhika Fox. *Closing the Water Access Gap in the United States: A National Action Plan*. Oakland, CA: US Water Alliance, 2019. http://uswateralliance.org/sites/uswateralliance.org/files/publications/Closing%20the%20Water%20Access%20Gap%20in%20the%20United%20States_DIGITAL.pdf.

McGreal, Chris. "How America's Food Giants Swallowed the Family Farm." *The Guardian*. March 9, 2019. https://www.theguardian.com/environment/2019/mar/09/american-food-giants-swallow-the-family-farms-iowa.

Medicaid and CHIP Payment and Access Commission. "Issue Brief: Medicaid and Rural Health." Washington, DC: MACPAC, April 2020. https://www.macpac.gov/wp-content/uploads/2021/04/Medicaid-and-Rural-Health.pdf.

Movement Advancement Project. *Where We Call Home: LGBT People in Rural America*. Boulder, CO: Movement Advancement Project, 2019. https://www.lgbtmap.org/file/lgbt-rural-report.pdf.

National Center for Frontier Communities. http://frontierus.org/ (accessed December 5, 2021).

Nayar, Preethy, Fang Yu, and Bettye A. Apenteng. "Frontier America's Health System Challenges and Population Health Outcomes." *The Journal of Rural Health* 29 (2013): 258–65.

Pecci, Alexandra Wilson. "How 2 Rural Hospitals Use Charities to Help Patients with Out-of-Pocket Costs." *Health Leaders*. July 27, 2021. https://www.healthleadersmedia.com/revenue-cycle/how-2-rural-hospitals-use-charities-help-patients-out-pocket-costs.

Peek-Asa, Corrine, Anne Wallis, Karisa Harland, Kirsten Beyer, Penny Dickey, and Audrey Saftlas. "Rural Disparity in Domestic Violence Prevalence and Access to Resources." *Journal of Women's Health* 20, 11 (2011): 1743–9. https://www.ncbi.nlm.nih.gov/pmc/articles/PMC3216064/.

Probst, Janice, Jan Marie Eberth, and Elizabeth Crouch. "Structural Urbanism Contributes to Poorer Health Outcomes for Rural America." *Health Affairs* 38, 12 (December 2019): 1976–84. https://npr.brightspotcdn.com/62/6c/fbb0dc5b4643a8b793eab7b09410/hlthaff.2019.00914.pdf.

Rowlands, DW, and Hanna Love. "Mapping Rural America's Diversity and Demographic Change." *The Brookings Institution*. September 28, 2021. https://www.brookings.edu/blog/the-avenue/2021/09/28/mapping-rural-americas-diversity-and-demographic-change/.

"Rural Faith Communities Play Anchoring Role." *NC State University Institute for Emerging Issues*. March 28, 2018. https://iei.ncsu.edu/2018/rural-faith-communities-as-anchor-institutions/.

Sacks, Peter. *Tearing Down the Gates: Confronting the Class Divide in American Education*. Berkeley: University of California Press, 2007.

Sharpe, Dayle, Maritza Bond, Kelly Cheek, and Holly Wolff. "Quality of Life Impacts Recruitment and Retention of Rural Health Care Providers." *National Rural Health Association*. February 2015. https://www.ruralhealth.us/getattachment/Advocate/Policy-Documents/QualityofLifeRecruitmentRetentionProvidersFeb2015.pdf.aspx?lang=en-US.

Siegler, Kirk. "The Struggle to Hire and Keep Doctors in Rural Areas Means Patients go Without Care." *NPR: National Public Radio*. May 21, 2019. https://www.npr.org/sections/health-shots/2019/05/21/725118232/the-struggle-to-hire-and-keep-doctors-in-rural-areas-means-patients-go-without-c.

TRIP: A National Transportation Research Nonprofit. *Rural Connections: Challenges and Opportunities in America's Heartland*. Washington, DC: TRIP, 2020. https://tripnet.org/wp-content/uploads/2020/05/TRIP_Rural_Roads_Report_2020.pdf.

Ullrich, Fred, and Keith Mueller. *COVID-19 Cases and Deaths, Metropolitan and Non-Metropolitan Counties Over Time (Update)*. Brief No. 2020-9. Iowa City, IA: RUPRI Center for Rural Health Policy Analysis, 2021. https://rupri.public-health.uiowa.edu/publications/policybriefs/2020/COVID%20Longitudinal%20Data.pdf.

Vogels, Emily A. "Some Digital Divides Persist between Rural, Urban, and Suburban America." *Pew Research Center*. August 19, 2021. https://www.pewresearch.org/fact-tank/2021/08/19/some-digital-divides-persist-between-rural-urban-and-suburban-america/.

White, Gillian B. "Rural America's Silent Housing Crisis." *The Atlantic*. January 28, 2015. https://www.theatlantic.com/business/archive/2015/01/rural-americas-silent-housing-crisis/384885/.

Wright, Aallyah. "Bus Driver Shortage Stresses Rural School Districts." *The Pew Charitable Trusts*. October 11, 2021. https://www.pewtrusts.org/en/research-and-analysis/blogs/stateline/2021/10/11/bus-driver-shortage-stresses-rural-school-districts.

Ziliak, James P. "Economic Change and the Social Safety Net: Are Rural Americans Still Behind?" *The Washington Center for Equitable Growth*. February 2019. https://equitablegrowth.org/working-papers/economic-change-and-the-social-safety-net-are-rural-americans-still-behind/

Chapter 11: Sexual and Gender Minority Populations

APA Working Group on Health Disparities in Boys and Men. *Health Disparities in Racial/Ethnic and Sexual Minority Boys and Men*. Washington, DC: American Psychological Association, 2018. www.apa.org/pi/health-disparities/resources/race-sexuality-men.aspx.

Bass, Brittney, and Hassan Nagy. "Cultural Competence in the Care of LGBTQ Patients." *StatPearls*. October 3, 2022. https://www.statpearls.com/ArticleLibrary/viewarticle/125326.

Bates, Nancy, Marshall Chin, and Tara Becker, eds. *Measuring Sex, Gender Identity, and Sexual Orientation*. Washington, DC: The National Academies Press, 2022.

Campus Pride. "The Worst List: The Absolute Worst Campuses for LBGTQ+ Youth." *campuspride.org*. www.campuspride.org/WorstList?gclid=EAIaIQobChMI_4SJlLWw_AIVl6_ICh3TJgVREAMYASAAEgKjhPD_BwE (accessed January 6, 2023).

Carrazana, Chabeli, and Orion Summler. "The Census Bureau's First Ever Data on LGBTQ+ People Indicates Deep Disparities." *PBS News Hour*. October 1, 2021. www.pbs.org/newshour/economy/the-census-bureaus-first-ever-data-on-lgbtq-people-indicates-deep-disparities.

Dawson, Lindsey, Ashley Kirzinger, and Jennifer Kates. "The Impact of COVID-19 Pandemic on LGBT People." *KFF: Kaiser Family Foundation*. March 11, 2021. www.kff.org/coronavirus-covid-19/poll-finding/the-impact-of-the-covid-19-pandemic-on-lgbt-people/.

Diaz, Jaclyn. "Trans Inmates Need Access to Gender Affirming Care. Often They Have to Sue to Get It." *NPR*. October 25, 2022. www.npr.org/2022/10/25/1130146647/transgender-inmates-gender-affirming-health-care-lawsuits-prison#:~:text=In%20a%20statement%20of%20interest,the%20treatment%20of%20gender%20dysphoria.

Eskridge, William N., Jr., and Christopher R. Riano. *Marriage Equality: From Outlaws to In-Laws*. New Haven, CT: Yale University Press, 2020.

Everett, Bethany G., Michelle A. Kominiarek, Stefanie Mollborn, Daniel E. Adkins, and Tonda L. Hughes. "Sexual Orientation Disparities in Pregnancy and Infant Outcomes." *Maternal and Child Health Journal* 23, 1 (2019): 72–81.

Gilchrist, Tracy E., and Daniel Reynolds. "17 LGBTQ Tropes Hollywood Needs to Retire." *Advocate*. August 29, 2017. www.advocate.com/arts-entertainment/2017/8/29/17-lgbt-tropes-hollywood-needs-retire#media-gallery-media-9.

Gomez, Scarlett Lin, Christine Duffy, Jennifer J. Griggs, and Esther M. John. "Surveillance of Cancer among Sexual and Gender Minority Populations: Where Are We and Where Do We Need to Go?" *Cancer* 125, 24 (December 15, 2019): 4360–2. www.ncbi.nlm.nih.gov/pmc/articles/PMC6891127/.

Kates, Jennifer, Usha Ranji, Alina Salganicoff, and Lindsey Dawson. "Health and Access to Care for Lesbian, Gay, Bisexual, and Transgender (LGBT) Individuals in the U.S." *KFF: Kaiser Family Foundation*. May 3, 2018. www.kff.org/report-section/health-and-access-to-care-and-coverage-lgbt-individuals-in-the-us-health-challenges/.

Kattari, Shanna K., Matthew Bakko, Lisa Langenderfer-Magruder, and Brendon T. Halloway. "Transgender and Nonbinary Experiences of Victimization in Healthcare." *Journal of Interpersonal Violence* 36, 23–4 (2021): NP13054–NP13076.

Liu, Michael, Sahil Sandhu, and Alex S. Keuroghlian. "Achieving the Triple Aim for Sexual and Gender Minorities." *New England Journal of Medicine* 387 (July 28, 2022): 294–7.

Mallory, Christy, Amira Hashenbush, and Brad Sears. "Discrimination and Harassment by Law Enforcement Officers in the LGBT Community." *The Williams Institute*. March 2015. https://williamsinstitute.law.ucla.edu/publications/lgbt-discrim-law-enforcement/.

Martin, Tracey, Scott M. Smukalla, Sunanda Kane, David P. Hudesman, Richard Greene, and Lisa B. Malter. "Receptive Anal Intercourse in Patients with Inflammatory Bowel Disease: A Clinical Review." *Inflammatory Bowel Diseases* 23, 8 (2017): 1285–92.

Martos, Alexander, Sheila Nezhad, and Ilan H. Meyer. "Variations in Sexual Identity Milestones among Lesbians, Gay Men, and Bisexuals." *Sexual Research and Social Policy* 12, 1 (2015): 24–33. www.ncbi.nlm.nih.gov/pmc/articles/PMC5042327.

McNair, Lindsay. "Making Clinical Research Inclusive: Strategies to Include the LGBTQIA+ Community in Research Trials." *WCG IRB*. https://wcgirb.com/wp-content/uploads/sites/2/2021/06/WCG-Making-clinical-research-inclusive.pdf (accessed November 28, 2022).

Medina, Caroline, and Lindsay Mahowald. "Collecting Data about LGBTQI+ and Other Sexual and Gender-Diverse Communities." *Center for American Progress*. May 24, 2022. www.americanprogress.org/article/collecting-data-about-lgbtqi-and-other-sexual-and-gender-diverse-communities/.

Meyers, Laurie. "LGBTQ Issues across the Lifespan." *Counseling Today*. March 24, 2017. http://ct.counseling.org/2017/03/lgbtq-issues-across-life-span/.

Migdon, Brooke. "Here Are the States Where You Can (and Cannot) Change Your Gender Designation on Official Documents." *Changing America*. May 31, 2022. https://thehill.com/changing-america/respect/diversity-inclusion/3507206-here-are-the-states-where-you-can-and-cannot-change-your-gender-designation-on-official-documents/.

Mittleman, Joel. "Intersecting the Academic Gender Gap: The Education of Lesbian, Gay, and Bisexual America." *American Sociological Review* 87, 2 (2022): 303–35.

Nowakowski, Alexandra C.H., J.E. Sumerau, and Nik M. Lampe. *Transformations in Queer, Trans, and Intersex Health and Aging*. Lanham, MD: Lexington Books, 2020.

Nowaskie, Dustin Z., and Anna C. Roesler. "The Impact of COVID-19 on the LGBTQ+ Community: Comparisons between Cisgender, Heterosexual People, Cisgender Sexual Minority People, and Gender Minority People." *Psychiatry Research* 309 (2022). www.ncbi.nlm.nih.gov/pmc/articles/PMC8743502/pdf/main.pdf.

Palmer, Neal A., Emily A. Greytak, and Joseph G. Kosciw. *Educational Exclusion: Drop Out, Push Out, and School-to-Prison Pipeline among LBGTQ Youth*. New York, NY: GLSEN, 2016. Available: www.glsen.org/sites/default/files/2019-11/Educational_Exclusion_2013.pdf.

Patterson, Charlotte J., Martín-José Sepúlveda, and Jordyn White, eds. *Understanding the Well-Being of LGBTQI+ Populations*. Washington, DC: National Academies Press, 2020.

Pratt-Chapman, Mandi L., Kristen Eckstrand, Amorie Robinson, Lauren B. Beach, Charles Kamen, Alex S. Keuroghlian, Scott Cook, Asa Radix, Markus P. Biddell, and Liz Margolies. "Developing Standards for Cultural Competency Training for Health Care Providers to Care for Lesbian, Gay, Bisexual Transgender, Queer, Intersex, and Asexual Persons: Consensus Recommendations for a National Panel." *LGBT Health* 9, 5 (2022): 340–7.

Rafei, Leila. "How LGBTQ Voices Are Being Erased in Classrooms." *ACLU*. June 27, 2022. www.aclu.org/news/lgbtq-rights/how-lgbtq-voices-are-being-erased-in-classrooms-censorship.

Ramchand, Rajeev, Megan S. Schuler, Michael Schoenbaum, Lisa Colpe, and Lynsay Ayer. "Suicidality among Sexual Minority Adults: Gender, Age, and Race/Ethnicity Differences." *American Journal of Preventative Medicine* 62, 2 (February 1, 2022): 193–202. www.ajpmonline.org/article/S0749-3797(21)00443-8/fulltext.

Reis, Elizabeth. *Bodies in Doubt: An American History of Intersex*. Baltimore, MD: Johns Hopkins University Press, 2009.

Romero, Adam P., Shoshana K. Goldberg, and Luis A. Vasquez. "LGBT People and Housing Affordability, Discrimination, and Homelessness." *The Williams Institute*. April 2020. http://williamsinstitute.law.ucla.edu/publications/lgbt-housing-instability/.

Rothblum, Esther D., ed. *The Oxford Handbook of Sexual and Gender Minority Health*. New York: Oxford University Press, 2020.

Sears, Clare. *Arresting Dress: Cross-Dressing, Law, and Fascination in Nineteenth-Century San Francisco*. Durham, NC: Duke University Press, 2015.

Shover, Chelsea L., Michelle A. DeVost, Matthew R. Beymer, Pamina M. Gorbach, Risa P. Flynn, and Robert K. Bolan. "Using Sexual Orientation and Gender Identity to Monitor Disparities in HIV, Sexually Transmitted Infections, and Viral Hepatitis." *American Journal of Public Health* 108 (2018): S277–S283.

Siers-Poisson, Judith. "The Complexity of LGBT Poverty in the United States." Policy Brief No. 53-2021. *Institute for Research on Poverty*. June 2021. www.irp.wisc.edu/resource/the-complexity-of-lgbt-poverty-in-the-united-states/.

Steed, Heather, Brandon Stratford, and Alexander Gabriel. "Only 17 States and DC Report LGBT-Inclusive Sex Ed Curricula in at Least Half of Schools, Despite Recent Increases." *Child Trends*. October 6, 2021. www.childtrends.org/blog/only-17-states-and-dc-report-lgbtq-inclusive-sex-ed-curricula-in-at-least-half-of-schools-despite-recent-increases.

Substance Abuse and Mental Health Services Administration (SAMHSA). *Top Health Issues for LGBT Populations Information & Resource Kit*. HHS Publication No. (SMA) 12–4684. Rockville, MD: U.S. Department of Health and Human Services, 2012.

The Trevor Project. *Research Brief: Eating Disorders among LGBTQ Youth*. February 17, 2022. www.thetrevorproject.org/research-briefs/eating-disorders-among-lgbtq-youth-feb-2022/#:~:text=In%20alignment%20with%20results%20on,.%2C%202011)%20and%20young%20adults.

Townsend, Megan, and Raina Deerwater. *Where We Are on TV: 2021-2022*. New York, NY: GLAAD, 2022. www.glaad.org/sites/default/files/GLAAD%20202122%20WWATV.pdf.

Truman, Jennifer L., and Rachel E. Morgan. "Violent Victimization by Sexual Orientation and Gender Identity, 2017-2020." *U.S. Department of Justice Statistical Brief #NCJ 304277*. Washington, DC: Bureau of Justice Statistics, June 2022. https://bjs.ojp.gov/content/pub/pdf/vvsogi1720.pdf.

Williams, Keisha, RaShawn Hawkins, Raina Nelson, Courtney Stanford, and Linda Ochoa. *Corporate Equality Index 2022: Rating Workplaces on Lesbian, Gay, Bisexual, Transgender, and Queer Equality*. Washington, DC: Human Rights Campaign Foundation, 2022. https://reports.hrc.org/corporate-equality-index-2022?_ga=2.93285149.1202849102.1668976238-1580286318.1668263625.

Zaliznyak, Michael, Catherine Bresee, and Maurice M. Garcia. "Age at First Experience of Gender Dysphoria among Transgender Adults Seeking Gender-Affirming Therapy." *JAMA Open Network*. March 16, 2020. http://jamanetwork.com/journals/jamanetworkopen/fullarticle/2762788.

Chapter 12: Veterans

Alexandra, Rae. "How On-Screen Depictions of Veterans So Often Betray Them." *KQED*. January 16, 2019. https://www.kqed.org/pop/107528/how-on-screen-depictions-of-veterans-so-often-betray-them.

Borsari, Brian, Ali Yurasek, Mary Beth Miller, James G. Murphy, Meghan E. McDevitt-Murphy, Matthew P. Martens, Monica G. Darcy, and Kate B Carey. "Student Service Members/Veterans: Challenges for Reintegration." *American Journal of Orthopsychiatry* 87, 2 (2017): 166–75. https://www.ncbi.nlm.nih.gov/pmc/articles/PMC5319708/.

Centeno, José A., Duane A. Rogers, Gijsbert B. van der Voet, Elisa Fornero, Lingsu Zhang, Florabel G. Mullick, Gail D. Chapman, et al. "Embedded Fragments from U.S. Military Personnel—Chemical Health Analysis and Potential Health Implications." *International Journal of Environmental Research and Public Health* 11 (2014): 1261–78. https://www.ncbi.nlm.nih.gov/pmc/articles/PMC3945537/pdf/ijerph-11-01261.pdf.

Committee to Review the Health Effects in Vietnam Veterans of Exposure to Herbicides. *Veterans and Agent Orange.* 11th Biennial Update. Washington, DC: National Academies Press, 2018. https://nap.nationalacademies.org/read/25137/chapter/1.

Cormack, Lindsey. *Congress and U.S. Veterans: From the GI Bill to the VA Crisis.* Santa Barbara, CA: Praeger, 2018.

Crowell-Williamson, Gavin A., Martina Fruhbauerova, Christopher R. DeCou, and Katherina A. Comtois. "Perceived Burdensomeness, Bullying, and Suicidal Ideation in Suicidal Military Personnel." *Journal of Clinical Psychology* 75, 12 (2019): 2147–59.

Faraji, Elahe, Mostafa Allami, Nafiseh Feizollahi, Amir Karimi, Amir Yavari, Mohammedreza Soroush, and Majid Moudi. "Health Concerns of Veterans with High-Level Lower Extremity Amputations." *Military Medical Research* 5, 36 (2018). https://mmrjournal.biomedcentral.com/articles/10.1186/s40779-018-0183-4.

Fischer, Hannah. *A Guide to U.S. Military Casualty Statistics: Operation Freedom's Sentinel, Operation Inherent Resolve, Operation New Dawn, Operation Iraqi Freedom, and Operation Enduring Freedom.* Washington, DC: Congressional Research Service, 2015. https://sgp.fas.org/crs/natsec/RS22452.pdf.

Hayes, Jared. "'Forever Chemicals' Contamination at Defense Department Sites Threatens Chesapeake Bay Fish." *EWG: Environmental Working Group.* August 11, 2021. https://www.ewg.org/news-insights/news/2021/08/forever-chemicals-contamination-defense-department-sites-threatens?auHash=B9crbTXRJQLoQuXvOnR3b4KUP0Z5pnpQXqe1-HruWxo.

Hirschfield, Andrew. "For Veterans, Bad Financial Choices While on Active Duty Can Spiral Into Decades of Debt." *The American Homefront Project.* December 28, 2021. https://americanhomefront.wunc.org/2021-12-28/for-veterans-bad-financial-choices-while-on-active-duty-can-spiral-into-decades-of-debt.

Inoue, Catarina, Evan Shawler, Cristopher H. Jordan, and Christopher A. Jackson. "Veteran and Military Mental Health Issues." *PubMed.* January 2022. https://pubmed.ncbi.nlm.nih.gov/34283458/.

Jones, Audrey L., Michael J. Fine, Peter A. Taber, Leslie R.M. Hausmann, Kelly H. Burkitt, Roslyn A. Stone, and Susan L. Zickmund. "National Media Coverage of the Veterans' Affairs Waitlist Scandal: Effects on Veterans' Distrust of the VA Health Care System." *Medical Care* 59 (2021): S322–S326. https://journals.lww.com/lww-medicalcare/Fulltext/2021/06001/National_Media_Coverage_of_the_Veterans_Affairs.14.aspx.

Jowers, Karen. "Trouble's Brewing for the Post-Pandemic VA Health Care System, Top Doc Says." *Military Times.* December 10, 2020. https://www.militarytimes.com/pay-benefits/2020/12/10/troubles-brewing-for-the-post-pandemic-va-health-care-system-top-doc-says/.

Kintzle, Sara, Mary Keeling, Elizabeth Xintarianos, Kamil Taylor-Diggs, Chris Munch, Anthony M. Hassan, and Carl A. Castro. *Exploring the Economic and Employment Challenges Facing U.S. Veterans: A Qualitative Study of Volunteers of America Service Providers and Veteran Clients.* Los Angeles, CA: USC School of Social Work Center for Innovation & Research on Veterans & Military Families, 2015.

Kleykamp, Meredith, and Crosby Hipes. "Coverage of Veterans of the Wars in Iraq and Afghanistan in the U.S. Media." *Sociological Forum* 30, 2 (June 2015): 348–68.

Lemmon, Gayle Tzemach. "Missing in Action: Why Are There So Few Cultural Portrayals of Women in Combat?" *The Atlantic.* August 4, 2015. https://www.theatlantic.com/entertainment/archive/2015/08/missing-in-action/400235/.

Miles, Shannon R., Deleen S. Menefee, Jill Wanner, Andra Teten Tharp, and Thomas A. Kent. "The Relationship between Emotional Dysregulation and Impulsive Aggression in Veterans with Posttraumatic Stress Disorder Symptoms." *Journal of Interpersonal Violence* 31, 10 (2015): 1795–816. http://citeseerx.ist.psu.edu/viewdoc/download?doi=10.1.1.1010.5739&rep=rep1&type=pdf.

Miralao, Sidney. "Military Recruiters Are Exploiting High School Students' Financial Insecurities." *Inequality.org*. August 14, 2020. https://inequality.org/research/military-recruiters-high-school/.

Molloy, Joseph M., Timothy L. Pendergrass, Ian E. Lee, Michelle C. Cervak, Keith G. Hauret, and Daniel I. Rhon. "Musculoskeletal Injuries and United States Army Readiness Part I: Overview of Injuries and Their Strategic Impact." *Military Medicine* 185, 9–10 (2020): e1461–e1471. https://academic.oup.com/milmed/article/185/9-10/e1461/5805225.

Moody, Josh. "What ROTC Programs Are and How They Work." *U.S. News & World Report*. August 12, 2020. https://www.usnews.com/education/best-colleges/what-rotc-programs-are-and-how-they-work.

Moyer, Melissa Wenner. "'A Poison in the System': The Epidemic of Military Sexual Assault." *The New York Times*. October 11, 2021. https://www.nytimes.com/2021/08/03/magazine/military-sexual-assault.html.

Ochinko, Walter, and Kathy Payea. "Brief #8: Veteran Student Loan Debt 7 Years after Implementation of the Post-9/11 GI Bill." *Veterans Education Success*. January 2019. https://vetsedsuccess.org/wp-content/uploads/2019/01/veteran-student-loan-debt-7-years-after-post-911-gi-bill-implementation.pdf.

Olenick, Maria, Monica Flowers, and Valerie J. Diaz. "US Veterans and Their Unique Issues: Enhancing Health Care Professional Awareness." *Advances in Medical Education and Practice* 6 (2018): 635–9. https://www.ncbi.nlm.nih.gov/pmc/articles/PMC4671760/.

Parker, Kim, Ruth Igielnik, Amanda Barroso, and Anthony Cilluffo. "The American Veteran Experience and the Post-9/11 Generation." *Pew Research Center*. September 10, 2019. https://www.pewresearch.org/social-trends/2019/09/10/the-american-veteran-experience-and-the-post-9-11-generation/.

Price, Jay. "The Defense Department Will Investigate U.S. Sites for PFAS Contamination." *NPR: National Public Radio*. March 9, 2022. https://www.npr.org/2022/03/09/1085355551/the-defense-department-will-investigate-u-s-sites-for-pfas-contamination#:~:text=Some%20other%20news%20now%20%2D%20the,do%20not%20break%20down%20easily.

Rabbitt, Matthew P., and Michael D. Smith. *Food Insecurity among Working-Age Veterans*. Economic Research Report Number 829. Washington, DC: Economic Research Service, U.S. Department of Agriculture, 2021. https://www.ers.usda.gov/webdocs/publications/101269/err-829.pdf?v=6067.

Salazar, Alexandra H. "How Building Features Impact Veterans with PTSD." *Texas A&M Today*. August 10, 2020. https://today.tamu.edu/2020/08/10/how-building-features-impact-veterans-with-ptsd/.

Semeah, Luz Mairena, Sherry Ahrentzen, Diane C. Cowper-Ripley, Leslie M. Santos-Roman, Julia O. Beamish, and Kristine Farley. "In Their Own Words: Veterans with Disabilities Share Their Housing Challenges." *Housing Matters*. March 13, 2019. https://housingmatters.urban.org/research-summary/their-own-words-veterans-disabilities-share-their-housing-challenges.

Sierra, Gabrielle. "Why It Matters: Sexual Assault in the U.S. Military." *Council on Foreign Relations*. September 30, 2021. https://www.cfr.org/podcasts/sexual-assault-in-the-us-military.

Sonderling, Keith E. "Opinion: Facing Down Discrimination against Vets." *The Atlanta Journal-Constitution*. July 23, 2021. https://www.ajc.com/opinion/opinion-facing-down-job-discrimination-against-vets/HKW2XLNIHRHFTC6EMSFBNSN2NI/.

Stafford, Kat, James Laporta, and Aaron Morrison. "AP Report: Deep-Rooted Racism and Discrimination Permeate U.S. Military." *PBS News Hour*. May 27, 2021. https://www.pbs.org/newshour/nation/ap-report-deep-rooted-racism-and-discrimination-permeate-u-s-military.

Stasha, Smiljanic. "How Many Veterans Are Homeless in 2022?" *Policy Advice*. March 5, 2022. https://policyadvice.net/insurance/insights/homeless-veterans-statistics/#:~:text=The%20decreasing%20rate%20has%20been,%2C%20state%2C%20and%20federal%20 authorities.&text=HUD%20reported%20a%20decline%20in,the%20streets%20in%20early%202018.

Tsilibary, Effie-Photini C., Eric P. Souto, Marian Kratzke, Lisa M. James, Brian E. Engdahl, and Apostolos P. Georgopolous. "Anthrax and Gulf War Illness (GWI): Evidence for the Presence of Harmful Anthrax Antigen PA63 in the Serum of Veterans with GWI." *Journal of Neurology and Neuromedicine* 4, 6 (2019): 1–9. https://www.jneurology.com/articles/anthrax-and-gulf-war-illness-gwi-evidence-for-the-presence-of-harmful-anthrax-antigen-pa63-in-the-serum-of-veterans-with-gwi.pdf.

United States Department of Agriculture, Economic Research Service. *Rural Veterans at a Glance.* Economic Brief Number 25. Washington, DC: United States Department of Agriculture, November 2013. https://www.ers.usda.gov/webdocs/publications/42891/40612_eb25.pdf?v=8124.7.

United States Environmental Protection Agency. "Health and Environmental Effects of Particulate Matter." https://www.epa.gov/pm-pollution/health-and-environmental-effects-particulate-matter-pm#:~:text=Exposure%20to%20such%20particles%20can,nonfatal%20heart%20attacks (accessed April 21, 2022).

U.S. Department of Defense. *Hazing Prevention and Response in the Armed Forces.* Washington, DC: U.S. Department of Defense, 2018. https://diversity.defense.gov/Portals/51/Documents/2018%20Hazing%20Report.pdf?ver=owYztvdR8oINv_zgUyg8ew%3D%3D.

U.S. Department of Veterans Affairs. "Veteran Health Issues Related to Service History." *Veterans Affairs.* https://www.va.gov/health-care/health-needs-conditions/health-issues-related-to-service-era/ (accessed April 12, 2022).

Wilkie, Robert L., and Matthew P. Donovan. *DoD Instruction 1020.03: Harassment Prevention and Response in the Armed Forces.* Washington, DC: U.S. Department of Defense, February 8, 2018. https://www.esd.whs.mil/Portals/54/Documents/DD/issuances/dodi/102003p.PDF?ver=DAAzonEUeFb8kUWRbT9Epw%3D%3D.

Chapter 13: Women and Girls

American Association of University Women. "The STEM Gap: Women and Girls in Science, Technology, Engineering, and Math." https://www.aauw.org/resources/research/the-stem-gap/ (accessed November 17, 2021).

Caiazza, Amy, April Shaw, and Misha Werschkul. *Women's Economic Status in the States: Wide Disparities by Race, Ethnicity, and Region.* Washington, DC: Institute for Women's Policy Research, 2004. https://iwpr.org/wp-content/uploads/2020/12/R260.pdf.

Carroll, Jamie M., Evangeleen Pattison, Chandra Muller, and April Sutton. "Barriers to Bachelor's Degree Completion among College Students with a Disability." *Sociological Perspectives*, March 5, 2020. https://journals.sagepub.com/doi/10.1177/0731121420908896.

Charles, Kerwin Kofi, Jonathan Guryan, and Jessica Pan. "The Effects of Sexism on American Women: The Role of Norms v. Discrimination." Working Paper No. 2018-56. *Becker Friedman Institute for Economics.* August 2018. https://bfi.uchicago.edu/wp-content/uploads/WP_2018-56.pdf.

Children's Defense Fund. *The State of America's Children 2021.* Washington, DC: Children's Defense Fund, 2021.

Christ, Amber, and Tracey Gronniger. "Older Women and Poverty: Special Report." *Justice in Aging.* December 2018. https://justiceinaging.org/wp-content/uploads/2020/08/Older-Women-and-Poverty.pdf.

Colby, Glenn, and Chelsea Flowers. "Data Snapshot: IPEDS Data on Full-Time Women Faculty and Faculty of Color." *American Association of University Professors.* December 2020. https://www.aaup.org/sites/default/files/Dec-2020_Data_Snapshot_Women_and_Faculty_of_Color.pdf.

DeChants, Jonah, Amy E. Green, Myeshia N. Price, and Carrie Davis. *Measuring Youth Sexual Orientation and Gender Identity.* West Hollywood, CA: The Trevor Project, 2021.

Available: https://www.thetrevorproject.org/research-briefs/measuring-youth-sexual-orientation-and-gender-identity/.

Dittmar, Kelly, Kira Sanbonmatsu, and Susan J. Carroll. *A Seat at the Table: Congresswomen's Perspectives on Why Their Presence Matters*. New York: Oxford University Press, 2018.

Duquaine-Watson, Jillian M. *Mothering by Degrees: Single Mothers and the Pursuit of Postsecondary Education*. New Brunswick, NJ: Rutgers University Press, 2017.

Duquaine-Watson, Jillian M., ed. *Women's Health: Understanding Issues and Influences*. Santa Barbara, CA: ABC-CLIO/Greenwood Press, 2022.

Fins, Amanda. "National Snapshot: Poverty among Women & Families, 2020." *National Women's Law Center*, December 2020. https://nwlc.org/wp-content/uploads/2020/12/PovertySnapshot2020.pdf.

Flores, Laura E., Walter R. Frontera, Michele P. Andrasik, Carlos Del Rio, Antonio Mondríguez-González, Stephanie A. Price, Elizabeth M. Krantz, Steven A. Pergam, and Julie K. Silver. "Assessment of Inclusion of Racial/Ethnic Minority, Female, and Older Individuals in Vaccine Clinical Trials." *JAMA Open Network*. February 19, 2021. https://jamanetwork.com/journals/jamanetworkopen/fullarticle/2776562.

Frederikson, Brittni, Usha Ranji, Alina Salganicoff, and Michelle Long. "Women's Experiences with Health Care during the COVID-19 Pandemic: Findings from the KFF Women's Health Survey." *KFF: Kaiser Family Foundation*. March 22, 2021. https://www.kff.org/womens-health-policy/issue-brief/womens-experiences-with-health-care-during-the-covid-19-pandemic-findings-from-the-kff-womens-health-survey/.

"Gender Matters: Women Disproportionately Report Sexual Harassment in Male-Dominated Industries." *CAP: Center for American Progress*. August 6, 2018. https://www.americanprogress.org/article/gender-matters/.

Georgetown Institute for Women, Peace, and Security. *The Best and Worst States to Be a Woman: Introducing the U.S. Women, Peace, and Security Index 2020*. Washington, DC: Georgetown Institute for Women, Peace, and Security, 2021. https://giwps.georgetown.edu/wp-content/uploads/2020/10/The-Best-and-Worst-States-to-Be-a-Woman.pdf.

Ginder, Scott A., and Janice E. Kelly-Reid. *Postsecondary Institutions and Cost of Attendance in 2017-18; Degrees and Other Awards Conferred: 2016-17; and 12-Month Enrollment: 2016-17: First Look (Provisional Data)*. Washington, DC: U.S. Department of Education, National Center for Education Statistics, 2018. https://nces.ed.gov/pubsearch/pubsinfo.asp?pubid=2018060rev.

Godsil, Rachel D., Jessica MacFarlane, and Brian Sheppard. *#PopJustice Volume 3: Pop Culture, Perceptions, and Social Change*. New York, NY: The Perception Institute, 2016. https://perception.org/wp-content/uploads/2016/05/PopJustice-Volume-3_Research-Review.pdf.

Hartley, Gemma. *Fed Up: Emotional Labor, Women, and the Way Forward*. New York: HarperCollins, 2018.

Harvard Medical School. "Women's Health" (website). Available: https://www.health.harvard.edu/topics/womens-health (accessed September 15, 2021).

Healthy People 2030. "Language and Literacy." https://health.gov/healthypeople/objectives-and-data/social-determinants-health/literature-summaries/language-and-literacy (accessed November 16, 2020).

Horowitz, Juliana Menasce, Kim Parker, and Renee Stepler. "Wide Partisan Gaps in U.S. on How Far the Country Has Come on Gender Equality." *Pew Research Center*. October 18, 2017. file:///C:/Users/jilli/Downloads/Gender-Equality-Report-FINAL-10.18.pdf.

Institute for Women's Policy Research. "Status of Women in the States." 2021. https://statusofwomendata.org/explore-the-data/state-data/united-states/.

Jeung, Russell, Aggie Yellow Horse, Tara Popovic, and Harold Lim. *Stop AAPI Hate National Report*. San Francisco, CA: Stop AAPI Hate, 2021. https://secureservercdn.net/104.238.69.231/a1w.90d.myftpupload.com/wp-content/uploads/2021/03/210312-Stop-AAPI-Hate-National-Report-.pdf.

Knoll, Benjamin R., and Cammie Jo Bolin. *She Preached the Word: Women's Ordination in Modern America*. New York: Oxford University Press, 2018.

Kukura, Elizabeth. "Obstetric Violence." *The Georgetown Law Journal* 106 (2018): 721–801. https://www.law.georgetown.edu/georgetown-law-journal/wp-content/uploads/sites/26/2018/06/Obstetric-Violence.pdf.

Levine, Elana, ed. *Cupcakes, Pinterest, and Ladyporn: Feminized Popular Culture in the early Twenty-First Century*. Chicago, IL: University of Illinois Press, 2015.

Lucchesi, Annita, and Abigail Echo-Hawk. *Missing and Murdered Indigenous Women & Girls: A Snapshot of Data from 71 Urban Cities in the United States*. Seattle, WA: Urban Indian Health Institute, 2018. https://www.uihi.org/wp-content/uploads/2018/11/Missing-and-Murdered-Indigenous-Women-and-Girls-Report.pdf.

Milestone, Katie, and Anneke Meyer. *Gender and Popular Culture*. 2nd ed. Cambridge, UK: Polity Press, 2021.

Nagle, Rebecca. "Media Representations of Native Women: Invisibility, Stereotypes, Whitewashing." *Women's Media Center*. June 12, 2018. https://womensmediacenter.com/news-features/media-representation-of-native-women-invisibility-stereotypes-whitewashing.

National Eating Disorders Association. https://www.nationaleatingdisorders.org/ (accessed November 20, 2010).

National Institute of Mental Health. "Child and Adolescent Mental Health." https://www.nimh.nih.gov/health/topics/child-and-adolescent-mental-health (accessed October 23, 2021).

Office on Women's Health. www.womenshealth.gov (accessed September 15, 2021).

Palmer, Neal A., Emily A. Greytak, and Joseph G. Kosciw. *Educational Exclusion: Drop Out, Push Out, and the School-to-Prison Pipeline among LGBTQ Youth*. New York: GLSEN, 2016. https://www.glsen.org/sites/default/files/2019-11/Educational_Exclusion_2013.pdf.

Porterfield, Carlie. "A Lot of PPE Doesn't Fit Women—and in the Coronavirus Pandemic, It Puts Them in Danger." *Forbes*. April 29, 2020. https://www.forbes.com/sites/carlieporterfield/2020/04/29/a-lot-of-ppe-doesnt-fit-women-and-in-the-coronavirus-pandemic-it-puts-them-in-danger/?sh=3a908fae315a.

Quinlan, Casey. "The Particular Struggles of Rural Women." *The Atlantic*. June 12, 2013. https://www.theatlantic.com/sexes/archive/2013/06/the-particular-struggles-of-rural-women/276803/.

RAINN: Rape, Assault, and Incest National Network. https://www.rainn.org/ (accessed November 30, 2021).

Ranji, Usha, Caroline Rosenzweig, Ivette Gomez, and Alina Salginicoff. "Overview: 2017 Kaiser Women's Health Survey." *KFF: Kaiser Family Foundation*. March 13, 2018. https://www.kff.org/womens-health-policy/issue-brief/overview-2017-kaiser-womens-health-survey/.

Richards, Misty, and Maureen Sayres Van Niel. "Mental Health Disparities: Women's Mental Health." *American Psychiatric Association*. 2017. https://vibdoc.com/0-mental-health-womenb40723da2f01424e830fb400998875e08472.html.

Shibu, John, and Prerna Singh. "Female Education and Health: Effects of Social Determinants for Economic Growth and Development." *International Journal of Research Foundation of Hospital and Healthcare Administration* 5, 2 (December 2017): 84–8. https://www.researchgate.net/publication/323731896_Female_Education_and_Health_Effects_of_Social_Determinants_on_Economic_Growth_and_Development.

Smith, Sharon G., Xinjian Zhang, Kathleen C. Basile, Melissa T. Merrick, Jing Wang, Marcie-jo Kresnow, and Jieru Chen. *National Intimate Partner and Sexual Violence Survey: 2015 Data Brief—Updated Release*. Atlanta, GA: National Center for Injury Prevention and Control, Center for Disease Control and Prevention, 2018. https://www.cdc.gov/violenceprevention/pdf/2015data-brief508.pdf.

Sun, Shengwei. *Young Women Workers Still Struggling a Decade after the Great Recession: Lessons for the Pandemic Recovery*. Policy Brief #C499. IWPR: Institute for Women's Policy Research, May 2021. https://iwpr.org/wp-content/uploads/2021/05/Brief_Young-Women-Workers_Lessons-for-Pandemic-Recovery_2021-05-26_FINAL.pdf.

Terrell, Cynthia Richie, and Courtney Lamendola. *2020 Gender Parity Index*. Takoma Park, MD: Represent Women, 2020. https://fairvote.app.box.com/s/zec83ir42w87xrlgbuunwprzm28b9wzb.

U.S. Bureau of Labor Statistics. "Women in the Labor Force: A Databook." Report #1092. April 2021. https://www.bls.gov/opub/reports/womens-databook/2020/home.htm.

U.S. Department of Justice, Civil Rights Division, Interagency Working Group on Limited English Proficiency. "Education." https://www.lep.gov/education (accessed November 16, 2021).

U.S. Food and Drug Administration. "Women's Health Topics" (website). Available: https://www.fda.gov/consumers/women/womens-health-topics (accessed September 15, 2021).

Washington, Harriet. *Medical Apartheid: The Dark History of Medical Experimentation on Black American from Colonial Times to the Present*. New York: Harlem Moon, 2008.

Williams, Kimberlé Crenshaw, Priscilla Ocen, and Jyoti Nanda. *Black Girls Matter: Pushed Out, Overpoliced, and Underprotected*. New York: African American Policy Forum, 2015. https://www.law.columbia.edu/sites/default/files/2021-05/black_girls_matter_report_2.4.15.pdf.

Wodon, Quentin, Claudio Montenegro, Hao Nguyen, and Adenike Onagoruwa. *Missed Opportunities: The High Cost of Not Educating Girls*. Washington, DC: The World Bank, 2018. https://www.globalpartnership.org/sites/default/files/2018-07-gpe-high-cost-of-not-educating-girls.pdf.

Women's Voices for the Earth. *Toxic Chemicals in Salon Products: What Salon Workers Need to Know*. Missoula, MT: Women's Voices for the Earth.. https://womensvoices.org/wp-content/uploads/2013/09/Ingredients-to-Avoid-in-Salon-Products_workers.pdf (accessed November 30, 2021).

Woolf, Steven H., Laudan Aron, Lisa Dubay, Sarah M. Simon, Emily Zimmerman, and Kim X. Luk. *How Are Income and Wealth Linked to Longevity? Income and Health Initiative*: *Brief One*. Washington, DC: Urban Institute, 2015. https://www.urban.org/sites/default/files/publication/49116/2000178-How-are-Income-and-Wealth-Linked-to-Health-and-Longevity.pdf.

World Economic Forum. *Global Gender Gap Report 2021*. Geneva, Switzerland (March 2021). https://www3.weforum.org/docs/WEF_GGGR_2021.pdf.

Zhou, Enyu, and Janet Gao. *Graduate Enrollment and Degrees: 2010 to 2020*. Washington, DC: Council of Graduate Schools, 2021.

INDEX

ABOUT THE AUTHOR

Jillian M. Duquaine-Watson, PhD, has taught in higher education for more than 25 years. Grounded in gender studies and medical/cultural anthropologies, her research and teaching focus on health inequities, reproductive health, cultural competence in healthcare, poverty, social change and development, and environmental sustainability. She is an award-winning educator who has taught a variety of courses in anthropology, sociology, gender studies, healthcare studies, and American studies. She is also an award-winning author with numerous book chapters, journal articles, books, and entries in academic reference volumes to her credit. Jillian currently serves as Dean of First-Year Students and Programs at Colby College in Waterville, Maine.